Biotech's

DICTIONARY *Of* Veterinary

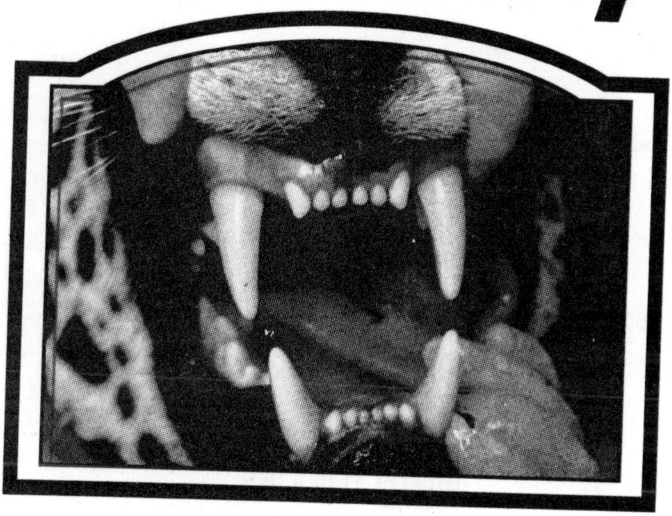

Compiled & Edited by

Dinesh Arora

BIOTECH

2004

BIOTECH BOOKS

DELHI - 110035

Biotech's

DICTIONARY *Of* Veterinary

Compiled & Edited by
Dinesh Arora

First Indian Edition 2004

ISBN 81-7622-123-6

Published by : **BIOTECH BOOKS**
1123/74, Tri Nagar,
Delhi - 110 035
Phone: 27382765
e-mail: biotechbooks@yahoo.co.in

Showroom : 4762-63/23, Ansari Road, Darya Ganj,
New Delhi - 110 002
Phone: 23245578, 23244987

Printed at : **Chawla Offset Printers**
New Delhi - 110 052

PRINTED IN INDIA

PREFACE

Veterinary medicine today is without doubt a challenging field. One significant difference between human and animal medicine is that veterinarians must be familiar with the anatomy and diseases of several different species. An appropriate treatment for one species might be ineffective or harmful if applied to another. Veterinarians must be proficient in both medicine and surgery, and be well versed in areas such as paediatrics, obstetrics, anaesthesiology, dentistry, dermatology, geriatrics, and orthopaedics. They must deduce problems without sharing a single spoken word with the patient. Many veterinarians, therefore, are acute diagnosticians with top-notch powers of observation and intuition.

The primary purpose of this dictionary is to provide veterinary practitioners, veterinary students, and veterinary technologists with a concise knowledge of the infectious and parasitic diseases of almost all domestic animals like cats, dogs and horses. Included are the diseases caused by bacteria, fungi, viruses, protozoa, helminths, and external parasites. Some other terms used in this dictionary include various medical terms used for the treatment of a particular disease and the equipments used in the process.

The material in this dictionary is organised and presented for quick reference in a user-friendly manner and is therefore also useful to laboratory technicians, and veterinary students.

- **acey-deucy**

uneven stirrups, popularised by jockey Eddie Arcaro, who rode with his left (inside) iron lower than his right to achieve better balance on turns.

- **acid**

a fluid containing a high proportion of hydrogen ions, giving the liquid a sour taste. Measured by pH units, with 1 themostacid and 14 the least acid. Chemical reactions in the body have to take place at or near neutrality, pH7.

- **acid detergent fibre (Abrev: ADF)**

the amount of residue (primarily cellulose, lignin and variable amounts of silica) left after boiling a feed sample in an acid detergent solution. The ADF value is used to predict the energy content (TDN, NE) of forages.

- **acne**

lesions seen most often on the chin. Acne may be a manifestation of a keratinisation disorder, a primary bacterial infection, dermatophytosis, secondary to allergic skin disease, demodicosis, Malassezia dermatitis, or secondary to systemic disorders.

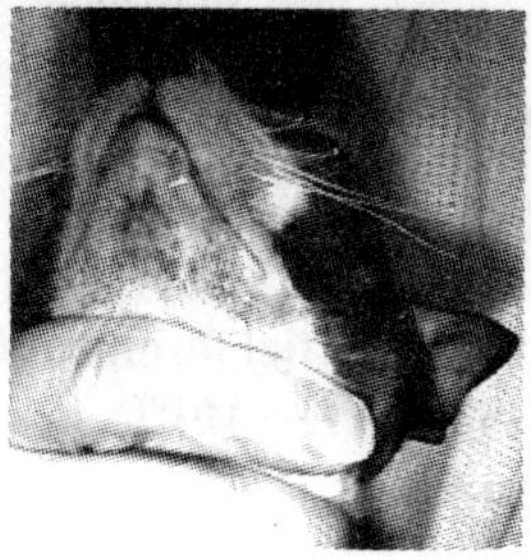

- **acquired**

a defect that happens after being born (contrasted to congenital).

- **acral lick dermatitis**

acral pruritic nodules – 'Lick granuloma'. Lesions caused by chronic licking.

- **acronym**

abbreviation for a phrase. MPL is the acronym for master problem list.

- **ACTH**

adreno cortico tropic hormone. A hormone, secreted by the pituitary gland, which stimulates the adrenal gland to work.

- **actinic**

the injurious effects of ultraviolet light.

- **action**

a horse's manner of moving.

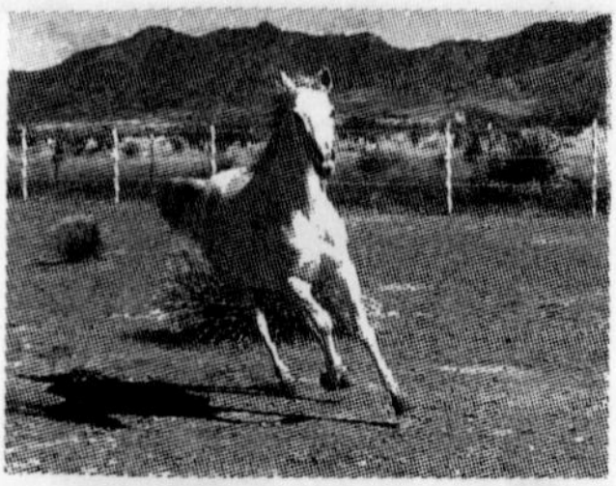

- **activated partial thromboplastin time (Abrev: APPT)**
  the time it takes for plasma to form a fibrin clot after the addition of calcium and a phospholipid reagent. APPT measures the intrinsic coagulation system.

- **activated charcoal**
  charcoal which has been treated to increase its adsorptive power(ability to have chemicals adhere to it). It is used to treat various forms of poisoning.

- **active immunity**
  immunity produced when an animal's immune system reacts to a stimulus, e.g., a virus or bacteria and produces antibodies and cells, which will protect it from the disease caused by the bacteria or virus.

- **acupressure**
  utilising stimulation on acupuncture points to treat an animal.

- **acupuncture**
  a centuries-old means of treating an animal or human through the use of needles, electrical current or moxibustion (heat and herbs) to stimulate or realign the body's electrical fields.

- **acute**
  1. single or short term exposure to a poison. Usually results in clinical signs and/or death.
  2. the sudden onset of signs of disease.

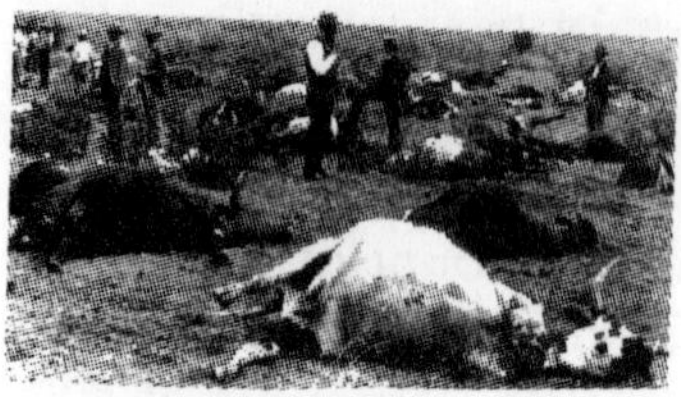

- **acute metritis**
  an infection of the uterus.

- **acute renal failure (Abrev: ARF)**
  an acute suppression of renal function. The most common causes of ARF are renal ischemia and nephrotoxicity.

- **acute tubular necrosis (Abrev: ATN)**
  acute death of the epithelial cells lining the renal tubules due to ischemia or toxins.

- **ad libitum (Abrev: ad lib)**
  feed offered free choice, allowing animals to eat as much as they desire.

- **added weight**
  a horse carrying more weight than the conditions of the race require, usually because the jockey exceeds the stated limit.

- **addison's disease**
  the pituitary gland produces a hormone that triggers the adrenal gland to produce corticosteroids. If there is a problem with the adrenal gland, or a pituitary tumour, the process breaks down and not enough corticosteroids are produced. Characterised by weakness, weight loss, anorexia, and fatigue.

- **adenocarcinoma**
  a form of cancer that occurs in the prostate gland.

- **adequan**
  brand name for polysulfated glycosaminoglycan, used in the treatment of certain arthritic conditions.

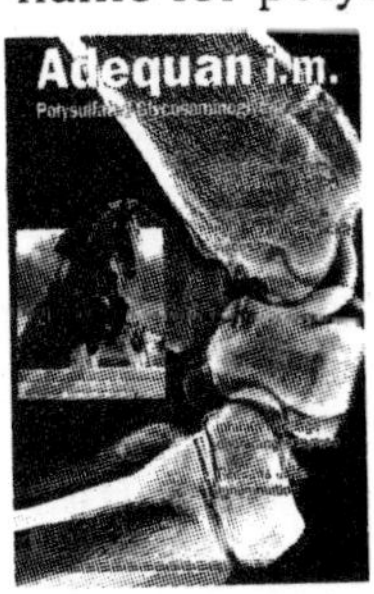

- **adhesions**
  when structures that are not normally bound together become stuck to one another.

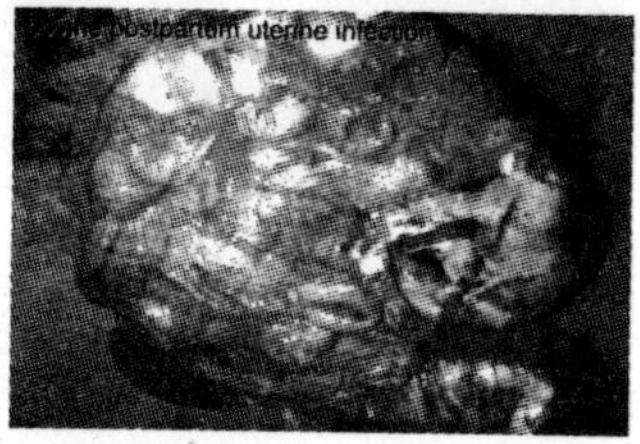

- **adjuvants**
  aluminum derivatives that are added to killed vaccines to generate more of an immune response than the killed vaccine alone would.

- **adnexa**
  structures bound to the skin such as sebaceous and apocrine glands.

- **adontia**
  absence of a tooth or multiple teeth - also called hypodontia or oligodontia

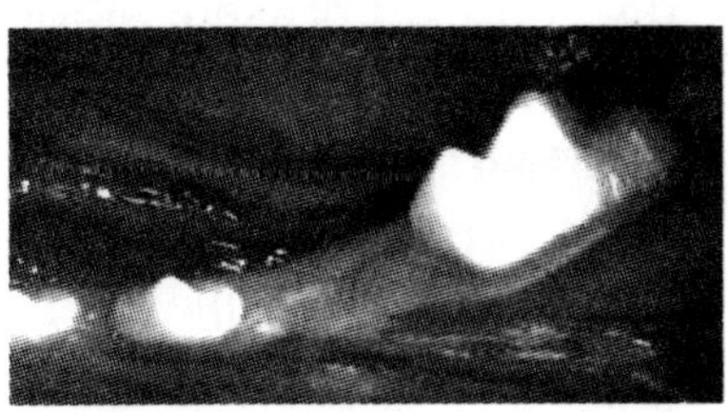

- **adrenal gland**
a gland located close to the kidneys that produces several hormones including cortisol.

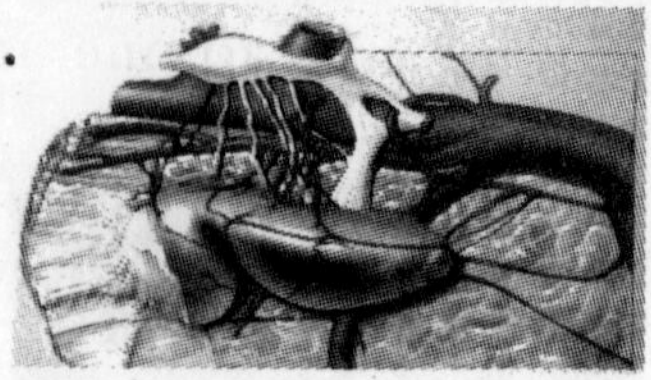

- **adrenaline**
a hormone produced by the adrenal glands that elevates heart and respiration rates, also called 'epinephrine.'

- **adrenergic**
communication between the nerves and muscles that uses epinephrine as the messenger. Adrenergic stimulation is what is involved in the 'flight or fight' response, which means the body is alerted to a danger of some sort and prepares to run or fight. Adrenergic stimulation results in an increased heart rate, sweating, and increased blood pressure.

- **adsorbent**
solid substance which attracts other molecules to its surface.

- **adulticide**
medication formulated to kill adult forms of a parasite.

- **adv**
advise or advice

- **adverse event**
any undesirable occurrence, either injury or death, following the use of an immunobiological product.

- **adverse reaction to food**
an abnormal clinical response attributed to an ingested food or food product.

- **aerobic**
needing oxygen to live.

- **aerobic bacteria**
bacteria that grow only when oxygen is present.

- **afghan hound**
the great windhound of Afghanistan.The Afghan Hound also runs in large numbers along the Boderland and in Northern India, where it is known as the Barakzai, Kurram Valley Hound. It is not clear how these greyhound types made their way from the Middle East into northern Afghanistan, the country that provides its present

name. Also referred to as Tazi and Baluchi Hound, the Afghan Hound, as we know him today, is one of the most ancient of dogs and, many believe, is the dog that Noah granted visa on his Ark. Although the whole truth may never be told, the Afghan's pedigree is without a doubt pre-Christian in age. Portraits of the Afghan's ancestors appear engraved upon cuneiform pillars and tablets. Native Indian and Asian hunters prize their individual strains and guard them with jealous care. In Afghanistan, the breed is used to guard sheep and cattle and to hunt deer, wolves' gazelles and foxes. The leopard and the panther are the Afghan Hound's most impressive game - it has been known to hunt and kill big cat single-handedly. Its approach to hunting is not the typical courser's - the breed is more inclined to slay its prey, although it can be trained not to.

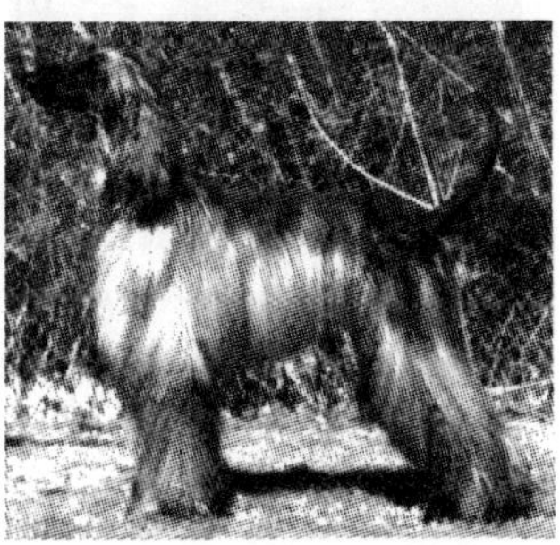

- **ag**
  anal glands
- **age**
  all thoroughbreds celebrate their birthday on august 1st.
- **age specific data base**
  the minimum amount of information that is planned to be collected on all patients of a certain age; for example pediatric or geriatric databases.
- **agglutination**
  an abnormal clumping of red blood cells. Often seen in patients with immune-mediated anaemia.

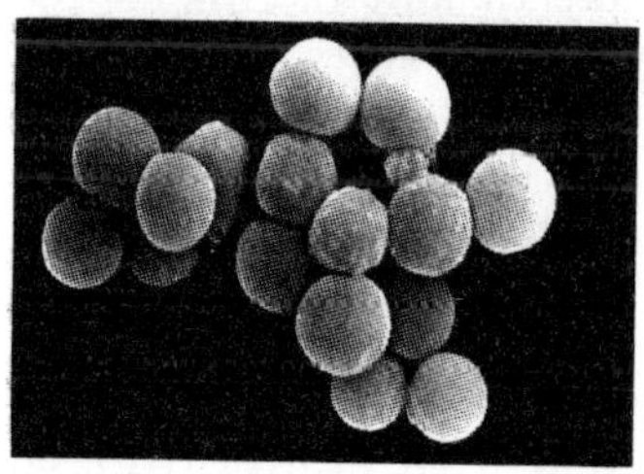

- **agonist**
  a drug which when attached to a receptor causes an effect.

- **agouti**
  the colour between the stripes of a Tabby cat. In non-agouti cats there is no contrast, producing a solid (self) coat.

- **AIDS defining diseases**
  if a person is HIV+ and is diagnosed with one of several disease conditions, by definition the person has AIDS. Included among the AIDS defining diseases are several zoonotic diseases (toxoplasmosis, cryptosporidiosis).

- **aiha**
  auto-immune haemolytic anaemia.

- **ailurophile**
  a person who loves cats.

- **ailurophobe**
  a person with an intense dislike or fear of cats.

- **airing**
  not running at best speed in a race.

- **ankylosis**
  fusion of cementum with alveolar bone

- **akbash dog**
  a native flock-guarding breed of Turkey, the Akbash Dog is a durable and tremendously resourceful component of the agricultural life of that country. Thousands of years ago, the dog's prototypes were embraced by local shepherds and adapted to their specific needs. These dogs are said to have accompanied wandering Eastern travellers to Turkey and to be a cross-pollination of Eastern mastiffs and sight hounds. The breed's ranginess and acute eyesight (assumedly the contribution of the long-legged fleet hounds) along with the Akbash's white coat, which enables the shepherd to distinguish between dog and predator, make the Akbash a vital part of the shepherds' well-being in Turkey.

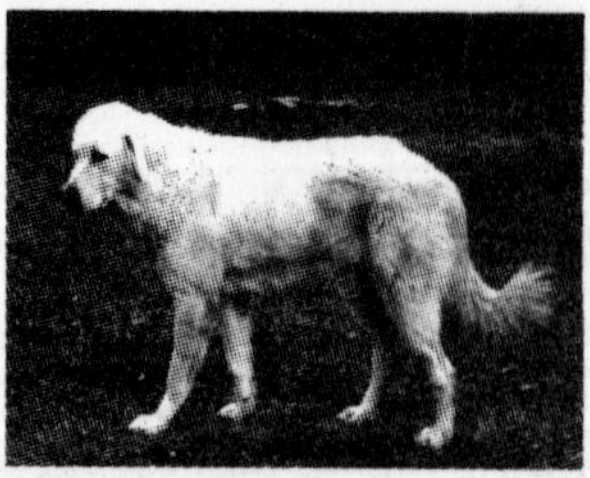

- **alanine aminotransferase (Abrev: ALT)**
  also known as serum alanine aminotransferase

(SALT). An enzyme found in hepatocytes (liver cells), released with cellular injury including cellular hypoxia.

- **albino**
  an animal that is completely white because it lacks the ability to make pigment. Its eyes are pale blue or pink.

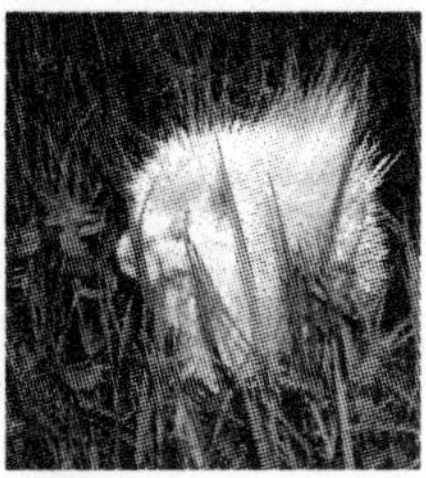

- **albumin**
  a small protein in blood that acts like a 'sponge' to keep fluid within the blood vessels. If albumin is low, fluid leaks out of the blood vessels and causes edema.
- **aldosterone**
  a hormone produced by the adrenal gland that is responsible for salt and water balance in the body.
- **alimentary**
  another term for the gut or intestinal tract. The alimentary tract runs from the mouth, through the oesophagus to the stomach, duodenum, small intestine, large intestine, rectum, and anus.
- **alkaline**
  a substance with very few hydrogen ions and a pH over 7. Lye is strongly alkaline.
- **alkaline phosrhatase(Abrev: AP SAP)**
  also known as serum alkaline phosphatase (SAP). An enzyme found in many tissues but most often elevated in serum in response to cholestasis, bone remodelling or glucocorticoid excess.
- **all in, all out management system**
  a management system where the entire population is removed from a single area, the area is thoroughly cleaned and disinfected, and then the pigs are moved back in.
- **allergen**
  any inanimate or living object that creates an allergic reaction in an animal,e.g., pollen.
- **allergic contact dermatitis (Abrev: ACD)**
  dermatitis caused by caustic or irritating substances. No prior sensitisation is required.

• **allergy**
immunological hypersensitivity to certain foreign antigens.
anaemia reduction of red blood cells or haemoglobin. The red cells contain the protein 'haemoglobin' which binds oxygen in the red blood cell. This allows the transport of oxygen from the lungs to the tissues. Symptoms include weakness, reluctance to exercise, pale mucous membranes, and tachycardia (abnormally rapid heart rate).

• **allodynia**
pain from a stimulus that would normally be non-painful.

• **alopecia**
loss of hair or baldness.

• **alopecic syndrome**
colour dilution alopecia. Deficiency of hair, caused by a failure to grow or regrow after loss. Signs may include bacterial folliculitis, scaling and hair loss. Caused by the dilution gene at the D locus.

• **alsike clover**
alsike clover is indeed toxic to horses. It can manifest as either photosensitisation or neurologic impairment. Both are due to compounds, which affect the liver.

• **altered**
a cat that has had its reproductive organs removed (either spayed females or neutered males).

• **aluminum hydroxide**
an adjuvant which is a common component of killed vaccines, included to increase the ability of the vaccine to stimulate an immune response.

• **alveolar sacs**
the tiny microscopic areas of the lungs where the exchange of oxygen and carbon dioxide into and out of the blood occurs. Also called alveolus.

• **American Eskimo**
The American Eskimo is a member of the spitz family, a family that traces its lineage back six millennia to the Peat Dog of the New Stone Age lake dwellers. Remains of these protoypes have been uncovered in various European countries. The American Eskimo resulted from Americans breeding white German

Spitz and promoting the variety. Initially these dogs were larger than the Standard American Eskimo that stands only 19 inches (48 cm) high.

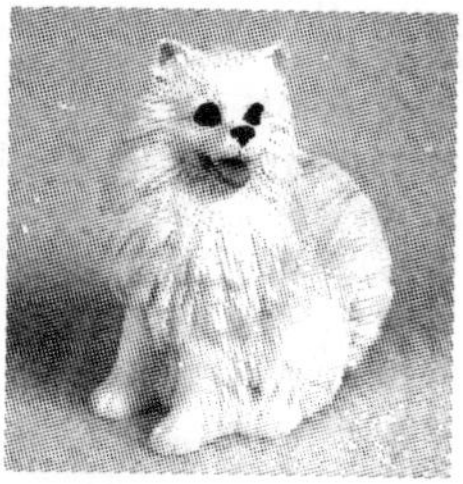

- **amino acids**
  nitrogen-containing compounds that are the building blocks from which proteins are made.
- **aminoglycoside**
  a class of antibiotics, which act by interfering with bacterial protein synthesis in the bacteria, which results in the death of the bacteria. Antibiotics in this class include gentamicin (Gentocin), kanamycin, neomycin, streptomycin, tobramycin, and amikacin. Many of these antibiotics are not well absorbed from the animal's digestive system so they are often administered as injections or used topically.
- **amiodarone**
  a class III antiarrhythmic drug.
- **amitraz**
  a treatment for demodectic mange. Mechanism of action is unknown, probably a monamine oxidase inhibitor.

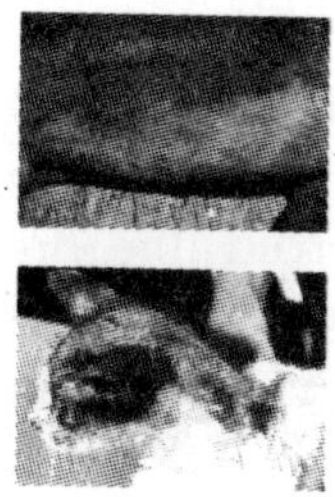

- **amlodipine**
  a long-acting calcium channel blocker that is the drug of choice for management of hypertension in cats.
- **amnion**
  the inner most layer of the membrane surrounding the embryo in the uterus. The sac formed by this membrane contains amniotic fluid.
- **amniotic vesicle**
  another name for the embryonic vesicle.

- **amphotericin B**
  systemic antifungal drug.

- **amylase**
  digestive enzyme, produced by the pancreas which breaks down carbohydrates and starches.

- **amylopectin**
  a branched chain of glucose molecules

- **anabolic steroid**
  a type of steroid (not a corticosteroid like prednisone, cortisone, or dexamethasone) which promotes the building of tissues like muscle.

- **anaemia**
  a condition caused by iron deficiency.

- **anaerobic bacteria**
  a bacteria that grows only when oxygen is not present.

- **anagen**
  the phase of the hair cycle during with the hair is synthesised.

- **analgesia**
  refers to the absence of pain in the presence of stimuli that would be expected to be painful. In clinical practice we use the term analgesia to mean a reduction in pain.

- **analgesic**
  a drug administered to reduce the perception of pain.

- **anamnestic response**
  the immune response produced by an animal who has previously encountered that specific antigen. Memory cells are responsible for this more efficient response.

- **anaphylaxis**
  a severe hypersensitivity reaction often resulting in bronchoconstriction and hypotension.

- **anaphylaxis (anaphylactic shock)**
  anaphylaxis is a rare, life threatening, immediate allergic reaction to something ingested or injected. If untreated, it results in shock, respiratory and cardiac failure, and death.

- **anatomy**
  the physical structure of the body.

- **ancylostomiasis**
  hookworm dermatitis. The etiological agents are migrating 3rd stage larvae of

Ancylostoma canium or *Uncinaria stenocephala*.

- **androgen**
hormone which produces male sexual characteristics e.g., testosterone.

- **anaemia**
anaemia is a decrease in PCV or haemoglobin resulting in decreased oxygen carrying capacity of the blood.

- **anesthesia**
loss of sensation induced by a drug. This can be loss of sensation in a body part, which is called local anesthesia, or loss of consciousness with general anesthesia.

- **angiography**
the x-ray of vessels after injecting a contrasting fluid.

- **angiotensin-converting enzyme (ACE) inhibitor**
drug, which decreases the function of this particular enzyme. The angiotensin-converting enzyme changes a compound called angiotensin I to angiotensin II. Angiotensin II is a potent blood vessel constrictor. ACE inhibitors have the effect of dilating blood vessels since less angiotensin II is produced.

- **angular limb deformity**
a limb that is not conformationaly correct because of developmental problems in the angles of the joints.

- **anhydrosis**
inability to sweat in response to work output or increases in body temperature. Also known as a 'non-sweater.' Most are athletic horses though frequently the condition appears in pasteured horses not being ridden. Most commonly occurs when both the temperature and humidity are high. Horses raised in temperate regions and then transported to hot climates are most prone to develop the condition but even acclimated horses can be at risk. Clinical signs include inability to sweat, increased respiratory rate, elevated body temperature and decreased exercise tolerance. The condition can be reversed if the horse is moved to a more temperate climate.

- **animal baiting**

animal baiting prevailed in seventeenth-century Europe. This now illegal activity is markedly one of the most demented and illustriously cruel undertakings of modern mankind. Bull, bear, and boar baiting were the first of these 'sports' to be enjoyed. Baiting was popular with all classes of society. The dogs were intended to lay the baited animal by the ears, eventually grappling the animal by the snout or nose becaoe increasingly popular. Thus the smaller dogs were favoured and received the most tumultuous approval of the spectators. A bulldog was considered to be any dog that could function in the 'sport' of bullbaiting. Those bulldogs bred in England during the early 1800s were more specifically of mastiff origins, selected for particular traits. The Bulldog of Britain, one of the world's most distinctive and admired canines, while no longer possessing the ability to function in a sporting capacity, does maintain the short legs and undershot jaw for which many of the bulldog types were bred. Bullbaiting was the most widespread of the animal baiting 'sports.' Like these other sports, bullbaiting was a terrible, frighteningly brainless diversion: 'it is the most cruel and infernal practice that ever entered the mind of man, under the prostituted appellation of sport to the multitude.'

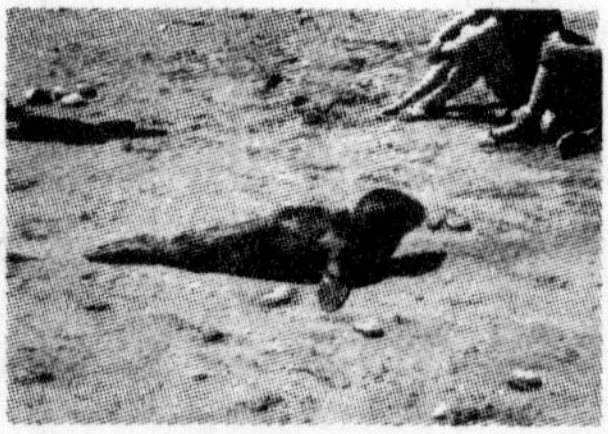

- **animal reservoir**

an animal with an inapparent infection that is also transmitting the agent.

- **animal rights**

a ideology defined by the belief that in addition to meeting the basic needs of an animal, taking into account their species specific behaviours and some other criteria, society has a moral obligation to make sure that those animals are appropriately cared for and handled.

- **animal well being**
a state in which the animal is existing within a range of acceptable environmental and psychological specifications.

- **animals rights**
a belief in the total elimination of use of animals in our society, period. Human life is equated to animal life.

- **anisocoria**
pupils that are unequal in size. The problem may be caused by diseases of the eye or the nerves to the eyes.

- **anisocytosis**
varied sizes of red blood cells. May be an indicator of regenerative anaemia.

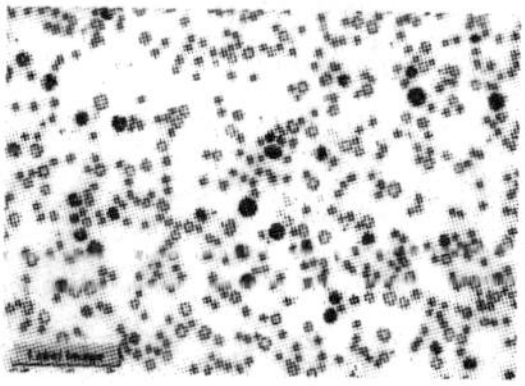

- **anoestrus**
the period of inactivity in the female cat's reproductive cycle.

- **anorexia**
lack of appetite. May be partial or total.

- **antagonist**
a drug which when attached to a receptor blocks the receptor from being stimulated by an agonist drug.

- **anterior**
positioned in front of another body part, or towards the head of the animal. Opposite of posterior.

- **anterior chamber**
space between the cornea and iris and filled with aqueous.

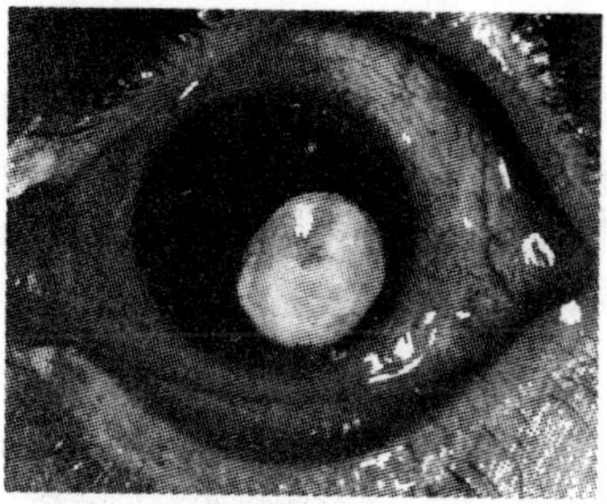

- **anterior enteritis**
acute inflammation of the small intestine producing signs of abdominal distress, such as colic and diarrhoea.

- **anterior uveitis**
inflammation of the iris and ciliary body.

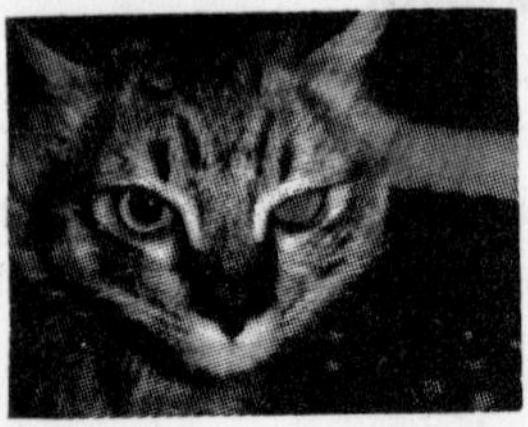

• **anthelmintic**
medication which kills certain types of intestinal worms, dewormer.

• **anthropomorphism**
projecting human needs or wants on to an animal.

• **antibiotic**
a class of drug usually produced by living organisms (molds, bacteria or green plants), which can inhibit or kill undesirable bacteria. Example: penicillin.

• **antibody**
a protein produced by the immune system to protect the body from disease caused by infectious agents (bacteria, viruses).

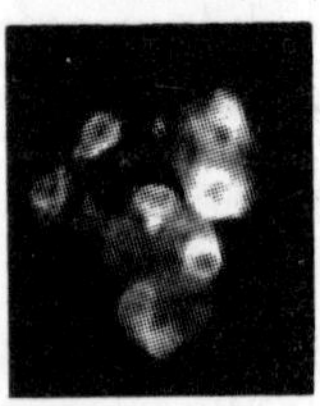

• **an antibody titer**
a measurement of the amount of antibodies in the blood. The test to measure antibodies is usually performed by making a number of dilutions of the blood and then measuring at what dilution there is sufficient antibody to react in the test. For example, a titer of 1:8 (one to eight) means the blood can be diluted to one part blood and seven parts saline and still produce a positive reaction in the test. The higher the titer (1:16 is higher than 1:8), the more antibody is present.

• **anticholinergic**
stopping the communication between certain nerves and muscles of the body including those of the gastrointestinal tract and heart. These nerves are called parasympathetic nerves and do such things as constrict the pupils of the eye, stimulate contractions of the muscles in the intestine, and slow the heart rate. Anticholinergic drugs have the effect of dilating the pupils, slowing contractions of the intestines, and increasing the heart rate.

• **anticholinesterase**
a drug that blocks the enzyme acetylcholinesterase; this results in stimulation of the parasympathetic nervous system.

• **anticoagulants**
drugs that reduce the ability of the blood to clot. Also called blood thinners.

• **anticoagulation**
stopping the blood clotting process.

• **anticonvulsant**
a drug used to prevent or decrease the severity of convulsions.

• **antidiuretic hormone (Abrev: ADH)**
a hormone produced in the brain that acts on the kidney causing it to save water and to produce less urine.

• **antiemetics**
drugs administered to reduce vomitting.

• **antifungal**
a drug used in the treatment of a disease caused by a fungus.

• **antigen**
a molecular structure on surfaces of such particles as bacteria and viruses. This structure is recognised by the body as 'foreign' and stimulates the body to produce special proteins called antibodies to inactivate this foreign invader.

• **antiprotozoal**
an agent that kills protozoa, which are one-celled organisms such as Giardia.

• **antipruritic**
relieves itching.

• **antipyretics**
drugs that suppress a fever in an attempt to bring the temperature to normal.

• **antiseptic**
a substance which inhibits the growth of bacteria but does not kill them.

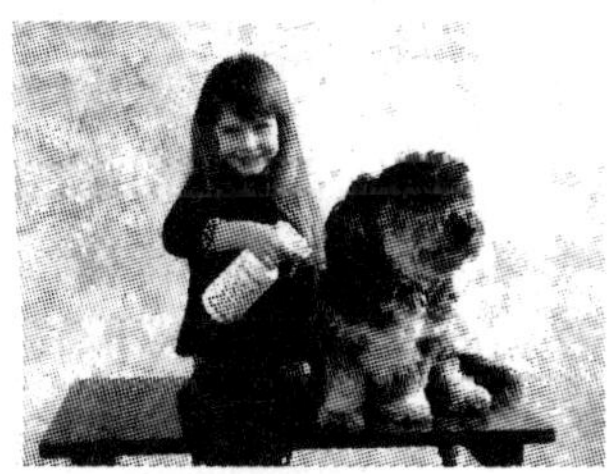

• **antispasmodic**
an agent that relieves or decreases spasms in muscle. The muscle could include 'smooth muscle' which is the type of muscle in intes-

tines that causes them to contract and move food through the digestive system.

- **antitussive**
cough suppressant.

- **anuria**
the condition of complete failure of the function of the kidneys such that no urine is produced.

- **anus**
the muscular tissue at the end of the rectum that keeps stool in the rectum until the animal defecates.

- **aon**
all others normal

- **apical (fracture)**

- **see sesamoids.**

- **aplastic anaemia**
a serious condition in which red blood cells, white blood cells, and platelets are not produced in sufficient quantity.

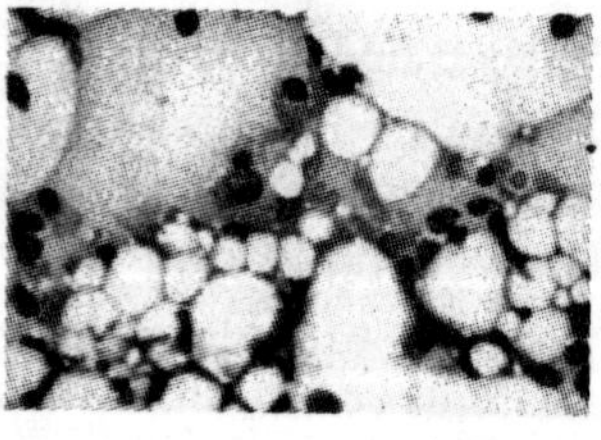

- **apron**
the (usually) paved area between the grandstand and the racing surface.

- **aquaculture**
The (usually commercial) captive raising of fish, corals, and other aquatic life for aquariums, food, and scientific purposes.

- **aqueous**
the clear liquid produced by the cells of the ciliary body which fills the anterior chamber (between the cornea and iris) and the posterior chamber (between the iris and lens).

- **aqueous humour**
the fluid found within the eyeball which provides nourishment to the interior eye structures and keeps the eyeball inflated.

- **arf**
apical repositioned flap - surgical procedure used to replace gingiva apically to eliminate periodontal pocket.

- **arrested development**
the parasites 'hibernate' in the host as a fourth stage

larva, and then in spring, they come out.

- **arrhythmia**
  a variation from normal heart rhythm.

- **arteries**
  blood vessels that carry blood from the heart to the organs and tissues. Arteries contain more oxygen and

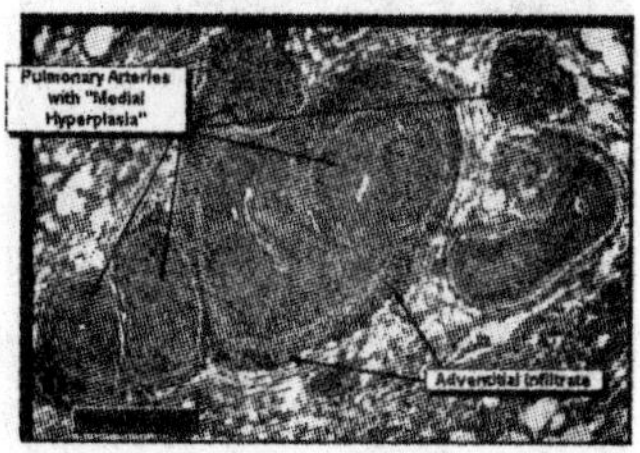

nutrients than veins and are under higher pressure.

- **arthritis**
  inflammation of a joint. An increase in the amount of synovial fluid in the joint is a result of this inflammation. Accumulation of synovial fluid in the fetlock joint is called a 'wind puff' or 'wind gall.' In young horses, a swelling in the fetlock joint, particularly on the front of the joint where the cannon and long pastern bones meet, is called a 'green osselet.' This swelling is a result of inflammation and reactive changes of the front edges of these two bones and adjacent cartilage. If the green osselet does not heal, a 'chronic osselet' might develop with a permanent build-up of synovial fluid in the joint and inflammation and thickening of the joint capsule over the damaged area with secondary bone changes following the initial inflammation.

- **arthroscope**
  a tiny tube of lenses used for viewing areas inside a joint. Usually attached to a small video camera.

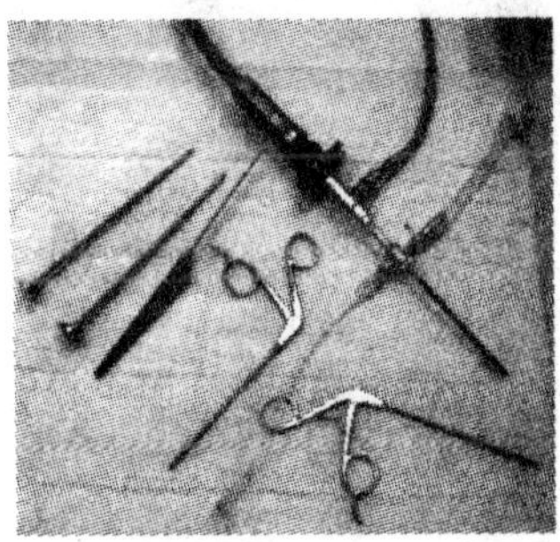

- **arthroscopic surgery**
  utilising an arthroscope to perform surgery, eliminating the need to open the joint with a large incision in order to view the damaged area.

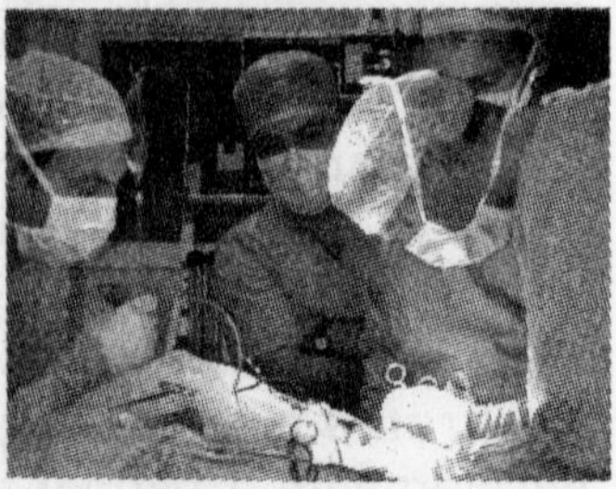

- **articular**
  pertaining to a joint.
- **articular cartilage**
  cartilage that covers the ends of bones where they meet in a joint.
- **artificial breeding**
  includes artificial insemination or embryo transfer (transplants).
- **artificial insemination (Abrev: AI)**
  the female is artifically inseminated with the male's sperm, breeding does not take place.
- **artificial vagina (Abrev: AV)**
  a rubber cone attached to a collection tube that is used to collect semen.
- **ARU**
  Animal Resources Unit
- **arytenoid cartilages**
  triangular cartilages in the upper part of the entrance to the larynx. Movements of the arytenoid cartilages control the diameter of the laryngeal opening.
- **as fed basis**
  an expression of feed nutrient content with moisture included. Nutrient content on an 'as fed' basis is always lower than on a 'dry matter' basis.
- **asap**
  as soon as possible
- **ascarid**
  roundworm.
- **ascites**
  the accumulation of fluid in the peritoneal cavity. Some define ascites as fluid of any type including blood, bile and other exudates. Others define ascites as including only pure transudates.

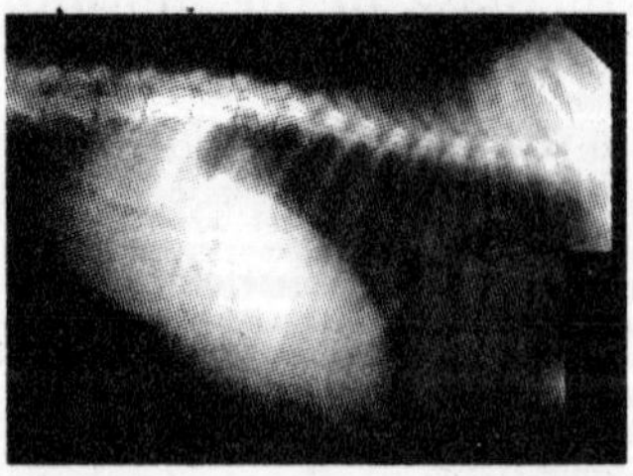

- **ash**
  the inorganic mineral elements of animals and plants, determined by burning off

the organic matter and weighing the residue (ash).

- **aspirate**
  withdrawing fluid or cells through the use of suctions. Usually the suction is produced by pulling back on the plunger of a syringe attached to a needle, which is inserted into the area to be sampled.

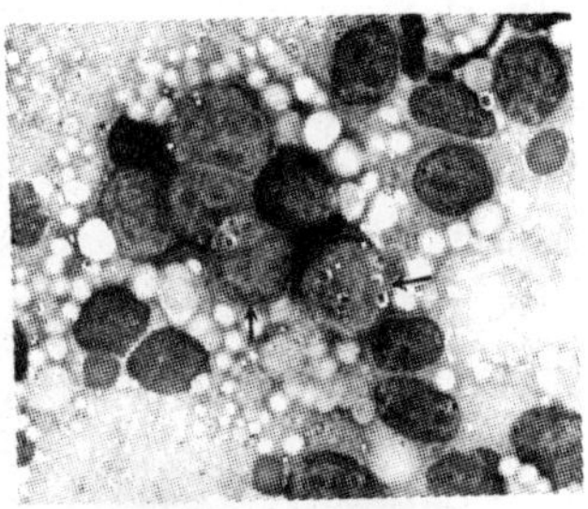

- **aspiration**
  inhaling food or other materials into the airways.

- **aspirin**
  a fair amount is known about the mechanism of action of acetylsalicilic acid and its nonsteriodal anti-inflammatory cousins. They inhibit the synthesis of prostaglandins, potent mediators of inflammation . Aspirin also has an inhibitory effect upon the release of PGE2 and F2 alpha from platelets, which quite nicely accounts for its anti-clotting activity. Aspirin inhibits local release of bradykinns, which decreases pain.

- **assessment**
  the interpretation of patient data. For example what is the significance of nucleated RBCs.

- **asthma**
  an allergic condition leading to wheezing and difficulty in breathing.

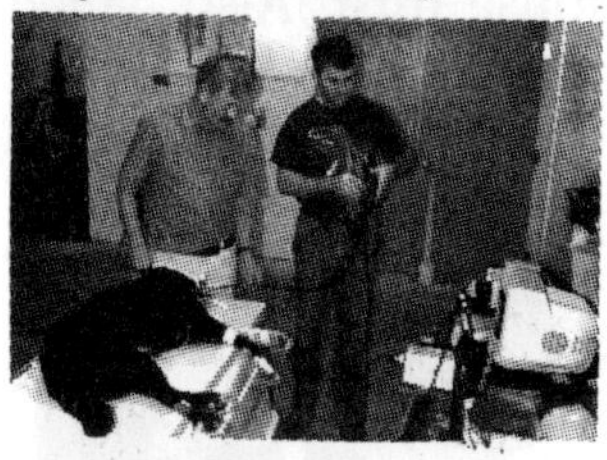

- **asymptomatic**
  a term used to decide a condition in which no symptoms are present.

- **asystole**
  cardiac arrest.

- **attrition**
  a pathological wearing away of the tooth caused by an opposing tooth

- **ataxia**
  a lack of muscle coordination usually causing an abnormal or staggered gait in a horse.

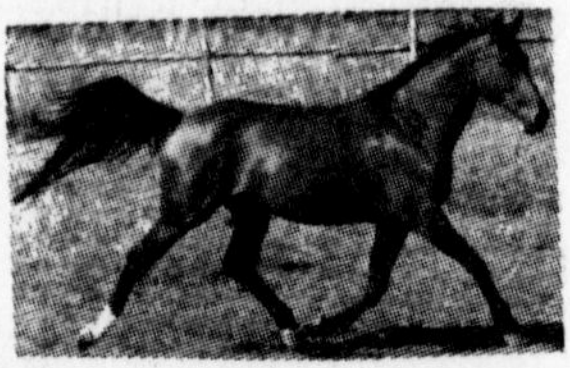

- **atoll**
  a coral island consisting of a reef surrounding a lagoon.

- **atopy**
  an allergy to something that is inhaled such as pollen or house dust. Also called inhalant allergy.

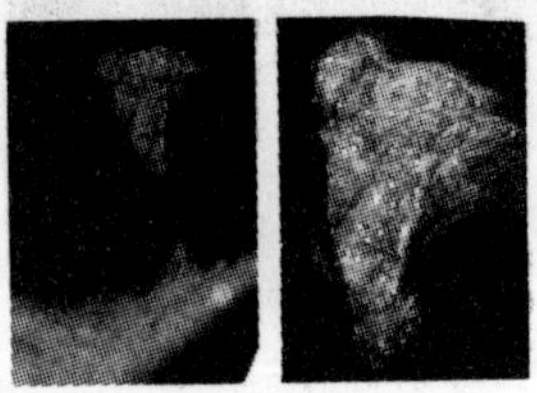

- **ATP**
  Adenosine triphosphate, a compound used for energy by cells.

- **atresia**
  regressing or shrinking in size.

- **atria**
  the heart has 4 chambers; the two chambers that make up the top of the heart are the atria.

- **atrial fibrillation/flutter**
  a heart condition in which the atria (chambers of the heart that receive the blood) contract rapidly, irregularly, and independently of the ventricles (the chambers of the heart that pump the blood). This greatly decreases the efficiency of the heart and its ability to move blood.

- **atrium (plural atria)**
  the two chambers of the heart that receive blood. The right atrium receives blood from the body. The left

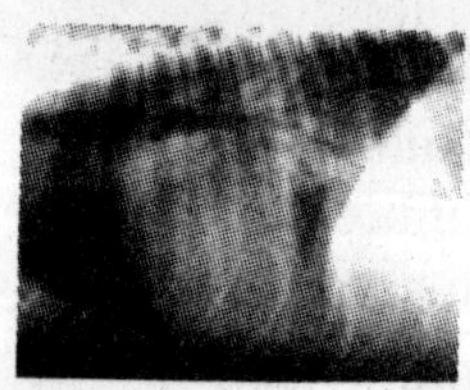

  atrium receives oxygenated blood from the lungs.

- **atrophy**
  to waste away, usually used in describing muscles.

- **atropine**
  a parasympatholytic drug which competitively blocks acetylcholine at muscarinic receptors and increases sinus node automaticity and atrial-ventricular conduc-

tion resulting in an increase in heart rate.

- **attack rate**
  The proportion of a defined population affected during an outbreak. Since the attack rate is based only on new cases of disease, it is comparable to incidence.

- **attenuated**
  weakened. An attenuated virus is one, which has been changed such that it will no longer cause disease. An attenuated virus would be used in a modified live vaccine.

- **attenuation**
  the reduction in virulence of an infectious agent.

- **auscultation**
  to listen with a stethoscope. The heart and lung sounds are heard by auscultation.

- **Australian cattle dog**
  the continent's pride and joy is the product of six decades of crossing and crisscrossing various breeds in an attempt to produce a herder stolid enough to work the rugged Australian environment. The Australian Cattle Dog, commonly called the Blue Heeler and also known as the Australian Queensland Heeler, carries the infusion of Bull Terrier, Dalmatian, Australian Kelpie, Red Deer Dingo, and two blue-merle, smooth-coated Collies. Exceedingly distressed with their dog's inability to work the wild native cattle of Australia, herdsmen began serious breeding programmes to produce an able dog. During the 1830, ambitious cattlemen crossed the Smithfield Collie with the wild dingo. The litter was known as Timmon's Biters they were more reserved and barked less than the overactive Smithfields but bit too hard for the job. Ten years later, Mr. Thomas Hall crossed two blue-merle, smooth-coated Collies with working dingoes. The half-breeds proved a notable success. Further crosses to Timmon's Biters and other experimental crossbreeds as well as the Dalmatian, Bull Terrier etc., yielded this silent, hard nipping but not distressing cattle herder. The breed has been bred true

since the year 1893. The Blue Heeler is so versatile that, in addition to cattle, he can work horses, goats, and even ducks with skill and panache. As a rule, the breed maintains a touch of the unruly and unrefined - all to his greater ability. He is 100% working dog, fearless and determined.

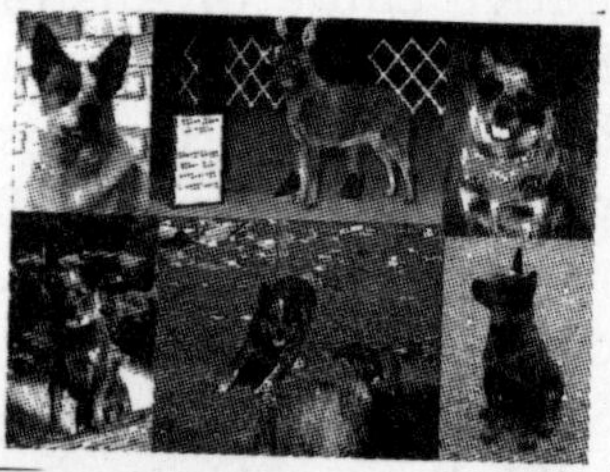

- **australian kelpie**

this native Australian breed developed from English North Country Collies of the Rutherford strain, which were well-built, thick-skulled, smooth-haired, semi-prick-eared dogs of stamina and courage. It is unlikely that many early herdsmen of Australia would have concerned themselves with the preservation of type. It is believed that they crossed the many Rutherford Collies with other proven herding dogs in the endless attempt to better the working dog, ending in the production of the Kelpie, known also as the Barb. Although many still assert that the Kelpie is a dingo cross, their position lacks supporting data. At most, dingo blood reached the Kelpie indirectly through crosses with native working dogs, which, although they are believed to have occurred, are suspected of happening only infrequently. Today nearly 100, 000 Kelpies are employed on the continent of Australia. Besides being outstanding herders of cattle, goats, poultry and reindeer, Kelpies also find work as search and rescue and detection dogs, which is surprising in consideration of their relatively small size.

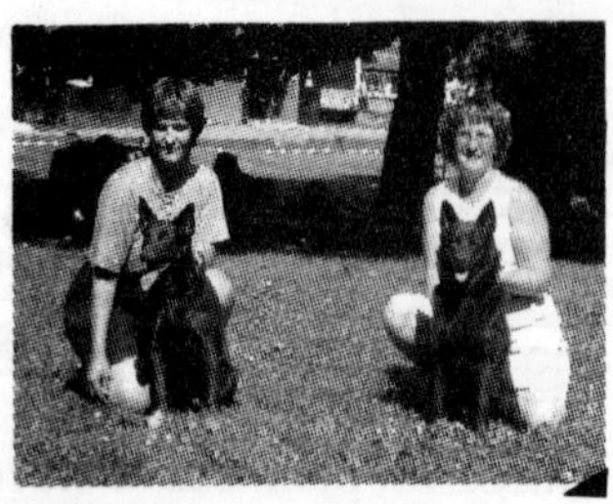

- **australian terrier**

the Australian Terrier, perhaps the only well-knwon

terrier breed (excluding the Silky Terrier) not created in Great Britain, was actually created by the British in Australia. As far back as the early nineteenth century, ten-pound blue and tan broken-coated terriers were popular in Australia as were sandy-colored dogs. The Australian Terrier was created from a blend of imported terriers from northern England and Scotland. Although the actual crossings are not recorded, Scottish Terrier, Cairn Terrier, Skye Terrier, Dandie Dinmont Terrier, Manchester Terrier and Irish Terrier are the usual suspects, each contributing individual traits to the creation of this Broken Coated Toy Terrier, as the Aussie was originally named. This little terrier was handy on rabbit and prized for his ability to handle snake. His feisty, jumping-bean approach allowed him the dexterity to spring into the air and manoeuvre himself behind the snake's neck in order to kill it. Of course, the Australian Terrier's confident attitude made him a terrific watchdog.

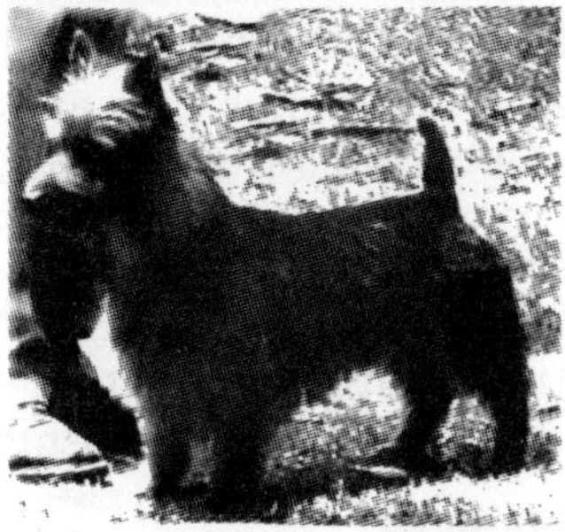

- **autoimmune**

condition in which in the immune system attacks the body's own tissues. To properly function, the immune system must identify foreign substances such as bacteria, viruses, parasites, slivers, etc., and it must be able to distinguish normal body tissue from these foreign substances. If the immune system fails to distinguish the difference, it attempts to destroy the tissue it wrongly identifies as foreign. For example, in autoimmune haemolytic anaemia, the body destroys its own red blood cells. In rheumatoid arthritis, the immune system attacks the cells in joints.

- **autoimmune haemolytic anaemia**

the body produces antibodies directed against its own red blood cells, causing their destruction. Many if not all of the autoimmune anaemias have antibodies that attack related, similar blood types.

- **autoimmunity**
  producing an immune response against normal or altered body components.

- **autosomal**
  any of the chromosomes other than the sex pair, the 'X' or 'Y' chromosomes.

- **auxiliary starting gate**
  a second starting gate used when the humber of horses in a race exceeds the capacity of the main starting gate.

- **avulsion**
  the separation of a tooth from its alveolus

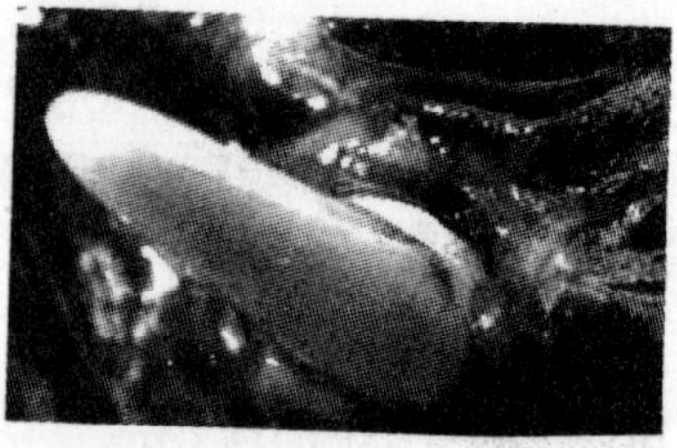

- **available protein**
  The portion of the crude protein that can be used by the animal.

- **average daily gain (Abrev: ADG)**
  the average daily live weight increase of a growing animal; usually expressed in kg, g or lb./day.

- **AEI (Average-Earnings Index)**
  a breeding statistic that compares racing earnings of a stallion or mare's foals to those of all other foals racing at that time. An AEI of 1.00 is considered average, 2.00 is twice the average, 0.50 half the average, etc.

- **awe**
  acute wet eczema

- **awn hair**
  Short, thick, bristly hair, which lies underneath a cat's topcoat.

- **ax**
  axial

- **axilla**
  armpit.

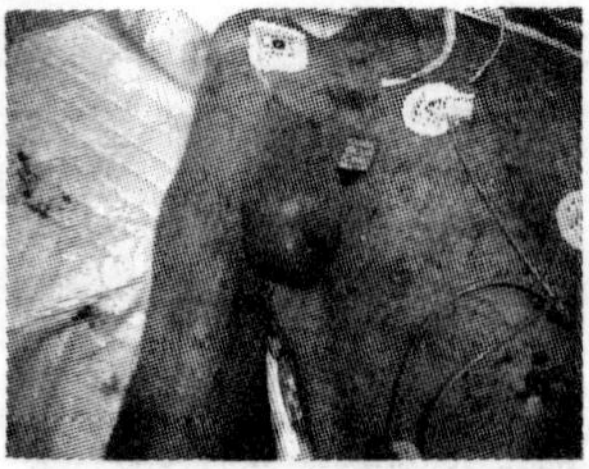

- **azathioprine**
  an immuno suppressive drug used in cancer chemotherapy and in treatment of immune mediated diseases.

• **azoospermia**
the complete absence of sperm in the ejaculate.

• **azotemia**
an increase in nitrogen containing waste products in the blood. Azotemia may be prerenal, renal or post-renal.

• **b**
booster

• **B cell**
also called B lymphocyte. The type of lymphocyte, which produces antibodies.

• **b.i.d.**
Twice a day. From Latin bis in die

• **B.V.M.S.**
Bachelor of Veterinary Medicine and Surgery.

• **B.V.Sc.**
Bachelor of Veterinary Science.

• **b/w**
black and white

• **back at the knee**
a leg that looks like it has a backward arc with its centre at the knee when viewed from the side.

• **bacterémias**
a bacterial population in the blood.

• **bacteria**
microscopic organisms that may be normal or may cause disease. The healthy body normally contains some bacteria.

• **bacterial or prokaryotes**
single celled organisms without a true nucleus.

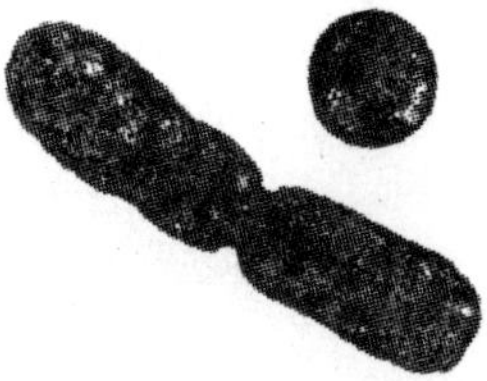

• **bacterin**
a vaccine made from a bacteria.

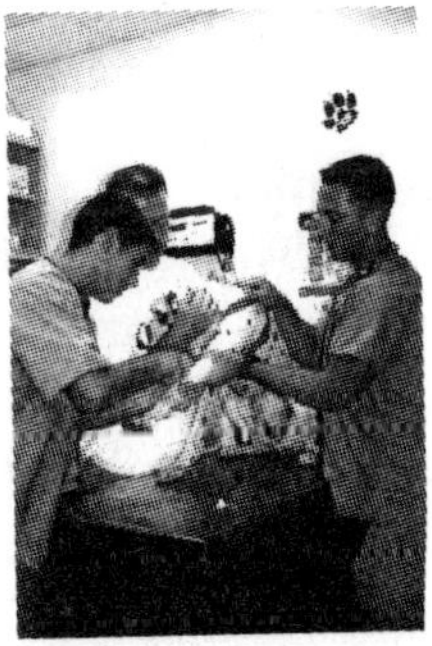

• **bacteriocidal**
a description of an agent that kills bacteria.

• **bacteriocide**
a substance that kills bacteria.

- **bacteriostat**
  a substance that inhibits or retards bacterial growth.

- **bacteriostatic**
  a description of an agent that stops the growth (reproduction) of bacteria, but does not kill them.

- **bacterium**
  microscopic organisms that lack nuclei and other organelles, pathogenic species cause disease, while non-pathogenic species are harmless.

- **bad doer**
  a horse with a poor appetite, a condition that may be due to nervousness or other causes.

- **balanced ration**
  a 24-hour feed allowance that provides an animal with appropriate amounts and proportions of all nutrients required for a given level of performance.

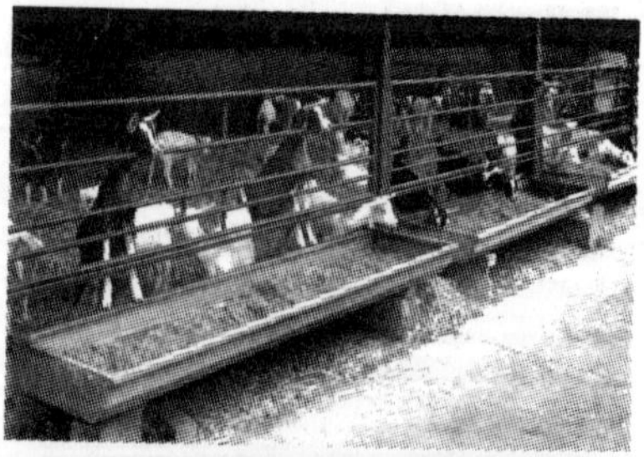

- **balanoposthitis**
  inflammation of the penis (balanitis) and prepuce (posthitis).

- **bandage**
  bandages used on horse's legs are three to six inches wide and are made of a variety of materials. In a race, they are used for support or protection against injury. 'Rundown bandages' are used during a race and usually have a pad under the fetlock to avoid injury due to abrasion when the fetlocks sink toward the ground during weight bearing. A horse may also wear 'standing bandages, ' thick cotton wraps used during shipping and while in the stall to prevent swelling and/or injury.

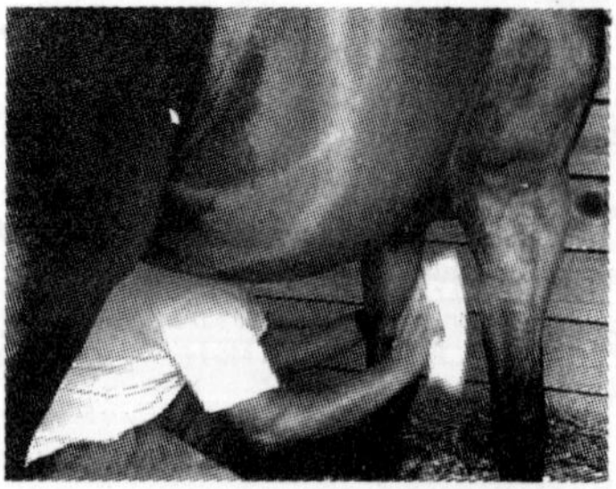

- **banding**
  distinct bands of colour in a cross-wise direction.

- **bar**
bright and responsive, or bright, alert, responsive

- **bar shoe**
a horseshoe closed at the back to help support the frog and heel of the hoof. It is often worn by horses with quarter cracks or bruised feet.

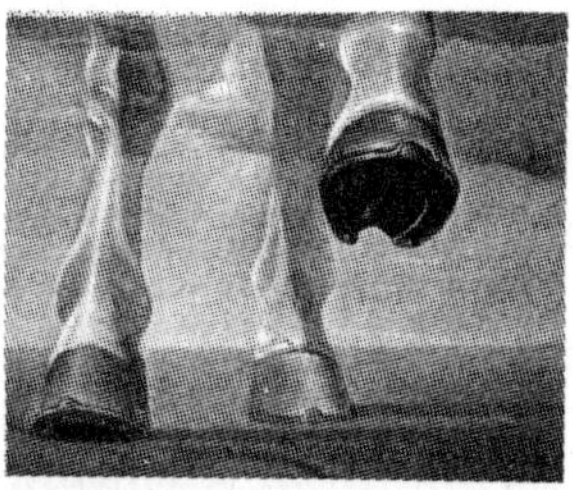

- **barb**
see Australian kelpie.

- **barh**
bright, alert, responsive, hydrated

- **barn ventilation**
most people overdo the warm and toasty bit to the detriment of the horse. Exhaust/air exchange fans are SOP in almost every cow and pig barn around, yet you rarely see them in a horse barn. Good rule of thumb is, if there's moisture condensing on the inside of your windows, you should be increasing your ventilation.

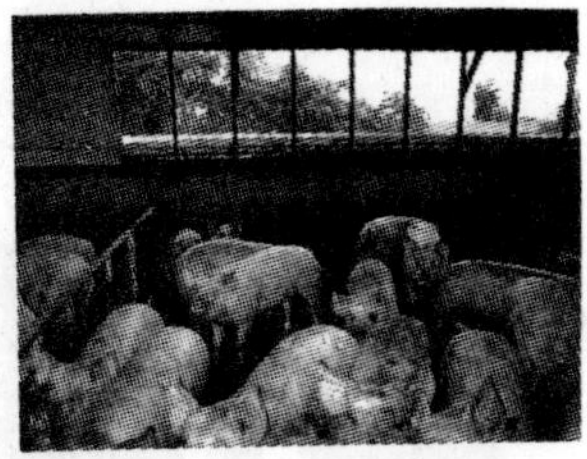

- **barren**
used to describe a filly or mare that was bred and did not conceive during the last breeding season.

- **barrier**
a starting device used in steeple chasing consisting of an elastic band stretched across the racetrack which springs back when released. Also known as a 'tape.'

- **basal fluid loss**
the basal fluid loss is the typical loss of fluids by both insensible and sensible routes. For a normal adult dog or cat, the net basal loss is about 20-30 ml/lb/day.

- **basilar (fracture)**
see sesamoids.

- **basset**
french term for a short-legged scent hound; equivalent to the German term

dachshund. The French have a number of basset types, which developed, in the Vendee, Bretagne, Normand and Gascogne regions.

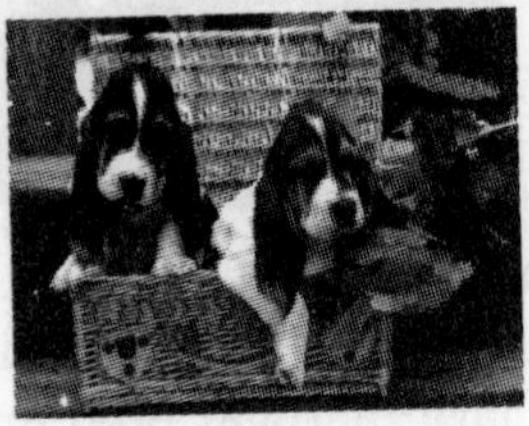

- **batch furrow system**

a management system where pigs are raised in batches from piglets to market hogs and as they mature the raising area they left is cleaned, disinfected, and left vacant until the next batch of pigs is purchased.

- **battery**

a term for an illegal electrical device used by a jockey to stimulate a horse during a race. Also known as a 'mahine' or 'joint.'

- **bay**

a horse colour that varies from a yellow-tan to a bright auburn. The mane, tail and lower portion of the legs are always black, except where white markings are present.

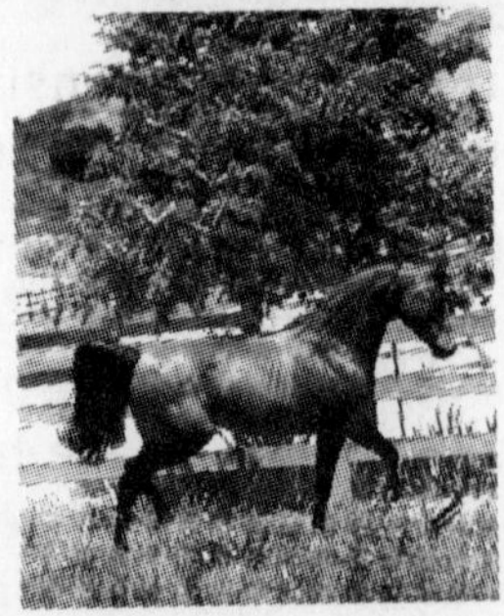

- **b-cells**

this cell population is derived directly from the bone marrow and is important because it gives rise to antibodies (humoral immunity).

- **BCU**

Biomedical Communications Unit

- **bearing in (or out)**

deviating from a straight course. May be due to weariness, infirmity, inexperience or the rider overusing the whip or reins to make a horse alter its course.

- **bedlington terrier**

the Bedlington Terrier, known in its pre-pedigree years as the Rothbury or Northumberland Fox Terrier, acquired its present name in 1825 when Mr. Joseph Ainsley referred to 'Piper' (undecidedly 'Young' or 'Old') as a Bedlington Terrier. The first dog documented as the predecessor of the Bedlington breed was owned by Squire Trevelyan and was whelped in 1782. One Northumbrian piper named James Allan was the original owner of Rothbury Terriers. This musically inadequate otter hunter belonged to the line of Yetholme gypsies, tinkers by trade. Allan's Rothburys were mercilessly game on otters, rats, and badger. 'Peachem' and 'Pincher' were Allan's two favourite terriers. As terrier crosses were common in the early nineteenth century, it is difficult to ascertain which of the British terriers were amalgamated to yield the Bedlington. If the Dandie Dinmont in fact predates the fixed Bedlington, it was likely a key ingredient, scholars disagree which breed came first. The Whippet and Otter Hound are the other two dogs generally thrown into the gene pool. Regardless, the result is a distinctive terrier with an assortedly sordid history. The Bedlington has not always been a well-groomed, soft show terrier, glowing with unsubtle ovinity, but was once a very hard game dog used by gypsies in northern England as a poacher and pit fighter. The dogs were fancied by many walks of life, including miners and pitmen, as hunters and ratters. The fast-paced industrialisation that swept Europe forced this overly snarly contender to mellow and concede to today's more fanciful fancier's type, which does not loathe the rat nor fancy dust-ups with his kind.

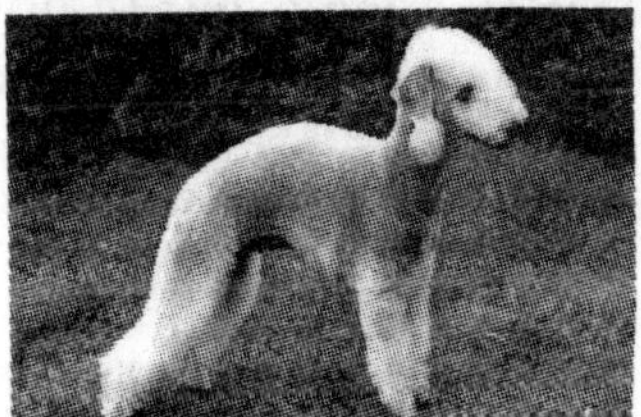

- **behaviour**

the act or manner in which animals conduct themselves.

- **benign**

a mild illness or a non-malignant form of a tumour. Benign tumours usually have well defined edges and tend to grow slowly.

- **benign prostate hypertrophy (Abrev: BPH)**
  a condition in which the prostate gland enlarges under the influence of sex hormones. BPH can lead to infection of the prostate gland.

- **benzoyl peroxide**
  topical antibacterial agent available as a gel and shampoo.

- **bernese mountain dog**
  the native Swiss dog to gain the most worldwide popularity and recognition. He remains, however, undeservingly sparse in number. An undoubtedly hardy dog of great strength and endurance, the Bernese can also be trained at a variety of canine tasks.

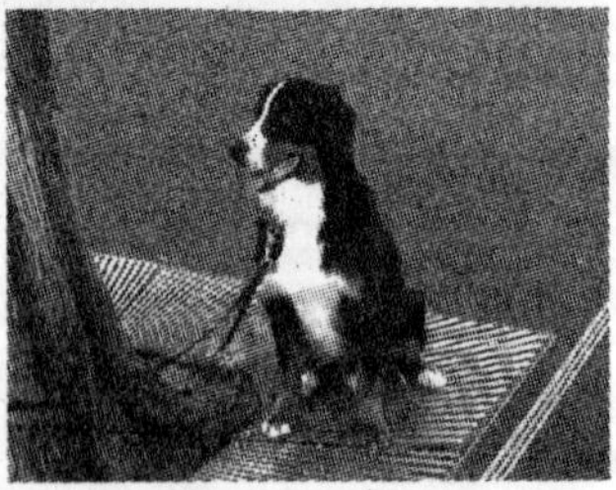

- **beta blockers**
  heart medications which block certain receptors in the heart called beta receptors. The beta-receptors receive signals, which generally increase the heart rate. If the heart rate is abnormally fast and uneven, beta-blockers will help stabilise the rate and rhythm of contractions.

- **beta carotene**
  a plant pigment which can be converted to vitamin A by many animals but not by cats.

- **beta lactamases**
  enzymes produced by some bacteria which inactivate certain types of penicillin thus making the bacteria resistant to them.

- **beyer number**
  a handicapping tool, popularised by author Andrew Beyer, assigning a numerical value (speed figure) to each race run by a horse based on final time and track condition. This enables different horses running at different racetracks to be objectively compared.

- **bib**
  the part of the ruff, or lengthened hair, around the chest area.

- **bicarbonate precursors**
  bicarbonate precursors are converted by the liver to bicarbonate and include Acetate, Gluconate, Lactate, and Citrate.

- **bicolour**
  a cat with more than two spots of colour on the torso, either white and one basic colour, or white with one tabby colour.

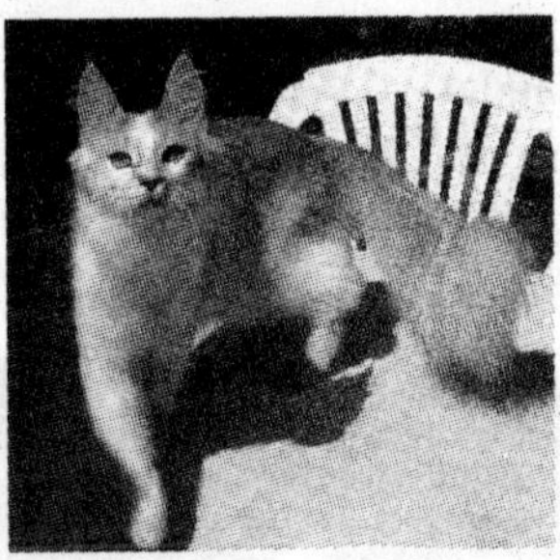

- **bifn**
  back if necessary

- **bilateral**
  involving both sides.

- **bile**
  a yellow fluid produced by the liver and stored in the gall bladder that helps in the digestion of fats.

- **bile acids**
  substances produced by the liver and secreted in the bile that aid digestion.

- **bilirubin**
  a substance produced when old red blood cells are destroyed in the body. Abnormal amounts of bilirubin cause jaundice and are caused by breakdown of large numbers of red blood cells or by disease of the liver or gall bladder.

- **biop**
  been in owner's possession

- **biopsy**
  surgical removal of a small amount of abnormal tissue, usually of tumours, for diagnosis.

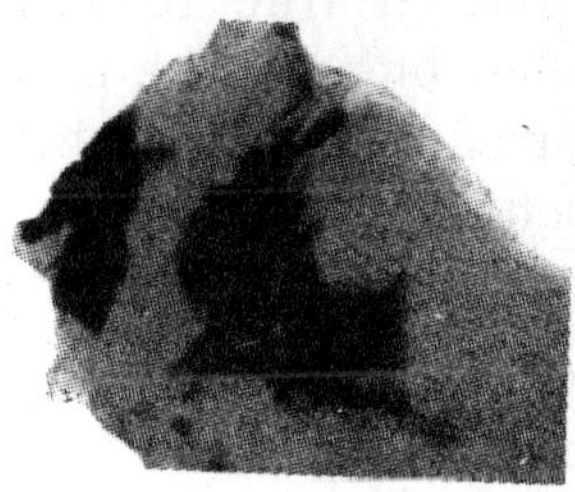

- **biotin**
  biotin will help wall regrowth only in those cases where there is a dietary deficiency or absorption.

- **bi-parietal diameter**
  the diameter of the skull as determined using ultrasound. This diameter can be used to determine age of the foetus.

• **bit**
a stainless steel, rubber or aluminum bar, attached to the bridle, which fits in the horse's mouth and is one of the means by which a jockey exerts guidance and control. The most common racing bit is the D-bit, named because the rings extending from the bar are shaped like the letter 'D.' Most racing bits are 'snaffled, ' (snaffle bit) which means the metal bar is made up of two pieces, connected in the middle, which leaves it free to swivel. Other bits may be used to correct specific problems, such as bearing in or out.

• **bitch**
another term for female dog.

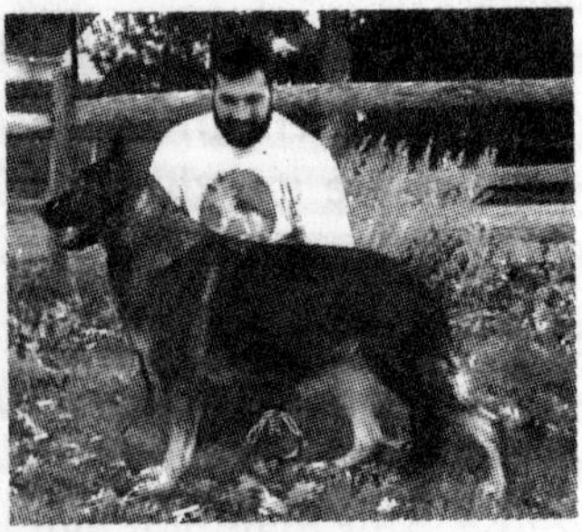

• **biw**
before if worried.

• **black**
a horse colour which is black, including the muzzle, flanks, mane, tail and legs unless white markings are present.

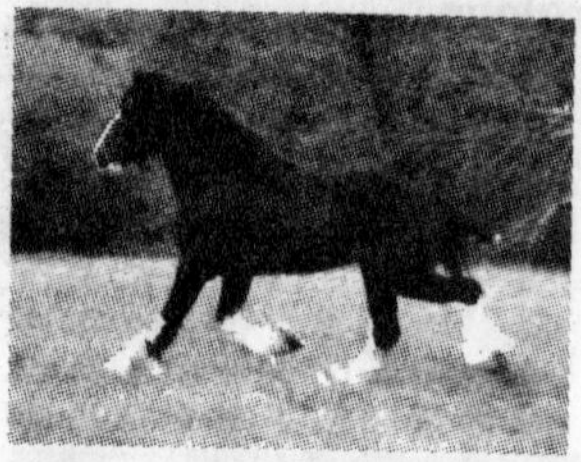

• **bladder**
the sac-like structure, which holds urine until the urine can be passed.

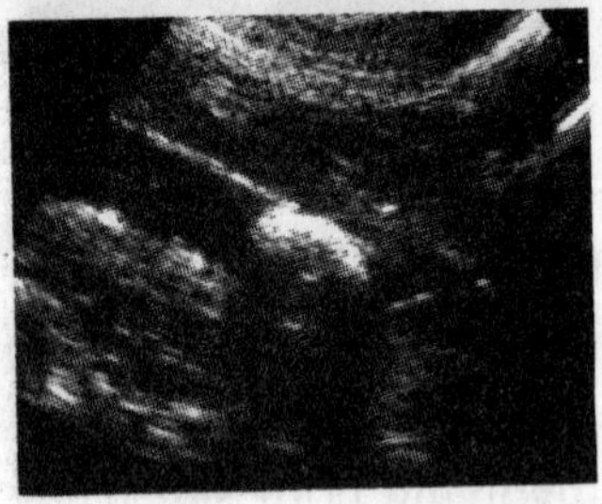

• **blaze**
a generic term describing a large, white vertical marking on a horse's face.

• **bleeder**
a horse that bleeds from the lungs when small capillaries that surround the lungs' air sacs (alveoli) rupture. The medical term is 'exercise-in-

duced pulmonary haemorrhage' (EIPH). Blood may be seen coming out of the horse's nostrils, known as 'epistaxis, ' although it is typically discovered by a fibre optic endoscopic examination after exercise. Hot, humid weather and cold are known to exacerbate the problem. The most common preventative treatment currently available is the use of the diuretic furosemide (Lasix). Less than one bleeder in 20 shows signs of epistaxis.

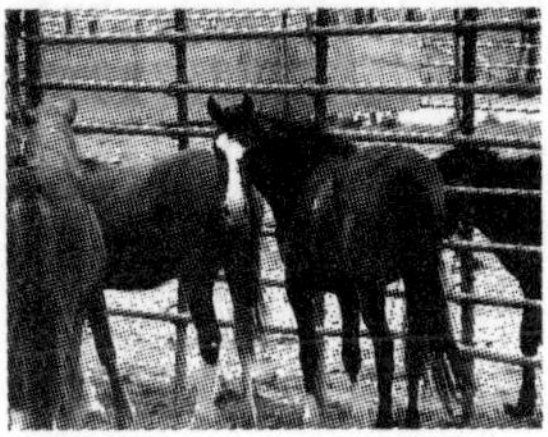

- **blepharitis**
  inflammation of the eyelids.

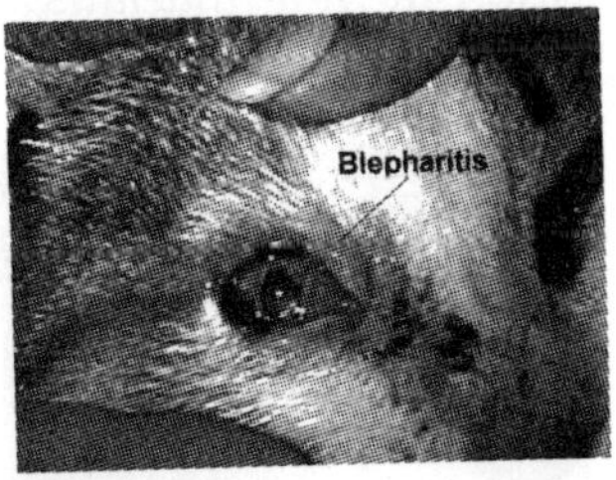

- **blepharospasm**
  spasm of the eyelids often resulting in complete closure of the lids due to eye pain such as seen with a scratch on the cornea.

- **blind switch**
  a circumstance in which a rider's actions cause him/her to be impeded during a race.

- **blinkers**
  a cup-shaped device to limit a horse's vision to prevent him from swerving from objects or other horses on either side of it. Blinker cups come in a variety of sizes and shapes to allow, as little or as much vision as the trainer feels is necessary.

- **blister**
  1. a thin walled structure containing fluid or air such as vesicles and bullae.
  2. counter-irritant causing acute inflammation used to increase blood supply, blood flow and to promote healing in the leg.

- **bloat**
  filling of the stomach with air.

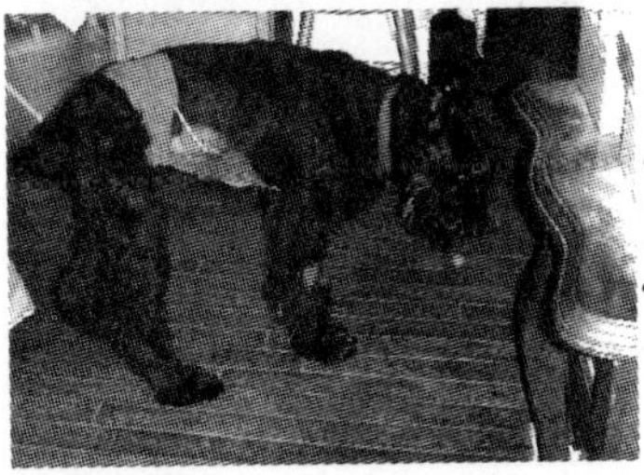

- **blood glucose (bg) or blood sugar (bs)**
  the concentration of glucose in the blood. Measured in milligrams per deciliter (mg/dL) in the US, and millimoles per litre (mmoles/L) in metric.
  Note: different countries use different units of measurement.

- **blood glucose profile (curve)**
  a graph of blood glucose levels over time. At the time of insulin injection, and at regular intervals throughout the day, the level of glucose in the blood is determined through laboratory testing.

- **blood gases**
  gases, such as oxygen or carbon dioxide, that are in the blood.

- **bloodline**
  a group of related animals.

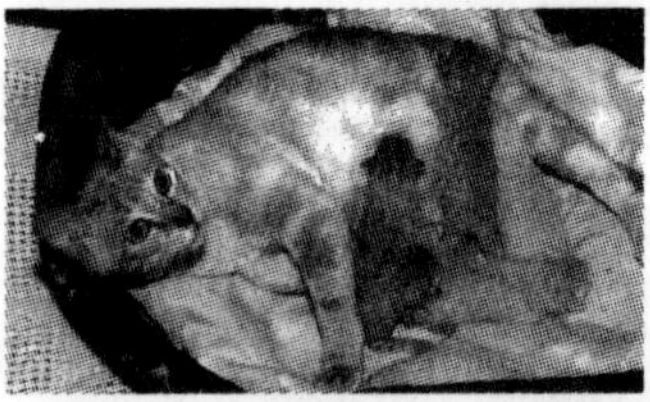

- **bloodstock agent**
  a person who advises and/or represents a buyer or seller of Thoroughbreds at a public auction or a private sale. A bloodstock agent usually works on commission, often five percent of the purchase price, and can also prepare a horse for sale.

- **blood-typing**
  a way to verify a horse's parentage. Blood-typing is usually completed within the first year of a horse's life.

- **blow-out**
  a short, timed workout, usually a day or two before a race, designed to sharpen a horse's speed. Usually three-eighths or one-half of a mile in distance.

- **blue eye**
  a post vaccination adverse event that has been reported by veterinarians vaccinating dogs with the

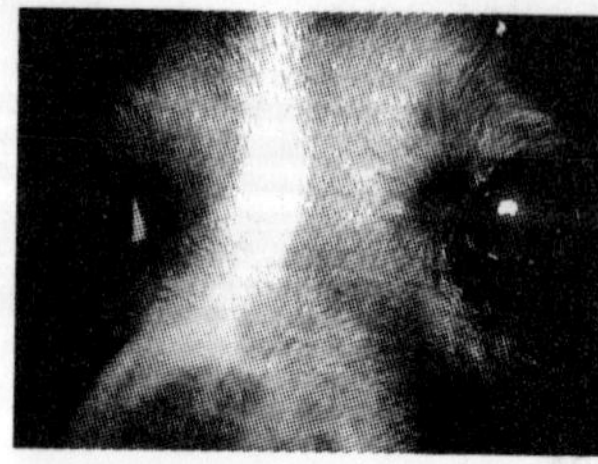

modified-live canine adenovirus-1 vaccine (CAV-1).

- **blue slip**
an application to register a cat of a registered litter.

- **blunt muzzle**
a truncated square muzzle typical of many breeds (e.g., Pointer, Mastiff).

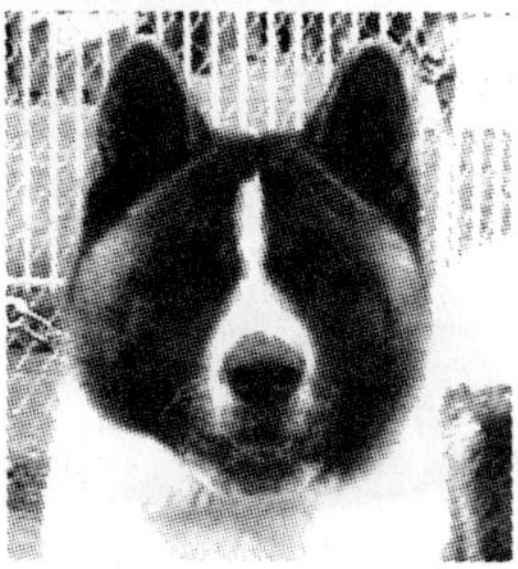

- **bnc**
base narrow canine.

- **body condition score (Abrev: BCS)**
a score based on a scale from 1 to 5 that asseses the amount of body fat on an animal. One is emaciated, three is ideal, and five is obese.

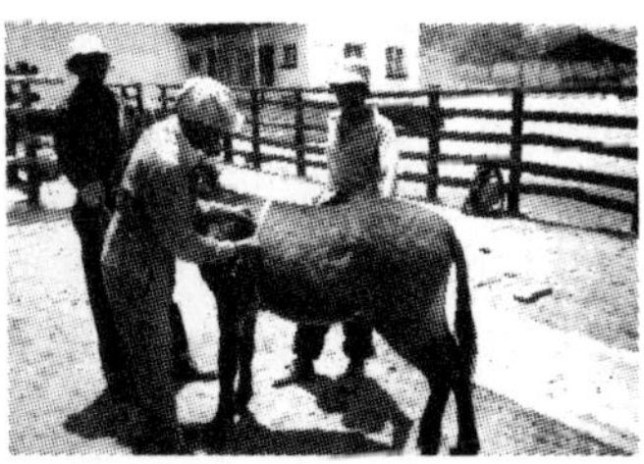

- **bog spavin**
a filling with excess synovial fluid of the largest joint of the hock called the 'tarsocrual joint.'

- **bolus**
the rapid administration of a fluid or drug over a short time period.

- **bone graft**
utilising bone taken from one part of the body to promote formation of bone in another region.

- **bone marrow**
the soft centre of bones. Blood cells are produced in the bone marrow.

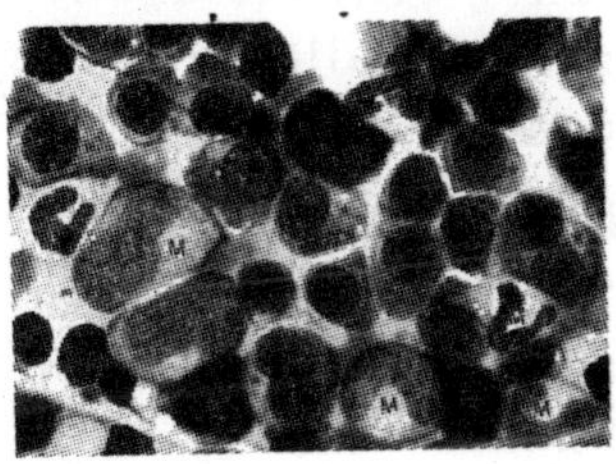

- **bone spavin**
arthritis of the hock joint. A bone spavin that has progressed to the point that the arthritis can be seen externally is called a 'Jack spavin.'

- **bone marrow**
a soft tissue composed of blood vessels and connective tissues found at the centre of bones. The primary

function is blood cell production.

- **bony orbit**
the bony fossa within the skull separating the eyes from the cranial cavity

- **book**
1. the group of mares being bred to a stallion in a given year. If a stallion attracts the maximum number of mares allowed by the farm manager, he has a full book.
2. a term used to describe a jockey's riding commitments with his agent: An agent handles a jockey's book.

- **borborygmus**
the sound of gas moving through the intestine bowel sounds.

- **border collie**
a strong-eyed herder of the old-type collie. The working collie, as he is commonly called, possesses the ability to manipulate a herd or a number of its members with his 'hypnotic' eyes. The Border Collie is deemed the closest purebred representative of the old collies of Scotland, believed to be the 'first' collies. The strong-eye characteristic is perhaps more developed in the Border Collie than in any other breed. His fine-focussed ability allows him to move, stop, steer, or otherwise guide a herd without the need to nip the heels or bark.

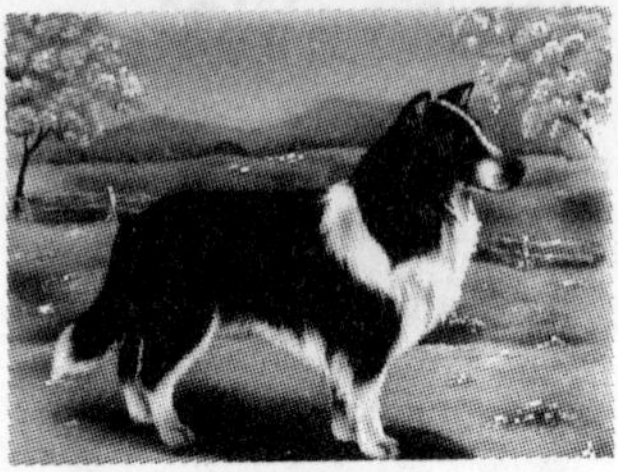

Besides consuming less physical energy, the strong eye is an advantage to the herder because nipping risks the receiving of a kick and the frightening of the herd.

- **border terrier**
the Border Terrier is the common working terrier used by hunters and farmers in the Border area between Scotland and England. In this region, the Border was used to destroy the burrowing and deceptive foxes, which preyed upon livestock. Appearance was never a concern of these workmen, strictly

function likewise, the Border Terrier's conformation is key to its functional abilities. The first written record of the breed dates back to 1880 - an article describing the terriers of Northumberland and Westmoreland. The Border Terrier described here, if not exactly the equivalent of today's standard, was of the general type desired today. Through the course of development, the breed has been called the Reedwater Terrier and the Coquetdale Terrier. Sufficiently legged to keep pace with the horses on the hunt yet squat and plucky enough to go to ground, the Border is truly an ideal worker. This dog's instincts are strong and cannot be ignored

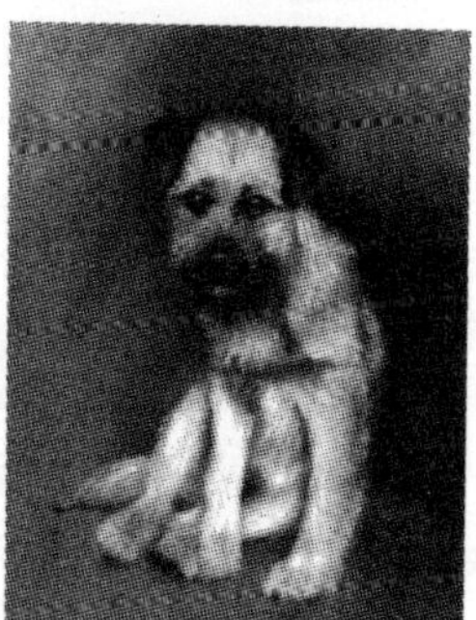

- **bottom**

stamina in a horse.

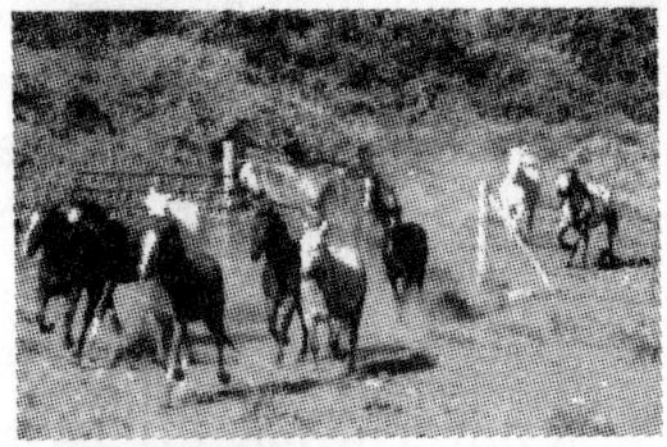

- **bottom line**

a Thoroughbred's breeding on the female side. The lower half of an extended pedigree diagram.

- **bounce**

a poor race run directly following a career-best or near-best performance.

- **bowed tendon**

a type of tendinitis. The most common injury to the tendon is a strain or 'bowed' tendon, so named because of the appearance of a bow shape due to swelling. The most common site of injury is in the superficial flexor tendon between the knee and the ankle. Despite aggressive treatment with anti-inflammatory drugs, physical therapy and rest, horses commonly reinjure the tendon when they go back into competition. Two surgeries are felt to aid horses to come back to racing: tendon splitting at the lesion site to release accumulated fluid and blood, and superior check ligament desmotomy. The latter surgery is designed to reduce forces on the tendon when the horse returns to training and racing.

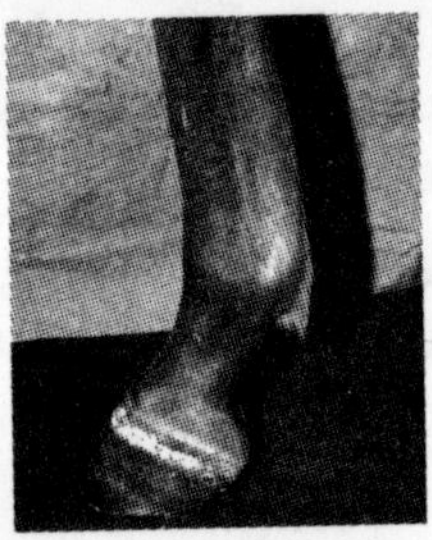

- **boxed (in)**
  to be trapped between, behind or inside of other horses.
- **brace**
  paired dogs of a kind. Braces are used in field trials, sled-dog races, obedience trials, as well as conformation competition.
- **brace-mate**
  each paired dog in bird-dog field trials is called a 'brace-mate' of the other.
- **brachiocephalic**
  a short skull. Used to describe breeds such as Pugs, Bulldogs and Pekingnese dogs.

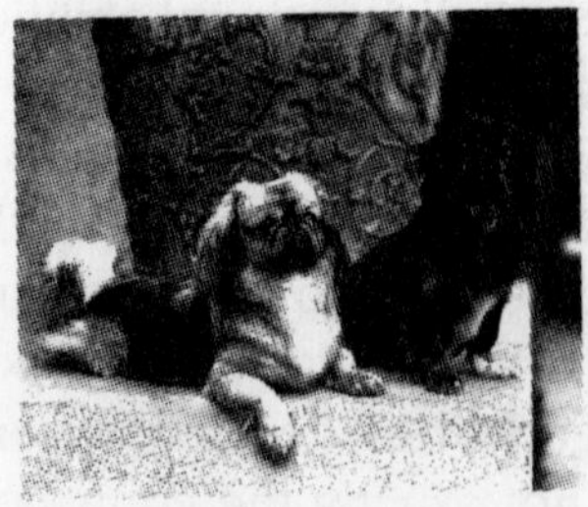

- **bradycardia**
  an abnormal slowing of the heart rate.
- **breakdown**
  when a horse suffers a potentially career-ending injury, usually to the leg: The horse suffered a breakdown. The horse broke down.
- **breech**
  area around the tail and back of hind legs.
- **breed standard**
  1. a written description of what the ideal specimen of a given breed should look like.
  2. the ideal characteristics for the breed, as agreed upon by a group of breeders.
- **breed true**
  to produce kittens that closely resemble the parents.

- **breeding**
  the process of reproduction; mating and giving birth to offspring.

- **breeding programme**
  a programme in which cats are mated together and kittens selected for breeding according to how close they come to an ideal.

- **breeding quality**
  a cat that meets its breed standard closely enough to be valuable to a breeding programme, but may not be competitive as a show cat.

- **breeding records**
  computerised or paper records that document the aspects of the reproductive life of an animal.

- **breeding soundness examination (Abrev: BSE)**
  a series of diagnostic tests performed on a male animal in order to evaluate his capabilities as a stud. The results of the tests are typically recorded in a standardised fashion on a specific form.

- **breed-suitable**
  a cat that meets strict breed criteria, proving its worthiness to reproduce.

- **breeze (breezing)**
  working a horse at a moderate speed, less effort than handily.

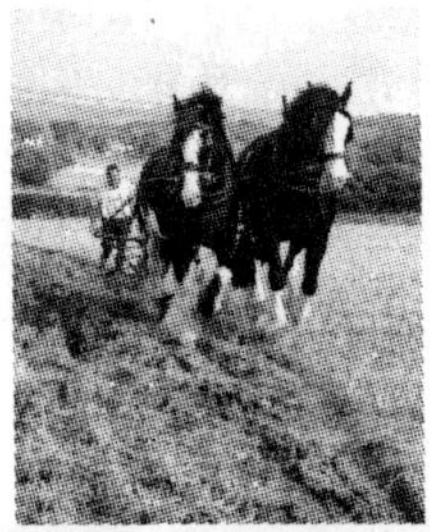

- **bretylium**
  a drug, which diminishes the release of norepinephrine from nerve endings with chronic oral dosing. It is used in treatment of ventricular fibrillation and ventricular tachycardia.

- **bridle**
  a piece of equipment, usually made of leather or nylon, which fits on a horse's head and is where other equipment, such as a bit and the reins, are attached.

- **brisket**
  most often used to refer to the breastbone or sternum, but sometimes referring to the chest itself.

- **brittany**
  a truly unique gundog possessing both setterlike and

spaniellike characteristics. Until 1982 the breed was referred to as Brittany Spaniel by the A.K.C. In its manner of working, however, the breed functions more like a setter. Though in size it is smaller than the typical setter, it is also leggier than the average spaniel.

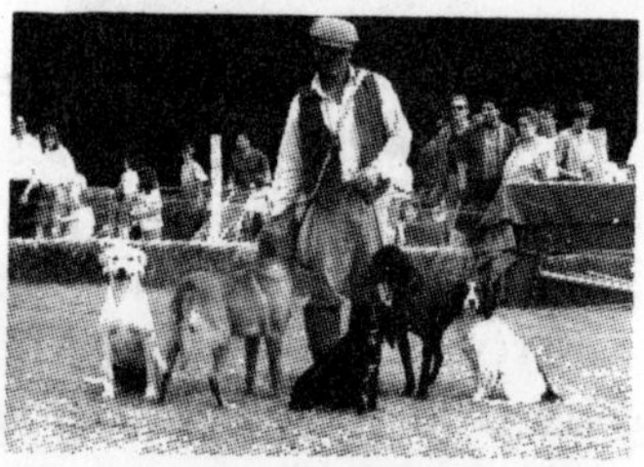

- **broken coat**

a crinkly wire coat, most often applied to terriers. A broken coat is comprised of a harsh outer coat and a dense, soft undercoat. The Stichelhaar or German Brokencoated Pointer has a coat, which is 1.5 inches (3-3.5 cm) in length, hard and bristly and lying close to the body. At full length, such a coat can resemble coconut matting. In the Jack Russell Terrier, the broken-coated variety is slightly different than the wire.

- **broken coated toy terrier**

original name of the Australian Terrier.

- **broken mouth**

a term describing a sheep which has lost one or more of its permanent incisors.

- **broken wind**

abnormality of the upper or lower respiratory tract causing loss of normal air exchange, generally resulting in reduced performance.

- **bronchi and bronchiole**

small tubular structures that lead from the trachea to the microscopic sac-like structures, alveoli, in the lungs.

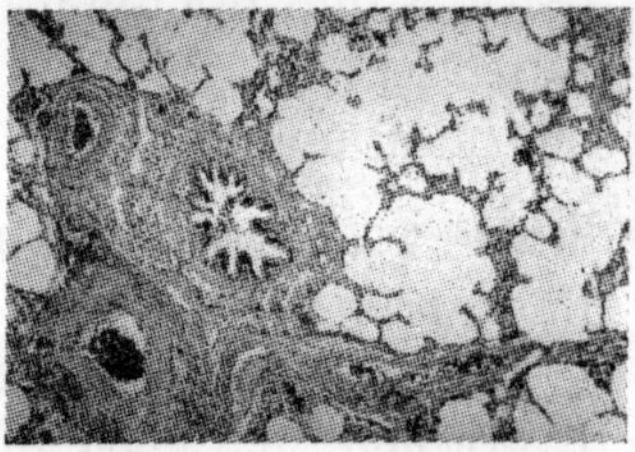

- **bronchodilator**

medication which opens up the main air passages to the lungs.

- **bronchoscope**

a stiff or flexible tube with a light that is used to look inside the airways.

• **bronchoscopy**
using a bronchoscope to look inside the trachea and large bronchi.

• **bronchospasm**
condition in which the muscles surrounding the air passages to the lungs contract, narrowing the passages.

• **broodmare**
a filly or mare that has been bred and is used to produce foals.

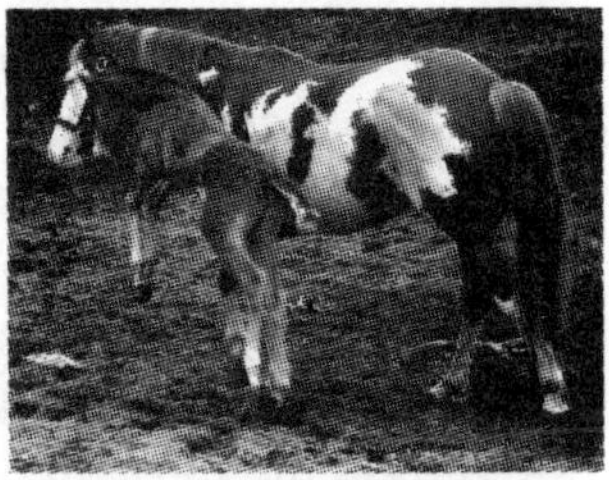

• **brush**
injury that occurs when one hoof strikes the inside of the opposite limb.

• **BS**
blood sample

• **BT**
blood test

• **bucked shins**
inflammation of the covering of the bone (periosteum) of the front surface of the cannon bone to which young horses are particularly susceptible. This is primarily a condition of the front legs.

• **buffer**
a substance used in livestock rations to help resist changes in the acidity of the digestive tract. Examples: sodium bicarbonate, bentonite.

• **bulbourethral glands**
an accessory sex gland of the male.

• **bulbs (of the heel)**
the two areas on either side of the back of the foot, similar to the heel of the hand.

• **bulbus glandis**
the rounded base of the penis.

• **bulk tank**
a refrigerated milk storage tank for each dairy herd.

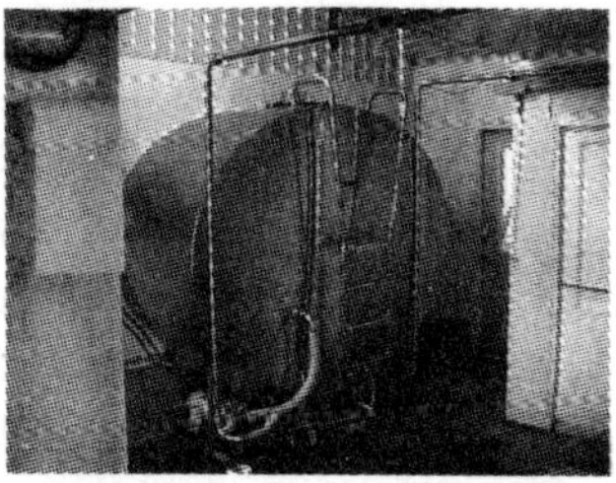

• **bull terrier**
in the 1850s, after years of experimentation, James

Hinks of Birmingham, England, thrust upon the world a new bull-and-terrier dog, one who further removed some of the undesireable traits of the then existing Bulldog (the roach back, the over-angulated legs, and the undershot jaw). The Bull Terrier was originally created in large part from crosses of bullbaiting bulldogs and the now extinct English White Terrier, possibly with later crossings to the Spanish Pointer to add size. These dogs were designed with a dual nature in mind: success at the show and slaughter in the pits. These two goals the Bull Terrier achieved. They are among the most refined of showmen and the most relentless of gladiators in the rat pits. In fact, the Bull Terrier has had a double history. It holds records for the most rats killed in minutes, hours, and other time parameters, and yet it quickly became the stylish breed of the English gentleman. Known also as the 'White Cavalier, ' these dogs were bred by gentlemen for gentlemen, to protect and serve unto death yet never to instigate a quarrel.

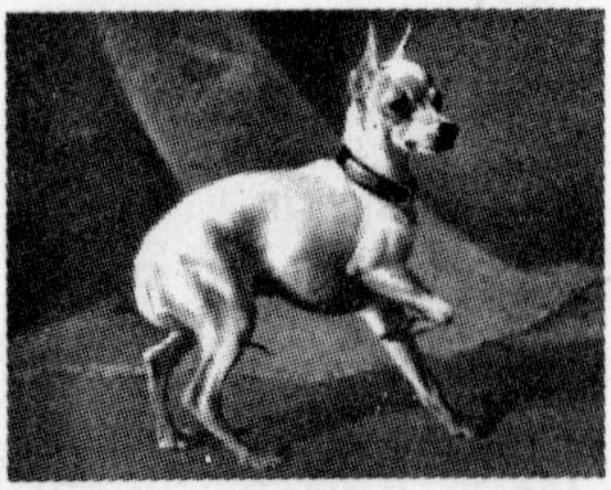

• **bulldog**

centuries ago, the probable crossing of the Old English Mastiff and feisty terrier types produced a dog with the courage, strength and tenacity to successfully combat a furious bull. These dogs – fast, fearless, and powerful – were the foundation stock for today's Bulldog breed. The sport of bullbaiting originated in Britain during the thirteenth century, though animal baiting was practised at least from the Roman era. The sport rose quickly to feverish heights, and the dogs of the sport, born on the British Isles, became the pride of the English people. Fanciers of the sport and of the dogs took no account of the beauty, type, or grace of the dogs. These dogs were bred to be able savages nearly insensitive to pain. In 1835, bullbaiting was made illegal, and the existence of the able-bodied bulldogs was threatened. Lovers of the breed then stepped in and attempted to preserve the breed. Today, though he retains the name, the Bulldog is a much-changed bulldog.

- **bullous pemphigoid**
an immune mediated skin disease in which autoantibodies are directed against antigens in basement membrane zone.

- **bullous retinal detachment**
the retina has detached from all points of contact except for around the periphery and at the optic disk.

- **bullring**
a small racetrack, usually less than one mile.

- **BUN**
short for 'blood urea nitrogen', a blood test that estimates kidney funtion.

- **buphthalmos**
enlarged eye caused by glaucoma.

- **buretrol**
buretrols are small plastic cylinders that are filled from a stock bottle, or bag, of fluids. It is much easier to see the residual volume of fluid in a rigid sided container than a flexible container.

- **burn(ed)**
commonly used in the term: burned heels.

- **bursa**
a sac containing synovial fluid (a natural lubricant). The purpose is to pad or cushion and thus facilitate motion between soft tissue and bone. Most commonly occurring where tendons pass over bones.

- **bursitis**
inflammation in a bursa that results in swelling due to accumulation of synovial fluid. Capped elbow is inflammation of the bursa over the point of elbow (olecranon process of the ulna). 'Capped hock' is inflammation of the bursa over the point of the hock (tuber calcis).

- **bute**
short for phenylbutazone, a non-steroidal anti-inflammatory medication that is legal in many racing jurisdictions. Often known by

the trade names Butazolidin and Butazone.

- **butterfly catheter**
  a style of catheter that has a rigid needle attached to a plastic finger grip that looks like 'wings' and then attached to a short piece of flexible tubing.

- **byproduct**
  feeds produced as a result of industrial manufacturing, plant or animal processing. Examples: distillers grains, beet pulp, meat and bone meal, fish meal.

- **C**
  cervical (vertebra - usually followed by a number to denote which one)

- **C**
  cough

- **C-**
  no cough

- **C/H**
  calculus heavy

- **C/MOD**
  calculus moderate

- **C/S OR C&S**
  culture and sensitivity

- **C/SL**
  calculus slight

- **C+**
  moderate cough

- **C++**
  severe cough

- **C7D**
  recheck in 7 days

- **CA**
  Carious Lesion
  crater-like lesion also called a cavity. Occurs mainly in the molar pits of large dogs

- **CAB**
  a new order of CPR in which chest compressions are first applied to cause circulation of blood, then airway for breathing is established. Used more commonly in humans and originated due to concerns of transmission of infectious diseases. In animals consider this order if the arrest is witnessed and it is known that the patient does not have underlying respiratory disease.

- **cachexia**
  extreme weight loss.

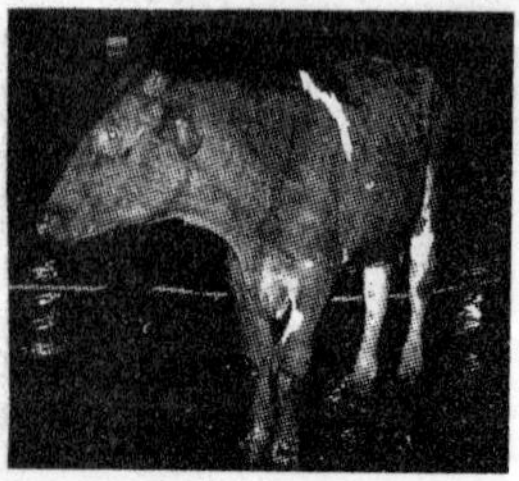

- **caesarian section (Abrev: C-section)**
surgical procedure to delivery feotuses.

- **CAH**
chronic active hepatitis

- **Cairn Terrier**
said to resemble the original Highland Terrier, today's Carn Terrier is the general stock from which arose the Scottish Terrier, Skye Terrier, Clydesdale Terrier, and West Highland White Terrier. The Highland Terrier lived to exterminate vermin: badgers, otters, foxes, setting the example for all his descendants. The Cairn Terrier is called such because of his smaller size and the ability it gave him to sniggle into cairns, the small openings in stone grave markers.

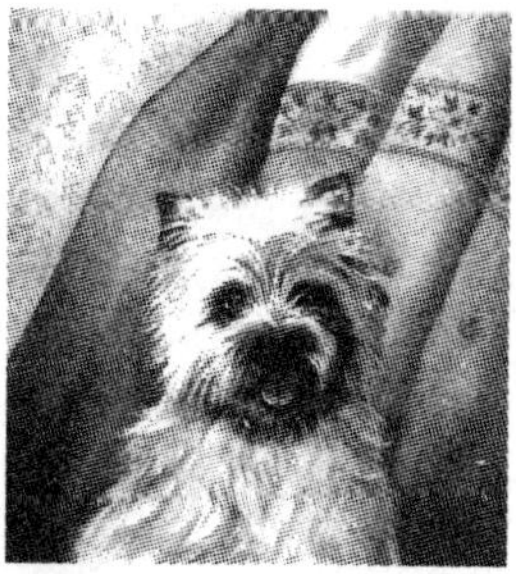

- **calcified**
the hardening of tissue through the influx of calcium, usually as a result of chronic inflammation.

- **calcinosis circumscripta**
deposits of calcium found in small lumps under the skin, in the tongue, or attached to tendons or in joint capsules.

- **calcinosis cutis**
hard crusts or white plaques in the skin of some patients with hyperadrenocorticism.

- **calcium channel blocker**
these drugs inhibit the movement of calcium ion across cell membranes. Calcium channel blockers are used in the treatment of certain heart conditions. In CPR, they may be used after resucsitation to protect the heart from the effects of calcium administered during CPR.

- **calculus/calculi**
abnormal stone like structure(s) usually composed of mineral salts e.g. a bladder calculus is the same thing as a bladder stone.

- **calf hutch**
individual housing unit for young calves assists in

blocking transmission of disease.

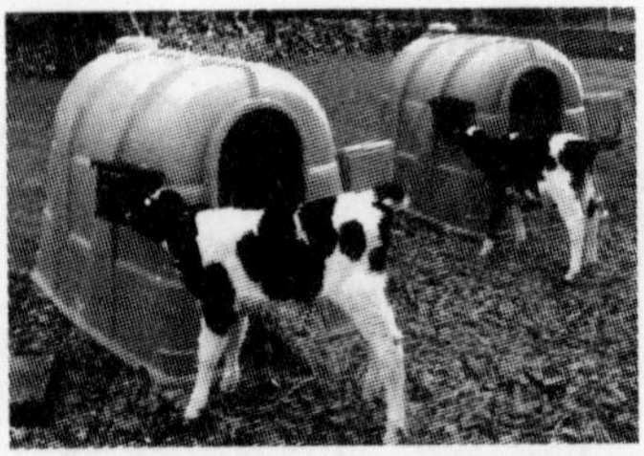

- **calf starter**
grain based mixes fed to young calves.

- **calicivirus**
a serious respiratory illness.

- **calipers**
a device used to measure the diameter of the testes.

- **calk**
a projection on the heels of a horseshoe, similar to a cleat, to prevent slipping, especially on a wet track. Also known as a 'sticker.' Sometimes incorrectly spelled 'caulk.'

- **calling**
the characteristic vocalisations (typically yowling, howling, or screaming) made by a cat in heat.

- **callus**
hypertrophy of the stratum corneum especially over pressure points such as the elbow.

- **cCalorie (Abrev: Kcal)**
a measure of energy, usually expressed as kilocalorie (Kcal) or megacalorie (Mcal). 1 cal = the amount of energy required to increase the temperature of 1 g of water 1 degree C.

- **calving interval**
the time between one calving and the next. Should not exceed 13 months.

- **camelids**
camelids are a large family including Old World camelids: camels and the bactrians, which are two-humped camels, and the New World camelids, llamas and alpacs.

- **cancer**
a group of diseases caused by transformation of normal cells into malignant ones. When these cells shed and travel to other areas of the body, the cancer is said to metastasise. As the cancerous growth draws nutrients, and the general lack of well-being diminishes the appetite, the resultant ema-

ciation is called cancer cachexia.

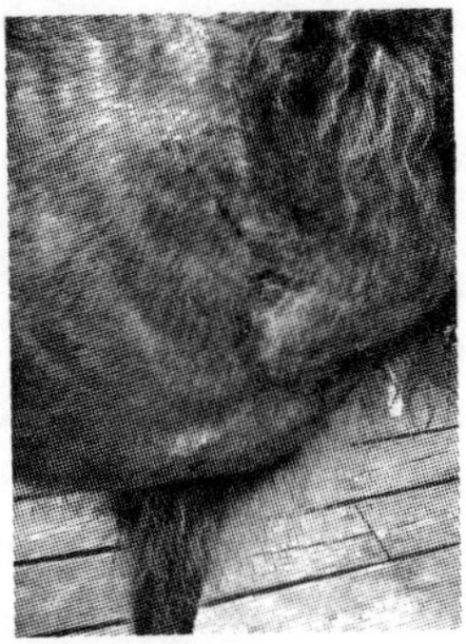

- **Candida**
  a certain genus of yeast which can cause disease in humans and animals, an infection with Candida is called candidiasis.

- **canine**
  a sharp-pointed tooth located next to the incisor teeth. The dog has four canine teeth, two uper and two lower also known as fangs.

- **canine adenovirus 2 (Abrev: CAV-2)**
  one of the agents causing 'kennel cough'. Also protects against CAV-1 (infectious canine hepatitis) when included in vaccines.

- **canine eosinophilic granuloma**
  possibly a hypersensitivity reaction resulting in oral lesions in young Siberian Husky dogs.

- **cannon bone**
  the third metacarpal (front leg) or metatarsal (rear leg), also referred to as the shin bone. The largest bone between the knee and ankle joints.

- **canthus**
  corner of the eye (medial and lateral).

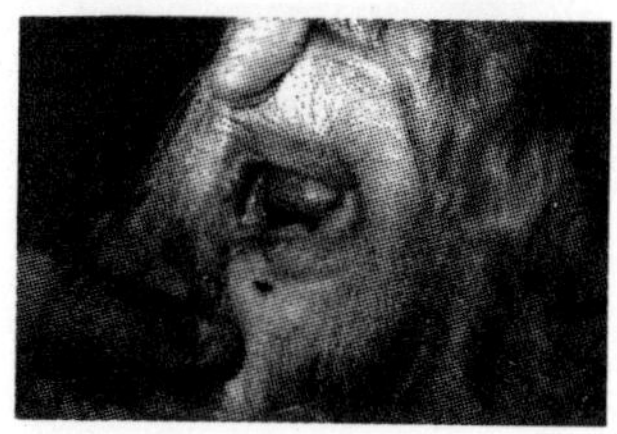

- **capillary refill time**
  the amount of time it takes for blood to return to capillaries after it has been forced out, normally two seconds. Usually assessed by pressing the thumb against the horse's gums. When the pressure is removed the gum looks white, but the normal pink color returns as blood flows into the capillaries.

- **capped elbow**
  inflammation of the bursa over the point of the elbow. Also known as a 'shoe boil.'

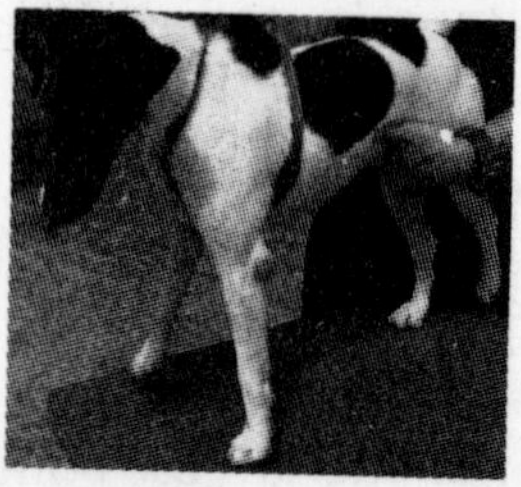

- **capped hock**
  inflammation of the bursa over the point of the hock.

- **caprine**
  goat.

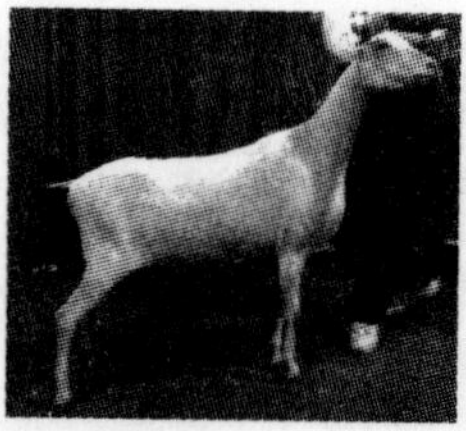

- **caprine arthritis-encephalitis (Abrev: CAE)**
  a disease characterised by the development of chronic arthritis and debility.

- **carapace**
  the upper shell of a turtle or tortoise.

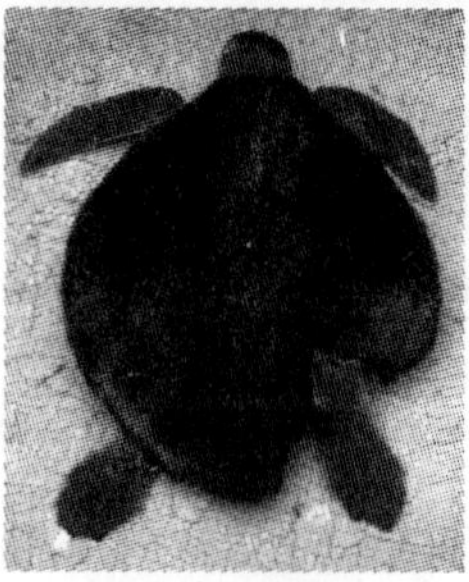

- **carbohydrate**
  compounds made up of chains of sugar units. Simple carbohydrates include table sugar (sucrose), milk sugar (lactose), and fruit sugar (fructose). Complex carbohydrates are very long chains held together by bonds that may not be digestible in the stomach and intestines of a carnivore. Starch is a digestible complex carbohydrate. Seed hulls such as oat bran are digestible by ruminants and horses but not carnivores.

- **carbonic anhydrase**
  an enzyme located in the eye and in the kidney tubules that is important in reabsorbing bicarbonate (kidney) and in the active secretion of aqueous in the eye.

- **carbonic anhydrase inhibitor**
  a drug that interfers with the action of the enzyme carbonic anhydrase. e.g. acetozolamide, dorzolamide (Truceopt). These drugs are used to reduce aqueous production in animals with glaucoma.

- **carbuncle**
  multiple cutaneous abscesses that are connected by sinuses.

- **carcinogen**
  a substance which causes cancer.

- **carcinoma**
  a type of cancer originating from epithelial cells. Example squamous cell carcinoma originates from cells of the skin and mouth, transitional cell carcinoma originates from the cells of the bladder.

- **cardiac**
  a synonym for heart.

- **cardiac pump theory (CPR)**
  in CPR, when the chest is compressed the heart underneath the chest wall is directly compressed as well, squeezing blood out into the major blood vessels so it can return to the heart and then go to the brain. CPR in animals weighing less than 7 kg is probably using the cardiac pump theory.

- **cardiomyopathy**
  diseases of the heart muscle does not include diseases of the valves of the heart or congenital defects.

- **cardiopulmonary**
  relating to the heart and lungs.

- **cardiopulmonary resuscitation (Abrev: CPR)**
  a life saving procedure that includes the external compression of the chest wall to stimulate blood flow and breathing (by mouth to mouth or other methods) to provide oxygen.

- **cardiovascular**
  the organ system that includes the heart and blood vessels.

- **carnivore**
  an animal whose natural diet includes meat.

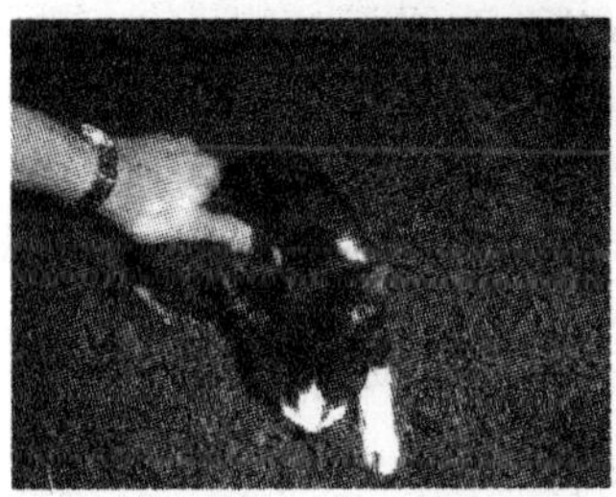

- **carpal pads**
  anti skid pads found on the wrists of the cat's front legs.

- **carpus**
  1. the wrist (front leg) of dogs and cats.

2. a joint in the horse's front leg, more commonly referred to as the knee.

• **carrier**
animal which harbours an infectious organism, such as a virus, bacteria or parasite. The animal does not appear ill but can still transmit the organism to other animals by direct contact or releasing the organisms (bacteria, protozoa, viruses) into the environment in the stool, urine, respiratory secretions, or vaginal discharges.

• **cast**
1. condition where full woolled sheep gets on its back and is unable to rise. Cast ewes are old ewes that are culled from the flock.
2. a horse, positioned on its side or back, and wedged against a wall, such that it cannot get up.

• **castration**
another term for neutering a male animal by removal of the testes.

• **catagen**
the transition phase of the hair cycle between growth (anagen) and cessation of growth (telogen).

• **cataracts**
loss of transparency of the lens of the eye. Can be genetic or acquired as the result of injury or diabetes, etc. Also associated with PRA which is inherited.

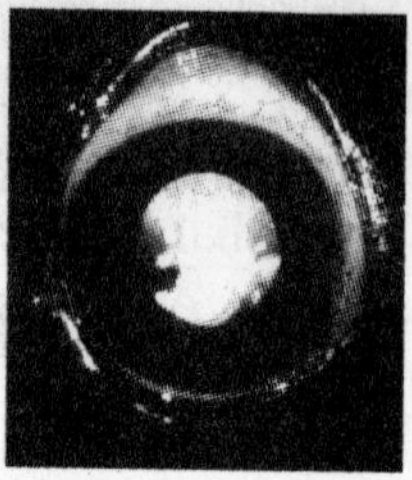

• **caudal**
refers to the rear or in a direction toward the rear of the animal. For example the abdomen is more caudal than the chest. The opposite term is cranial meaning closer to the head of the animal.

• **caval syndrome**
disease caused by large numbers of worms in the right side of the heart and venacava, which results in blood circulation problems in the liver leading to the break down of red blood cells, anaemia, weakness, and collapse.

• **CBA**
cat bite abscess

- **CBC**
  complete blood count (= routine haematology)

- **CC**
  coccygeal (vertebra - usually followed by a number to denote which one)

- **CCHF**
  chronic congestive heart failure

- **CD**
  caudal

- **CDRM**
  chronic degenerative radiculomyelopathy

- **CDS**
  cat and dog shelter

- **CCE**
  clinical examination

- **cecum**
  a blind sac that opens into the colon found in many animals.

- **cell mediated immunity**
  the immunity that is the result of either special lymphocytes directly killing foreign invaders, or lymphocytes (T cells) releasing special chemicals which activate macrophages to kill the invaders.

- **centre of distribution**
  a formula derived from the Dosage profile and a similar attempt to quantify speed and stamina.

- **central venous pressure (Abrev: CVP)**
  central venous pressure measures the ability of the right heart to accommodate the fluid load presented to it. Normal animals have a central venous pressure of less than 5 cm of water. Assuming there are no clots in the IV catheter, central venous pressures repeatedly above 10 cm of water are indicative of impending onset of edema and fluid overload. Measurement of central venous pressure requires that a central catheter (jugular catheter) be in place. CVP readings can be influenced by catheter position and patency.

- **CEP**
  ceporex

- **cerebellar degeneration**
  degeneration of the cerebellar portion of the brain.

- **cerebellum**
  a smaller portion of the brain responsible for balance.

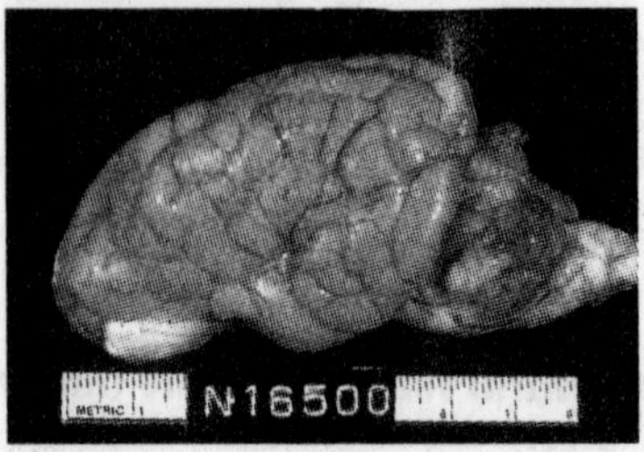

- **cerebral**
  relating to the part of the brain known as the cerebrum.
- **cerebrum**
  the major portion of the brain.
- **cerumen**
  waxy secretion of the apocrine glands of the ear.
- **ceruminolytic agents**
  agents that loosen and dissolve ear wax. Includes dioctyl sodium sulfosuccinate, squalene, propylene glycol, carbamide peroxide, and others.
- **cervical vertebral instability (wobblers)**
  compression of the cervical (neck) spinal cord caused by instability or malformation of the cervical vertebrae. Dogs show lack of muscle coordination in the back legs and possibly neck.
- **cervicitis**
  inflammation of the cervix.
- **cervix**
  part of the female reproductive tract located between the vagina and uterus.
- **cestodes**
  tape worms.
- **characteristic (typical - adj)**
  a distinguishing trait, quality or property.
- **chediak - Higashi syndrome**
  a macrophage deficiency.
- **cheeks**
  below the eyes, the skin regions beginning at the lips and reaching back to the masseter muscles area. Cheeks are often described in breed standards, and specific phraseology has developed. Developed musculation in the cheeks is termed fleshy in cheeks, structurally lean in the cheeks is known as clean in cheeks; coarse or prominent cheeks are referred to as cheeky.
- **cheeky**
  bulging in the cheeks sometimes the result of over-developed cheek muscles. This characteristic is desirable in

some breeds though undesired in others.

- **chelation**
binding of a substance to a metal.

- **cheloid**
a type of hypertrophied scar.

- **chemical defibrillator**
in the absence of an electrical defibrillator machine, certain drugs may be used in an attempt to reverse the cardiac arrhythmia of atrial fibrillation.

- **chemosis**
edema of the conjunctiva.

- **chemotherapy**
drugs used in the treatment of cancer.

- **cherry eye**
prolapse of the third eyelid gland.

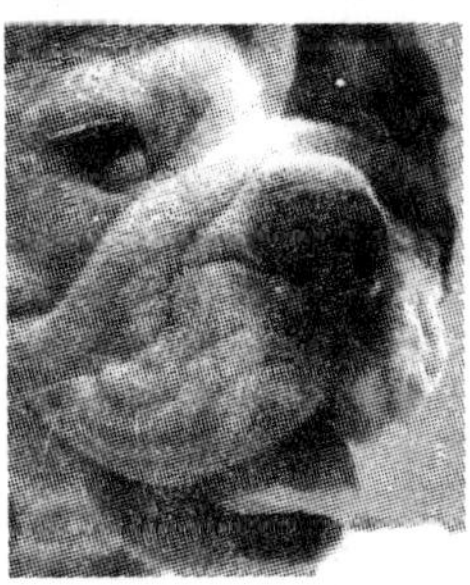

- **chest**
thorax, brisket. The anatomical region between the neck and abdomen. Composed of thirteen thoracic vertebrae above and thirteen ribs on either side, with the sternum below. Eight sternaebra or individual bones, attached by clocks of cartilage, comprise the sternum. This is the formation of the dog's chest or floor of the thorax.

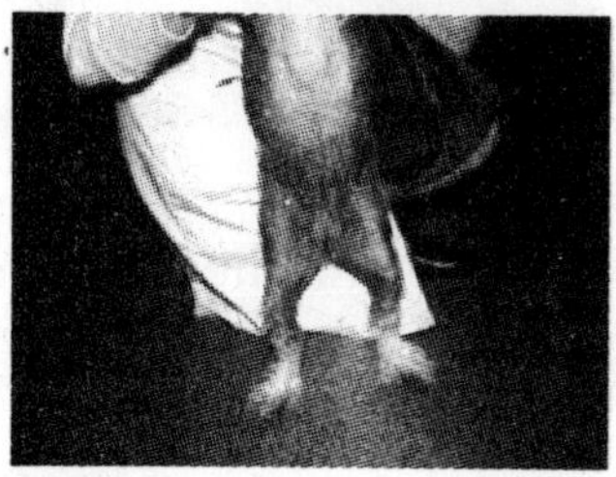

- **CHF**
congestive heart failure

- **CHF**
chronic heart failure

- **chiggers**
common name for Trombiculidiasis.

- **chihuahua**
the Chihuahua, named after the state in Mexico, is the smallest canine in recorded history, weighing in as little as one pound! Some sources trace the breed to South America. It is believed variously that the dog, or dogs

similar to it in size and type, was revered by the Aztecs as a sacred dog fostered by the ninth-century Toltecs when it was called Techichi, or developed and kept by the Incas.

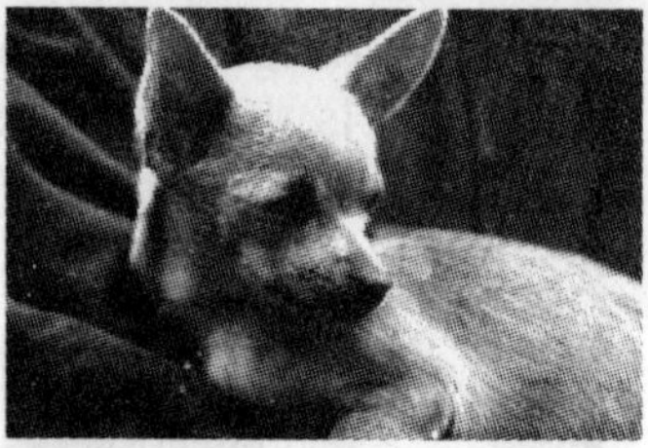

- **chiropractic**
  the use of bone alignment to treat specific or general health problems.

- **chlorhexidine**
  novalsan. Antibacterial, antifungal, and viricidal. Used primarily as soaks or in conjunction with whirlpool therapy.

- **chlorpheniramine**
  an antihistamine.

- **choanal atresia**
  a failure of a seperation to form between the nasal cavity and the nasopharnyx. A common birth defect in the crias.

- **choking down**
  dorsal displacment of the soft palate.

- **cholangio hepatitis**
  inflammation of the gall-bladder, bileducts, and liver

- **chondroprotective nutraceutical**
  a nutritional supplement that protects cartilage.

- **chorioditis**
  inflammation of the choroid.

- **chorioretinitis**
  inflammation affecting the choroid and retina causing choroidal, +/- retinal, blood vessels to become leaky and either transudative fluid or exudative fluid and cells to leak into the space between the choroid and retina, elevating the retina.

- **choroid**
  the posterior uvea lying between the sclera and retina, and joining the ciliary body anteriorly. The choroid provides nutrition to the outer layers of the retina and contains the tapetum.

- **chq**
  cheque

- **chronic**
  exposure to the poison occurs over a period of weeks, months, or years onset of

signs may be sudden and dramatic, or can be insidious like a slow loss in body condition or reduced productivity.

- **chronic interstital nephritis (Abrev: CIN)**
  chronic interstitial nephritis (CIN) is similar to the term end stage renal disease (ESRD) in that it is a non-specific histologic finding on renal biopsy and may be the end result of renal disease of any etiology.

- **chronic obstructive pulmonary disease**
  commonly known as 'COPD, ' a hyper allergenic response of the respiratory system that involves damage to the lung tissue, similar in many ways to human asthma. Affected horses may cough, develop a nasal discharge and have a reduced exercise tolerance. Respiratory rate is increased and lung elasticity is diminished.

- **chronic osselet**
  permanent build-up of synovial fluid in a joint, characterised by inflammation and thickening of the joint capsule over the damaged area. Usually attended by changes in the bone and cartilage.

- **chronic pain**
  persisting for a long time

- **chronic renal disease (Abrev: CRD)**
  irreversible renal disease caused by damage to a large part of both kidneys. Two thirds of both kidneys must be damaged before the animal loses the ability to concentrate and dilute urine and 75% of both kidneys must be destroyed before azotemia is observed.

- **chronic superficial keratitis**
  a chronic condition of the eye in which blood vessels grow across the cornea (the clear surface of the eye). The cornea looks hazy and sometimes reddened. It may eventually take on a dark pigment. This condition is also called pannus.

- **chronological records**
  records that are organised by arranging all the data in the record in the order in which it was collected.

- **chrysotherapy**
gold salt therapy used in treatment of immune mediated disorders.

- **cilia**
eyelashes.

- **ciliary body**
the section of uvea between the iris and choroid. It functions to produce aqueous and is the site of attachment for the lens zonules. Contraction of the ciliary body muscle results in lens accommodation for focussing.

- **cirrhosis**
a liver disease caused by placement of damaged cells with connective tissue. Severe scarring can eventually cause liver failure.

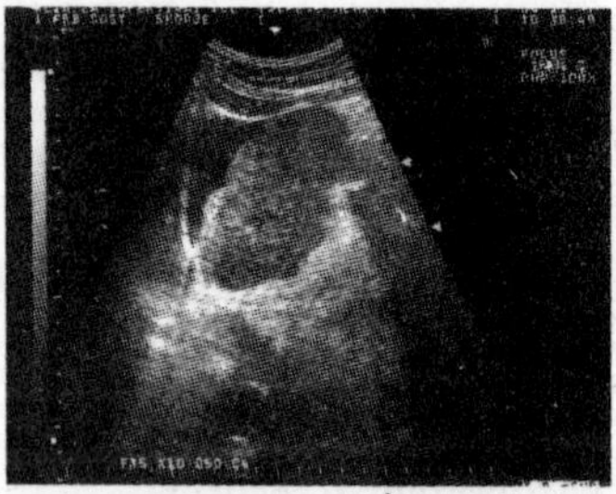

- **classic**
1. a race of traditional importance.
2. used to describe a distance A race at the American classic distance, which is currently 1quarter mile. The European classic distance is 1half mile.

- **clean wool**
wool after it has been 'scoured' to remove the dirt.

- **clear media**
includes the aqueous, lens and vitreous.

- **cleft palate**
a congenital split involving the hard or soft palate in the mouth. May cause nasal regurgitation in newborns. Known to be inherited in some breeds, may also be caused by environmental factors.

- **clerk of scales**
an official whose chief duty is to weigh the riders before and after a race to ensure proper weight is (was) carried.

- **climbing**
when a horse lifts its front legs abnormally high as it gallops, causing it to run inefficiently.

- **clinical study**
a clinical study or clinical trial is a test of a new drug or procedure that is being evaluated for effectiveness

in animals with naturally occurring disease. In some cases the effectiveness of the new drug or procedure is compared with currently available treatments.

- **clinimix**
  a pre-made solution used in partial parenteral solution.

- **cloaca**
  a tube like structure through which faeces, urine, and reproductive fluids/eggs pass in birds, turtles, and other lower vertebrates.

- **clone**
  the progeny of a single cell.

- **closed knees**
  a condition when the cartilaginous growth plate above the knee (distal radial physis) has turned to bone. Indicates completion of long bone growth and is one sign of maturity.

- **clostridium**
  a group of bacteria that produce spores. One type of clostridium causes tetanus.

- **clotting factors**
  protein components in the blood, which help the blood to clot. Clotting is a complex mechanism. In addition to platelets, clot formation is the result of a long chain of chemical reactions carried out by individual molecules called clotting factors. Each factor is numbered such that factor I leads to a reaction with factor II forming a new substance. This then reacts with factor III and so on to factor XII.

- **clutch**
  the uninterrupted series of eggs laid by a hen, usually 2-6 depending on the bird species.

- **CNS**
  central nervous system. Includes the brain, spinal cord, and the nerves leading from them.

- **coagulation**
  the process of clotting.

- **coagulopathy**
  a condition affecting the blood's ability to form a clot.

- **coat**
  the hair covering the dog's skin. Most breeds of dog have coats, and the majority of these are double-coated, that is, possess an outercoat and an undercoat. The outer coat, the

coat that is readily visible, is usually comprised of long, coarse, and/or standoffish hair; the undercoat is usually soft, short and smooth, providing the necessary insulation. Many smooth-coated breeds are single coated, but not all single-coated breeds are smooths. The Maltese, for instance, is a long but single-coated breed of dog.

- **cobby**
  describes a cat's body type characterised by a large bone structure and rounded shape.

- **coccidia**
  a one-celled parasite in the category of protozoa. In dogs and cats, coccidia are generally parasites of the intestinal tract.

- **coffin bone**
  the third phalanx (P3). The major bone that is within the confines of the hoof. Also called the 'pedal bone.'

- **cognitive dysfunction**
  a common medical condition in older dogs that results from abnormal brain function causing certain behavioural changes such as disorientation, house-breaking problems, and changes in sleeping patterns and interactions with others.

- **cognitive-evaluative dimension of pain**
  this relates to prior experience, level of anxiety, and conditioned responses that arise from the cerebral cortex and their influence on response to pain.

- **cold haemagglutination disease (Abrev: CHD)**
  a form of autoimmune haemolytic anaemia in which there is formation of cold acting anti-erythrocyte antibodies (IgM)resulting in agglutination of red cells in areas exposed to cold surface temperatures such as the extremities, ear margins and nose.

- **cold nursery**
  a nursery where piglets older than four weeks old are kept and the ambient temperature is around 65F.

- **cold-blooded**
  having a body temperature that is not regulated internally but varies with environmental temperature.

Turtles, lizards, and snakes are cold-blooded.

- **colic**
abdominal pain not necessarily associated with the digestive system any painful abdominal structure can cause colic.

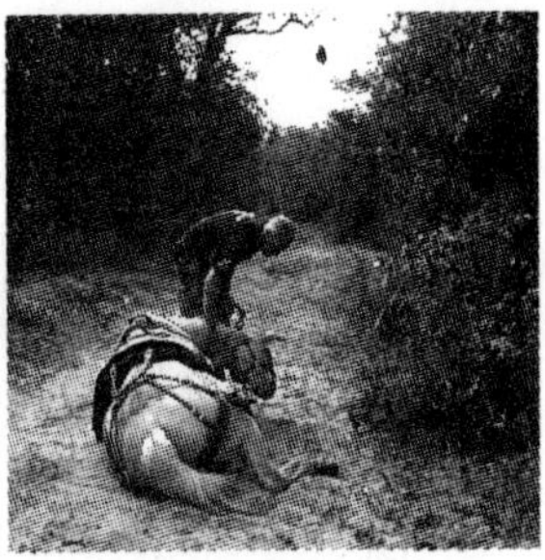

- **colic - gas**
depends on where in the GI tract the gas is. The pain receptors in the gut are all stretch receptors, by the way, so something as simple as gas can cause excruciating pain. And it is also the case that the gas filled loops of gut can be displaced from their normal position, making a simple gas colic a surgical case.

- **colisepticemic E. coli**
E. coli that spreads from the gut through the calf's body and causes abscesses in the brain, eyes, kidneys, and joints. This occurs when the newborn calf ingests it in manure, mud, or other material before or along with getting colostrum.

- **colitis**
an infection or inflammation of the colon.

- **collagenases**
enzymes secreted by certain bacteria that break down collagen and inhibit wound healing.

- **collie**
working type sheepdog, a generic term. Besides the Collie (Scotch Collie), there are the Border Collie, Shetland Sheepdog, Welsh Collie, and New Zealand Shepherd. The Collie is a member of the truly ancient herding 'race' which claims as its origin the country of Scotland. There are two varieties of the breed: the Rough and Smooth Collie, and both are sometimes referred to as Scotch Collies, suggestive of their native land. The title Collie is a derivative of the name Colley Dog which was given to the breed many years ago by the Scotch farmers who employed the dogs at herding the native moun-

tain-dwelling sheep called colleys, an ancient ovine which is the forebear of the renowned black-masked and black-footed Highland sheep of Scotland today. Originally primarily black in colour, the breed, even in its nineteenth-century heyday, scarcely presented the classic 'Lassie' colouration (sable/white).

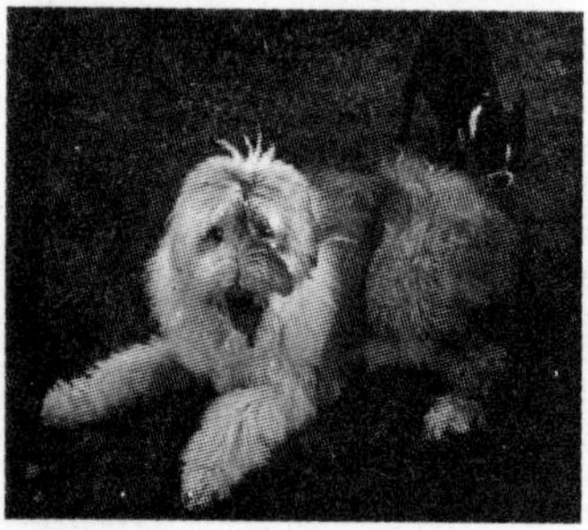

- **colloid**
microscopic particles suspended in a solution. The particles in a colloidal solution are large in molecular weight and can pull fluid into the intravascular space. Because the particles are large they stay in the vascular space longer than crystalloids and therefore exert their effect for a longer time.

- **colloidal solutions**
colloidal solutions are solutions that contain large particles. These large particles are either proteins or complex sugars, such as dextrans or hetastarches. Colloidal solutions because they are physically large molecules, will stay in the bloodstream and hold water in the bloodstream by their oncotic effect.

- **colon**
part of the large intestine.

- **colostrum**
the milk secreted by female mammals for the first few days after birth. It is particularly rich in nutrients and antibodies essential for newborn survival.

- **colt**
an ungelded (entire) male horse four-years-old or younger.

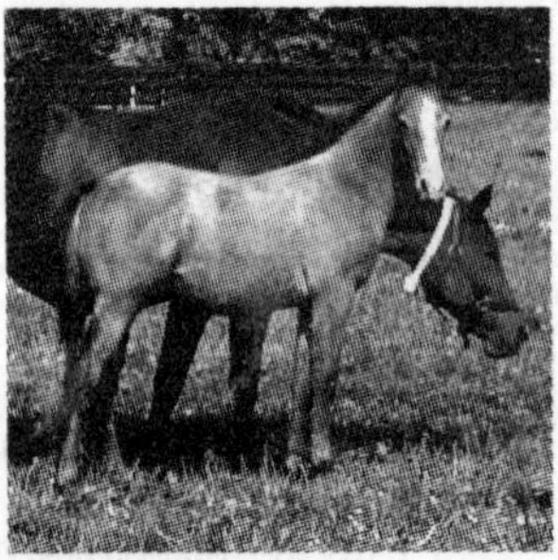

- **coma**
being in a state of unconsciousness.

- **combined immunodeficiency**
  found in Arabians and one or two Arab crosses. A simple recessive mode of inheritance. Results in affected foals having a deficiency of the immune system that results in serious infections and finally death as soon as maternal immunity wears off. Can be confirmed on post-mortem by examining thymus and lymph nodes. Can be inferred in neonates by obtaining a presuckle blood sample and assaying IgM. (which will be extremely low in affected foals.)

- **comedo**
  a blackhead, usually the result of a plugged gland within the skin.

- **commensalism**
  parasitic state in which the parasite lives with the animal without causing disease.

- **comminuted (fracture)**
  a fracture with more than two fragments.

- **commodity feed**
  a feed that has high energy, and often a high protein content.

- **comparable index (CI)**
  indicates the average earnings of progeny produced from mares bred to one sire when these same mares are bred to other sires. A CI of 1.00 is considered average, 2.00 is twice the average, 0.50 half the average, etc.

- **complement**
  a protein complex consisting of enzymes that facilitate the reaction of antibody with antigen resulting in destruction of cells or invading bacteria..

- **complete blood count (Abrev: CBC)**
  a blood test in which the number of red and white blood cells and platelets are counted.

- **complete feed**
  a thoroughly blended mixture of different feed ingredients formulated to meet specific nutrient requirements.

- **compound**
  to mix components following a 'recipe' or protocol.

- **compound (fracture)**
  a fracture where the damaged bone breaks through the skin. Also known as an 'open' fracture.

- **compounding**
  to create a medication by combining parts or to change the formulation of a drug, for example from tablet to liquid.

- **computerised tomography scan (Abrev: CT)**
  many x-ray pictures are taken during a CT scan. A computer is used to put the x-ray pictures together to obtain a 3-dimensional view of a structure.

- **concentrate**
  a classification of feedstuffs high in energy and low in fibre usually further divided into energy and protein concentrates. Often used interchangeably with supplement. Examples: corn, barley, soybeans.

- **conception**
  the onset of pregnancy, when the fertilized egg attaches to the uterus.

- **condylar (fracture)**
  a fracture in the lower knobby end (condyle) of the lower (distal) end of a long bone such as the cannon bone or humerus (upper front limb).

- **confirmed sire**
  one that has been used for breeding before and has known good fertility.

- **conformation**
  the outward appearance and physical formation of a canine, including the symmetry and balance of the composite of its parts. In canine terminology, conformation is applied to show ring competition and denotes the overall quality of a dog's structure, form, and arrangement of the parts.

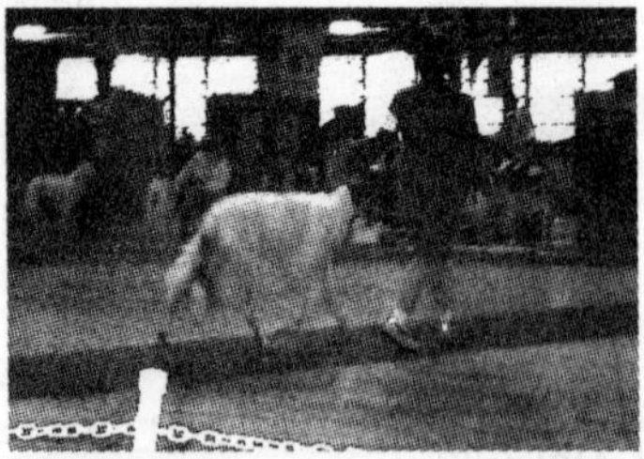

- **congenital**
  a defect that is present at birth. The defect may either be inherited or be caused by something during gestation.

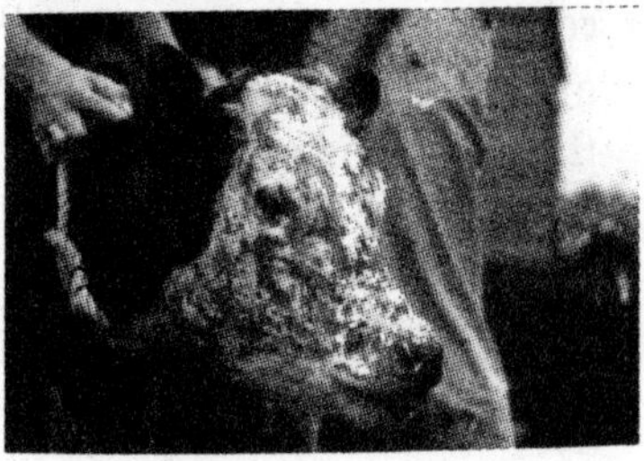

- **conjunctiva**
  the thin, moist, mucus membrane that lines the inside of the eyelids (palpebral conjunctiva) and curves around at the fornix to cover the eyeball up to the cornea (bulbar conjunctiva). Ventrally also it covers both sides of the nictitans

- **conjunctivitis**
  inflammation of the membrane on the inside surface of the eyes.

- **connections**
  persons identified with a horse, such as owner, trainer, rider and stable employees.

- **consolation double**
  a payoff to holders of daily double tickets combining the winning horse in the first race of the double with a scratched horse in the second.

- **constipation**
  a condition in which the movement of food through the digestive system is longer than normal often results in hard, dry stool.

- **contact dermatitis**
  inflammation of the skin from contact with an irritant.

- **contagious disease**
  a disease that is capable of being spread amongst animals by direct contact, e.g. **Pasteurella spp**. in nasal droplets.

- **contagious mastitis**
  aastitis that is caused by coagulated negative **Staphylococci**.

- **contrast agents**
  a substance given orally or injected into a patient that makes the affected tissue easier to identify on an x-ray.

- **controlled breeding**
  also called a timed breeding technique. Modification of the physiology of the ovaries in such a way that one can predict exactly when that female is going to be

ready and breed her only once.

- **contusion**
  an injury to underlying tissues without breaking the skin; a bruise.

- **convulsions**
  strong and involuntary contraction of the muscles.

- **cooling out**
  restoring a horse to normal temperature, usually by walking, after it has become overheated during exercise. All horses that are exercised are cooled out.

- **cop**
  cyclophosphamide/oncovin/prednisolone (chemotherapy protocol)

- **coprophagia**
  eating dung or faecal matter. Normal behaviour in some animals, such as rabbits.

- **copulation**
  insertion of the penis into the female reproductive tract.

- **core vaccine**
  a vaccine that should be administered routinely.

- **corn**
  an irritation on the sole of the foot, toward the heel.

- **cornea**
  the clear part of the front of the eye which allows light in.

- **corneal degeneration**
  after certain corneal or scleral injuries, lipid or cholesterol can be deposited in the cornea.

- **corneal reflex**
  used to assess corneal sensation.

- **corneal sequestrum**
  a focal area of collagen degeneration in the cornea with brown to black discoloration.

- **corneoscleral transposition**
  a surgical technique used to patch conjunctiva over a corneal ulcer.

- **cornification**
  the process of changes in vaginal epithelial cells under the influence of estrogen.

- **coronary band**
  the tissue right around the top of the hoof, similar to a fingernail cuticle.

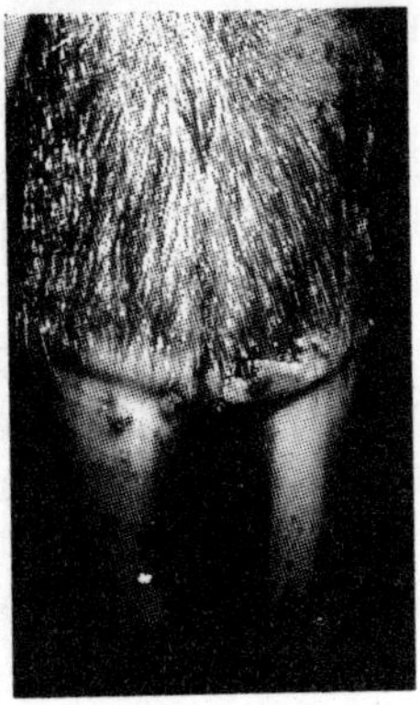

- **corona virus**
a single stranded RNA virus.

- **coronet**
see coronary band.

- **corpora nigra**
structures present mainly on the upper pupil margin in horses, upper and lower margins in the lamb. Quite obvious and elaborate on llamas and alpacas. Their function is not really known.

- **corpus hemorrhagicum**
a follicle that has been present on the ovary and has not been given the chance to ovulate so it will continue growing and become large and cyst-like and bleed inside.
Also called a haemorrhagic follicle.

- **corpus luteum**
a structure in the ovary that produces progesterone.

- **corticosteroid**
hormones produced by the adrenal gland which are important to almost every function of cells and organs. They are divided into two groups glucocorticoids and mineralocorticoids. Glucocorticoids regulate protein, carbohydrate, and fat metabolism. Mineralocorticoids regulate electrolyte balances.

- **cotyledonary type of placenta**
a type of placenta where the connection between the placenta and the foetus is based on buttons of tissue. Cattle and sheep have this type of placentation.

- **cough**
to expel air from the lungs in a spasmodic manner. Can be a result of inflammation or irritation to the upper airways (pharynx, larynx or trachea) or may involve the lower airways of the lungs (deep cough).

- **coumestan and coumestrol**
oestrogen-like substances produced by certain plants

such as alfalfa, types of phytoestrogen.

- **cover**
  a single breeding of a stallion to a mare.

- **cow hocks**
  abnormal conformation in which the points of the hocks turn in.

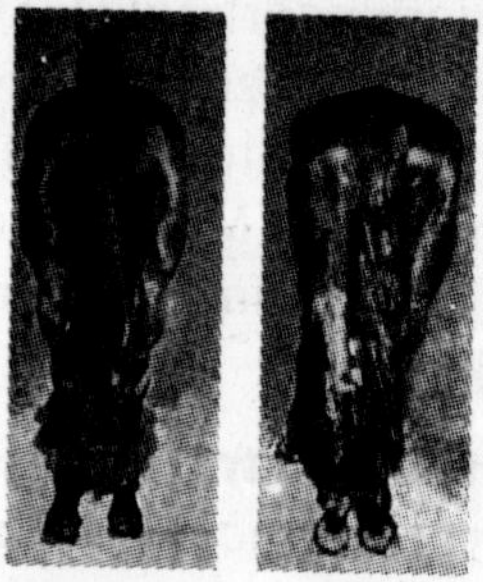

- **COX inhibitor**
  drugs that block cyclo-oxygenase and that are intended to relieve pain and inflammation.

- **CR**
  cranial

- **CR**
  crowding

- **cracked hoof**
  a vertical split of the hoof wall. Cracks may extend upwards from the bearing surface of the wall or downwards from the coronary band, as the result of a defect in the band. Varying in degrees of severity, cracks can result from injuries or concussion. Hooves that are dry and/or thin (shelly) or improperly shod are susceptible to cracking upon concussion. Corrective trimming and shoeing may remedy mild cracks but in severe cases, when the crack extends inward to the sensitive laminae, more extensive treatment is required, such as using screws and wires to stabilise the sides of the crack.

- **cranial**
  refers to the head or in a direction toward the front of the animal. For example the chest is more cranial than the abdomen. The opposite term is caudal meaning closer to the rear of the animal.

- **creep area**
  an area where newborn piglets crawl to, to keep warm and avoid being accidentally crushed by their mother.

- **creep feeder**
  a feed device designed to allow a foal to eat but keep

its dam out. Otherwise, the mare will eat the foal's food.

- **crepuscular (or Nocturnal)**
  active during twilight hours - dawn and dusk.
- **CRF**
  chronic renal failure
- **CRI**
  chronic renal insufficiency
- **CRI**
  constant rate infusion
- **cria**
  the term describing a llama from the age of birth to weaning (4-6 months).

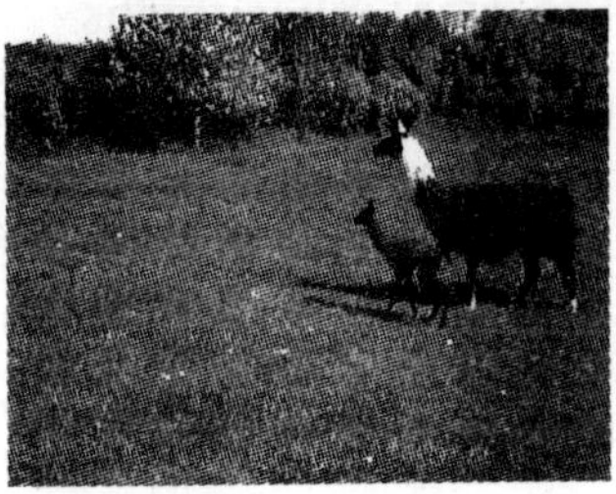

- **cribber**
  a horse that clings to objects with its teeth and sucks air into its stomach. Also known as a 'wind sucker.'
- **crimp**
  the 'wave' in the staple of wool.
- **crop**
  1. the number of foals by a sire in a given year.
  2. a group of horses born in the same year An average crop of three-year-olds.
  3. a jockey's whip.
- **crossbreed**
  the mating of animals of two different breeds. The offspring of such a mating is considered a hybrid.
- **CRT**
  capillary refill time
- **cruciate**
  shaped like a cross. Cruciate ligaments are found on the front (cranial or anterior) and the back (caudal or posterior) of the stifle ('knee') joint.
- **crude protein**
  an estimate of the total protein content of a feed determined by analysing the nitrogen content of the feed and multiplying the result by 6.25. Crude protein includes true protein and other nitrogen-containing substances such as ammonia, amino acids, nitrates.
- **crust**
  area of dried fluids or cells on the skin. The fluids may be blood, serum, pus, or medication.

- **crutching**
removing the wool from around the breech area.

- **cryoprotectant**
a substance such as glycerol which is added to semen to protect the sperm membrane from injury by ice crystals formed during the freezing and thawing process.

- **cryptorchid**
a condition seen in intact male animals where a testicle fails to descend into the scrotum.

- **crystalloids**
crystalloid solutions are solutions that contain small particles, particles with molecular weights of less than a few 100 molecular weight units. Examples of crystalloid solutions are lactated Ringer's solution, Ringer's, and the dextrose and saline containing solutions.

- **CS**
1. clinical signs
2. corticosteroids

- **CSK**
Chronic Superficial Keratitis (otherwise known as Pannus)

- **cull cow**
cow removed from a herd due to poor profitability. Generally due to poor production, reproduction, or mastitis.

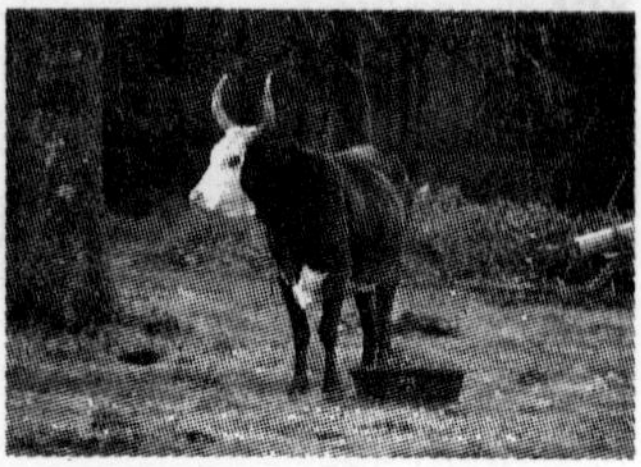

- **culotte**
the Shipperke's trousers - longish hair breeching at the rear upper thighs.

- **culture**
the process in which a sample of fluid or tissue is taken from an animal and placed in special media which allows the bacteria, virus, etc. to grow (reproduce) in the laboratory.

- **cup**
refers to the irregular occlusal surface of the tooth (the surfaces that meet when a horse closes its mouth) and is used as a visual method of determining age in a horse.

- **curb**
a thickening of the plantar ligament of the hock.

- **cush**
the laying down position of the female camelid during mating.

- **cushing's disease**
a disease of the adrenal gland that produces too much of the hormone cortisol. Too much cortisol causes signs including drinking, eating and urinating increased amounts and loss of hair on the body. Also called hyperadrenocorticism.

- **cut down**
horse suffering from injuries from being struck by the shoes of another horse. Or, due to a faulty stride, a horse may cut itself down.

- **cutaneous**
benign proliferation of nodules in or under the skin

- **cutaneous lupus erythematosus (Abrev: CLE)**
discoid lupus. A form of systemic lupus erythematosus which only involves the skin.

- **cutaneous vasculitis**
skin lesions caused by deposition and subsequent activation of soluble immune complexes along the basement membrane of blood vessels.

- **C-V or CV**
cardio-vascular

- **CVA**
cardiovascular accident

- **CX**
coccygeal (vertebra - usually followed by a number to denote which one)

- **cyanosis**
bluish or grayish colour to the skin and gums which occurs when the animal has insufficient oxygen.

- **cycle**
events that happen in the female such as ovulation, hormone production, receptivity, etc. In camelids the cycle does not follow regular time periods as it does in horses or cattle.

- **cyclitis**
inflammation of the ciliary body.

- **cyclo Oxygenase (Abrev: COX)**
an enzyme involved in the production of prostaglan-

dins from arachidonic acid in cell membranes. There are 2 forms, COX 1 & COX 2. COX 2 plays a greater role in inflammation.

- **cyclocryotherapy**
  a freezing probe is applied to sclera to destroy the underlying ciliary body in treatment of glaucoma.

- **cyclophosphamide**
  A chemotherapy drug also used in the treatment of immune mediated diseases.

- **cycloplegic**
  a drug that paralyses the ciliary muscle and helps reduce pain.

- **cyst**
  an abnormal sac-like structure that is lined with cells which produce a liquid or thick material.

- **cystic endometrial hyperplasia (Abrev: CEH)**
  morphological changes occurring in the uterus under the influence of progesterone secreted from the corpus lutei (CLs) of the ovaries during diestrus.

- **cystitis**
  inflammation of the urinary bladder.

- **cystocercus**
  the larval stage of a tapeworm encysted in muscle.

- **cythioate**
  an oral organophosphate.

- **cytokines/interleukins**
  regulatory proteins secreted primarily by lymphocytes to facilitate interaction between other lymphocytes and macrophages e.g., IL-2, IL-12, CSF, TNF.

- **cytology**
  the microscopic evaluation of cells removed from an organ or tissue.

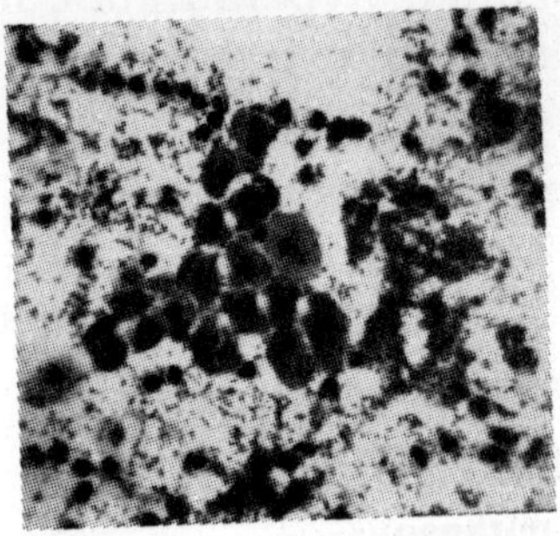

- **cytoplasm**
  substances which make up the inside of a cell and surround the nucleus of the cell.

- **cytoplasmic droplet**
  a round drop of cytoplasm that moves from the neck of the sperm down its tail and

is gone by the time normal sperm are ejaculated.

- **D-**
diarrhoea absent or diminished

- **dehisence**
absence of bone support around root.

- **D&D**
destroy and disposal

- **D.V.M.**
Doctor of Veterinary Medicine.

- **d/o**
1. drain out (removal of surgical drain)
2. dropped off (for treatment or examination)

- **D+**
diarrhoea

- **D++**
1. drinking increased
2. marked diarrhoea

- **D+++**
severe diarrhoea

- **dachshund**
German term for a short-legged scent hound used for badger, equivalent to the French basset and the Swiss niederlaufhund. Of course the Dachshund is the best example of this type of working dog. The Dachshund, known in Germany as the Teckel, has a long and much debated history. The word 'Tekal' from which the German Teckel derives can be found inscribed on the base of an ancient Egyptian sculpture - an Egyptian king seated with three rather curious, if not familiar, doglike animals. Apparently a race of long-backed, short-legged dogs existed in Egpyt at a very early date. These dogs were clumsy, egregiously eared 30-pounders and the said forebears of our current-day multi-talented Dachshund. In German, Dachshund translates as badger dog, reflecting the breed's original function.

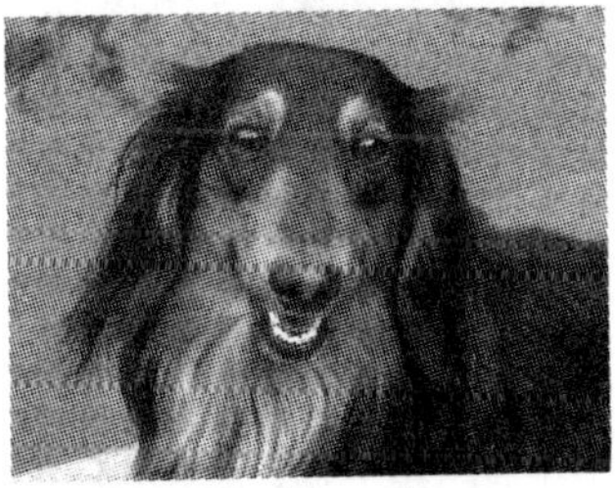

- **dacryocystitis**
inflammation of the lacrimal sac usually as a result of infection.

- **dacryocystorhinography**
a technique in which radiopaque contrast material is injected into the punctum and flushed through the nasolacrimal duct, followed by lateral and VD radiographic views of the skull, to evaluate the nasolacrimal system and surrounding bony structures.

- **dags**
breech wool that is coated with faeces. 'To dag' the sheep means to remove this wool by selective shearing or clipping with dagging shears.

- **dalmatian**
there is no doubt that the Dalmatian is an ancient breed of dogs. The Dalmatian has been known as a breed in England since the 1700s, but models of a spotted dog date back to ancient Greek friezes. E.C. Ash, the noted author of Dogs and Their History, refers to spotted dogs that appear on a tablet dated circa 2000 B.C. Authorities claim Dalmatia, (a southern region of Croatia), to be the birthplace of the breed.

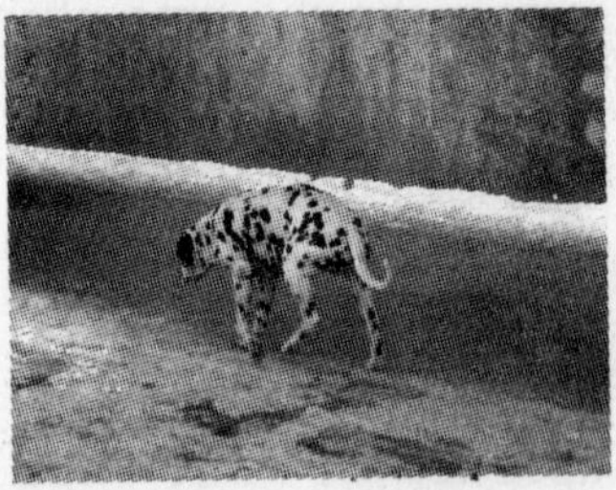

- **daltons**
a term used to indicate a unit of mass equal to 1/12 the mass of a carbon-12 atom.

- **dam**
the female parent of a foal.

- **DAMN IT acronym**
A method of looking at possible causes for a problem. D= degenerative A = anomalies or autoimmune M= metabolic N = neoplasia or nutritional I = inflammation or infectious or immune mediated or iatrogenic T= toxic or traumatic idiopathic.

- **dam's sire (broodmare sire)**
the sire of a broodmare. Used in reference to the maternal grandsire of a foal.

- **Dandie Dinmont Terrier**
this short-legged terrier was developed as an otter and badger specialist in seventeenth-century Great Britain - more specifically, in the

Cheviot Hills and Coquetdale. The Allans, also of Bedlington fame, are said to have kept this type of rough-coated Border Terrier. Farms in Lyndlea and in the Teviotdale Hills also had very similar terriers, and it was these terriers that so impressed Sir Walter Scott to influence their inclusion in his novel Guy Mannering, published in 1814. His character Dandie Dinmont gave its name to this breed of terrier. Whether selective breeding or pure blissful serendipity, the Dandie was derived from various running dogs and hounds. Often the Otter Hound is purported, but the physical characteristics would prove this largely erroneous The Dachshund and the Bedlington Terrier (if the prototype antecedes the Dandie's creation) would have provided a number of the Dandie traits that are unique: short, crooked legs, domed head, round eyes, scimitar-like tail, arch of loin, and the soft silky hair atop its head.

- **dapsone**

Diaminodiphenylsulfon, Alvosulfon. Used in the treatment of subcorneal pustular dermatosis.

- **database**

the database is information that is collected by the user of the medical record, either the veterinarian or a technician. In order to collect a similar amount of baseline information about all patients, and to avoid omissions, the minimum database should be defined in advance and should always be collected. The database may include laboratory tests, radiographs, or other diagnostic tests.

- **days in milk**

the number of days a cow has been milking in her current lactation, same as days since fresh.

- **days open**

the number of days between calving (parturition) and conception. Should be less than 120 days.

- **DBA**

dog bite abscess

- **DC**

diabetic cat

- **DCM**

dilated cardiomyopathy

- **DD**
  Diabetic dog
- **DD, DDX or DDXX**
  differential diagnosis
- **dead-end host**
  it cannot be transmitted from human to human. Example: brucellosis.
- **debride**
  to clean out dead or dying tissue from a wound.
- **deciduous teeth**
  non-permanent teeth (baby teeth)that will be shed and replaced with permanent adult teeth.
- **declawing**
  a surgical process that permanently removes the nails on an animal (British vets have unilaterally banned it by deciding they won't ever declaw except in cases of medical necessity, not to be encouraged elsewhere).

Onychectomy: "Declawing" - Feline Digital Amputation

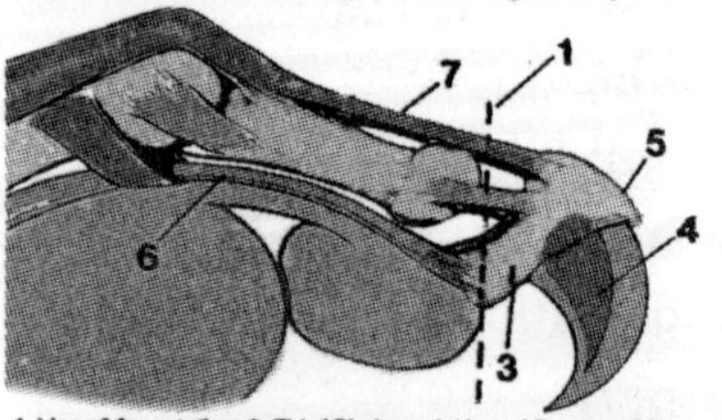

1. Line of Amputation; 3. Third Phalanx; 4. Ungual Process; 5.Ungual Crest; 6. Flexor Tendon; 7. Dorsal Ligaments - are all severed and amputated in the declawing surgery. Declawing involves 10 separate and painful amputations.

- **decontaminate**
  remove injurious material.
- **decubital ulcers**
  pressure sores, usually seen over bony prominences.
- **deep flexor tendon**
  present in all four legs, but injuries most commonly affect the front legs. Located on the back (posterior) of the front leg between the knee and the foot and between the hock and the foot on the rear leg. The function is to flex the digit (pastern) and knee (carpus) and to extend the elbow on the front leg and extend the hock on the rear leg. Functions in tandem with the superficial flexor tendon.
- **deep mycoses**
  diseases including Histoplasmosis, Blastomycosis, Coccidioidomycosis and Cryptococcosis.
- **defecation**
  to pass faeces, stool or manure.
- **definitive host**
  where sexual reproduction takes place.

- **degenerative joint disease (DJD)**
any joint problem that has progressive degeneration of joint cartilage and the underlying (subchondral) bone. Occurs most frequently in the joints below the radius in the foreleg and femur in the hind leg. Some of the more common causes include repeated trauma, conformation faults, blood disease, traumatic joint injury, subchondral bone defects (OCD lesions) and excessive intra-articular corticosteroid injections. Also known as osteoarthritis.

- **degradable intake protein (Abrev: DIP)**
portion of intake protein that is degraded (broken down) by rumen microbes to ammonia and amino acids. DIP is used for microbial synthesis.

- **dehydration**
loss of fluid from the bloodstream and tissues.

- **delayed wound closure**
this is a wound you will suture but not immediately; first you debride the wound several times through bandage changes to make it more amenable to closing.

- **demodectic mange**
skin disease characterised by hair loss particularly on the head, face, neck, shoulders and the front of the forelegs. Caused by the demodex mite, which is normally found on the skin of most dogs, but due to an abnormality of the immune system, the body overreacts to its presence. It can be treated, but it is occasionally resistant to treatment.

- **demodicosis generalised**
also called the pustular form. Many small focal areas of involvement or a diffuse generalized distribution. Lesions include generalized erythema, crusting, scaling and patching to diffuse alopecia.

- **demodicosis localised**
also called squamous. One or more well circumscribed areas of alopecia with mild scaling and erythema usually located on the forelimbs, face and on periocular skin.

• **dentition**
the canine dentition, which is the order and arrangemenet of the dog's teeth, consists of highly specialised structures designed for biting, tearing, cutting and grinding - basically the tool of a meat-eater. The outside of the dog's tooth is constructed of pearly white enamel. This outer exposed portion is known as the crown. Beneath the enamel is dentine, which comprises the bulk of the structure. The neck refers to the tooth at the gumline the root is the portion of the tooth that is embedded into the jawbone. Cementum covers the root. it is a thin bonelike substance. Composing the sensory nerves is soft tissue called pulp.

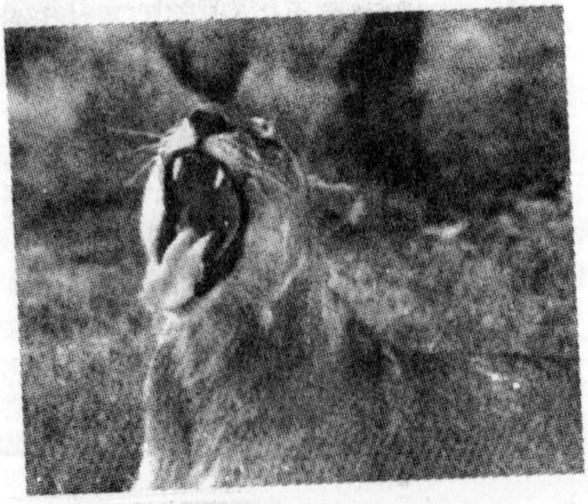

• **dermal**
relating to the skin.

• **dermatitis**
an inflammation of the skin.

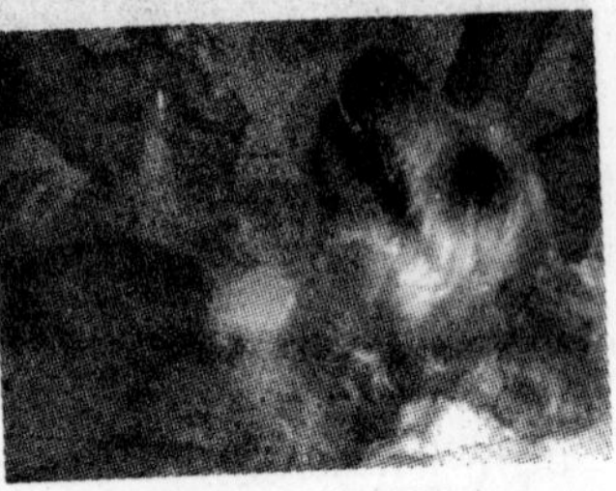

• **dermatitis herpetiformis**
a pruritic, vesiculoulcerative dermatitis, which is poorly documented in veterinary medicine and is associated with IgA deposition and gluten enteropathies in man.

• **dermatologic examination**
the dermatologic exam should include examination of the entire hair coat, careful palpation of the skin, careful examination of the skin surface over several areas of the body, visual examination (otoscopic) of the external ear canals, and inspection of the foot pads. In many cases it is helpful to clip hair from the patient so that specific lesions may be seen more clearly. It is also helpful to have a form for the medical record, or

which lesions may be drawn and recorded, as well as other information.

- **dermatomyositis**
  an immune-mediated, familial dermatopathy suggested to be a primary vasculopathy with secondary dermatitis and myositis. Breed predilection includes Collies and Shetland Sheepdogs.

- **dermatophilosis**
  pyoderma caused by the aerobic and facultative anaerobic actinomycete Dermatophilus congolensis. Also called Streptotricosis, rain scald, and streptothricosis (horses)

- **dermatophyte**
  fungus that causes ringworm include Trichophyton, Microsporum and Epidermophtyon.

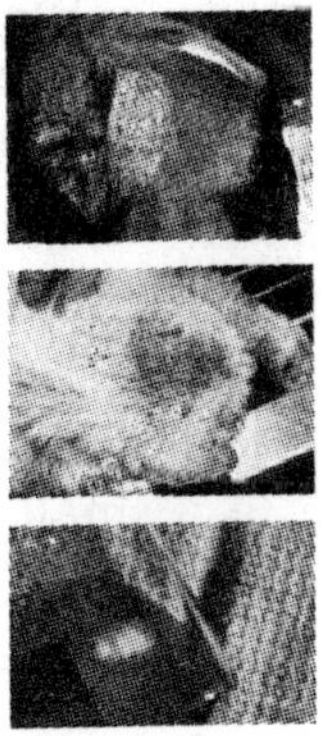

- **dermis**
  the dermal layer of the skin that contains blood vessels, hair follicles, sebaceous glands, erector pili muscles, and apocrine sweat glands.

- **dermoid**
  a piece of skin growing on the cornea.

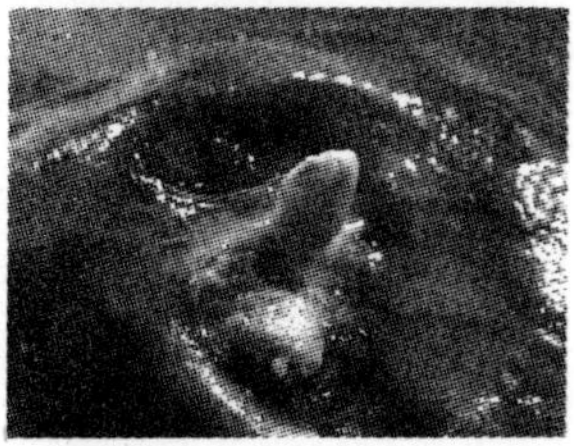

- **descemetocele**
  very deep ulcers right down to decemets membrane.

- **descemet's membrane**
  a clear membrane forming the inner boundary of the cornea.

- **descenting**
  the removal of the anal sacs of a carnivore to prevent the animal from releasing the very strong-smelling secretion.

- **desmitis**
  inflammation of a ligament. Often a result of tearing of any number of ligament fibrils.

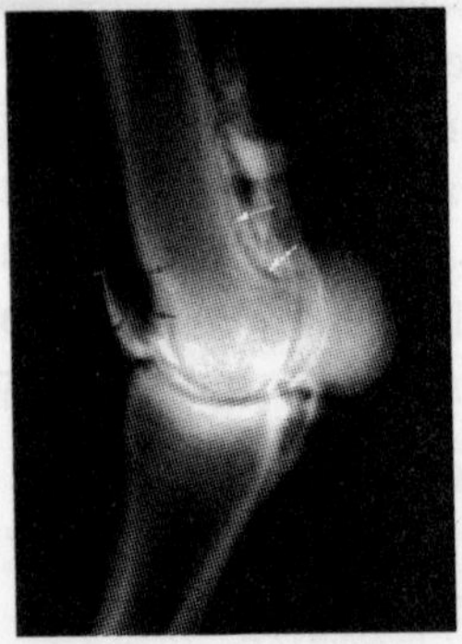

- **deworming**

  the use of drugs (anthelmintics) to kill internal parasites, often performed by oral paste or by passing a nasogastric tube into the horse's stomach.

- **dextran**

  high molecular weight polysaccharides used to expand blood volume. A colloid. Dextrans have an average molecular weight of 40, 000 daltons (Dextran 40) or 75, 000 daltons (Dextran 70).

- **dextrose 5% (Abrev: D5W)**

  5% dextrose is hypotonic relative to extra-cellular fluid. It contains only dextrose, no electrolytes. 5% dextrose is a constituent of most maintenance solutions. It can be used as sole fluid for rehydration for animals who cannot tolerate the administration of sodium, such as those with cardiac disease. More commonly, it is used as part of the rehydration solution in these sodium intolerant animals, used in combination with lactated Ringer's or sodium chloride.

- **dextrose hypertonic**

  hypertonic dextrose is any percentage of dextrose which has an osmolality in excess of extra-cellular fluid. Dextrose is available in several commercial strengths. Any concentration of dextrose can be created by adding additional dextrose to a commercial solution. The predominant use of hypertonic dextrose solutions is as a calorie source in total parenteral nutrition solutions. There is also an indication to promote urine flow in patients with oliguric acute renal failure. TPN solutions containing 50% dextrose are extremely hypertonic and can cause an irritation to the blood vessel if given in a small peripheral vein, such as cephalic or saphenous. Hypertonic solutions are typically given in larger veins such as the jugular vein in which blood flow is faster to dilute the hypertonicity of the infused solution and reduce irritation to the lining of the blood vessel.

- **DH**
  dead heat.

- **DHLPPI**
  distemper, hepatitis, Leptospirosis, parvovirus and parainfluenza: dog vaccine covering these diseases

- **DI**
  diabetes insipidus

- **diabetes**
  a metabolic disease caused by failure of the pancreas to produce insulin, a hormone that allows blood sugar (glucose) to be taken up by cells.

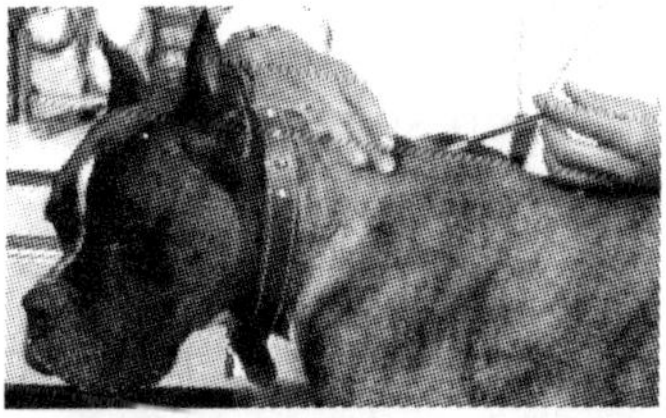

- **diabetes insipidus**
  inadequate secretion of, or resistance to the effects of, antidiuretic hormone (ADH or Vasopressin). This hormone stimulates the kidney to retain water in the body. Consequently, the dog passes a large volume of urine with a low specific gravity, and also exhibits great thirst. It may be acquired, inherited. Idiopathic mellitus may be due to a failure of the pancreas to produce sufficient insulin, or due to the cells' resistance to the effects of insulin the body is unable to properly process glucose. May require insulin injections, or may be controlled with diet.

- **diabetes mellitus**
  also known as sugar diabetes. An insufficient amount of insulin is produced by the pancreas resulting in a high blood sugar level.

- **diagnostic plans**
  diagnostic plans are made in order to determine if a certain disease is present. For example you may plan to perform bile acid analyses to determine if liver failure is present.

- **diagnostic tests**
  these are tests performed to find the cause of a pet's prob-

lem. Diagnostic tests may include analysis of blood, urine, and other body fluids x-rays (the correct term is radiographs) biopsies, etc.

- **dialysis**
  a process which involves removing waste products from the body.

- **diamond eyes**
  a combination of severe entropion and ectropion involving both upper and lower eyelids. Most commonly seen in Saint Bernard dogs.

- **diarrhoea**
  a condition in which the movement of food through the digestive system is faster than normal. It often results in the frequent passing of abnormally loose or watery stool.

- **DIC**
  disseminated intravascular coagulation

- **diestrus**
  a stage of the female reproductive cycle that follows the period of receptivity.

- **dietary history**
  this includes: the diet the animal is currently receiving and for how long? Have they ever home cooked a hypoallergenic diet (potato and pinto beans, lamb and rice)?

- **dietary indiscretion**
  eating what one should not. Dietary indiscretion would include eating garbage, dead fish, etc.

- **dietary scours**
  when the calf is getting so much nutrient intake they can not absorb it all and it is fermenting in the colon producing gassy, large volume, smelly diarrhoea.

- **differential diagnosis**
  differential diagnoses are also known as rule-outs and are possible causes for the problems displayed by a patient. For example, kidney failure is one possible cause for polyuria in a dog or cat.

- **DIFF-Quik stain**
  a 3-step staining process to stain cytology samples.

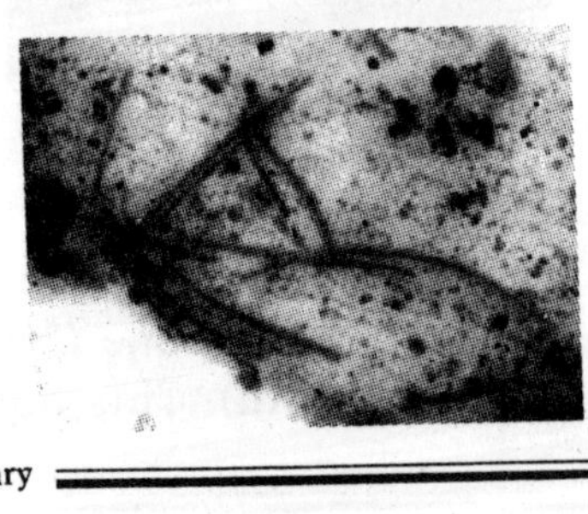

- **digestibility**
  expressed as a percent, is a measure of the content of food that is retained in the body after food is eaten. The difference between the weight of food eaten and the weight of stool produced, divided by the weight of the food.

- **digestible energy (Abrev: DE)**
  energy that is available to the animal by digestion, measured as the difference between gross energy content of a feed and the energy contained in the animal's faeces (gross energy minus faecal energy.)

- **digestion**
  the changes that occur to a feed within the animal's digestive tract to prepare it for absorption and use.

- **digestive system**
  an organ system that absorbs and digests food. The digestive system includes the oesophagus, stomach, intestine, liver and pancreas.

- **digital**
  the part of the limb below the ankle (fetlock) joint. Includes the long and short pastern bones and the coffin bone.

- **digital cushion**
  the area beneath the coffin bone in the back of the foot that separates it from the frog. The digital cushion serves as a shock absorber for the foot.

- **digital examination**
  using gloved fingers to examine. Usually refers to rectal or vaginal exams.

- **digital manipulation**
  manually stimulating the penis in order to obtain a semen sample for analysis.

- **digitalis glycosides**
  class of drugs including digitoxin and digoxin which are drugs derived from the Digitalis purpurea plant. Used in the treatment of congestive heart failure.

- **dihydrotestosterone (Abrev: DTH)**
  the form of testosterone used by the prostate gland.

- **dilated cardiomyopathy**
  a heart condition in which the heart enlarges but the heart muscle becomes thinner.

- **dimensions of pain**
  there are 3 dimensions of pain: sensory-discriminative, motivational-affective and cognitive-evaluative, which influence how an individual interprets and responds to a painful stimulus.

- **dimethyl sulfoxide (Abrev: DMSO)**
  an organic solvent used to deliver other substances that themselves are less soluble.

- **dingo**
  the Australian dingo, or warrigal, is a wild dog of great antiquity but not a native to Australia. It is believed that the dingo was brought by primitive man to the continent of Australia as a semi-domesticated feral dog.

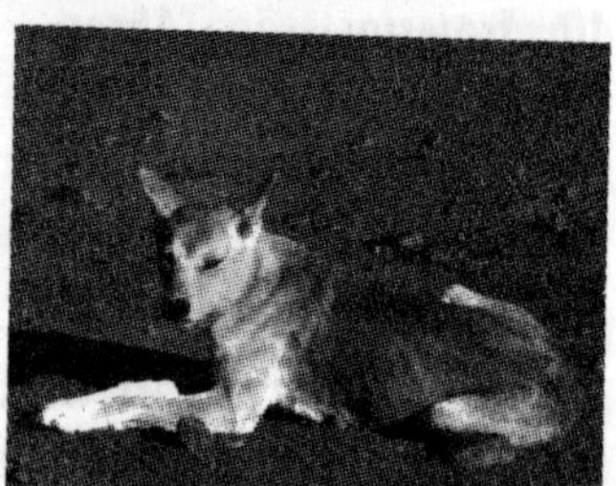

- **dinoflagellate**
  single-celledalgae, mainly marine and often with a cellulose shell some species may be luminescent, and some cause the red tides that are extremely toxic to marine life.

- **diphenhydramine HCL**
  Benadryl. An antihistamine.

- **direct lifecycle**
  there is a single host and the host animal is the animal that is being infected.

- **discharge summary**
  a description of a patient's workup. May include an overview in client terms of what tests were performed and test results as well as a description of treatment and care for the patient.

- **discoid lupus erythematosus (Abrev: DLE)**
  a form of systemic lupus erythematosus which only involves the skin.

- **disease triangle**
  interactions between the host, the pathogen, and the environment.

- **disinfectant**
  germicidal chemical that destroys micro-organisms and the potential infectivity of a material.

• **disinfection**
to destroy germs by using chemicals (disinfectants) or by physical means such as high temperature.

• **diskospondylitis**
infection of the interverte-bral disk with concurrent osteomyelitis of contiguous vertebrae.

• **disseminated intravascular coagulation (Abrev: DIC)**
concurrent stimulation of the clotting and fibrinolytic systems by a disease.

• **distaff**
a female horse.

• **distaff race**
a race for female horses.

• **distal**
away from a reference point. Usually refers to the limbs.

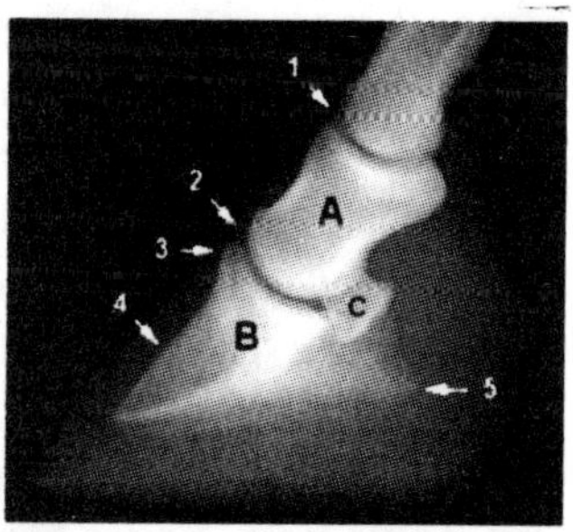

• **distal sesamoidean ligaments**
attaches to the bottom of the sesamoid bones, passing down and attaching to the long and short pastern bones.

• **distemper**
canine distemper is a viral disease that causes a severe and often-fatal system ill-ness in dogs and their close relatives. Distemper is also fatal in animals such as rac-coons, and mustelids includ-ing skunks, mink and ferrets.

• **distichiasis**
an extra row of cilia or eye-lashes grow from the meibomian gland openings on the eyelid margin.

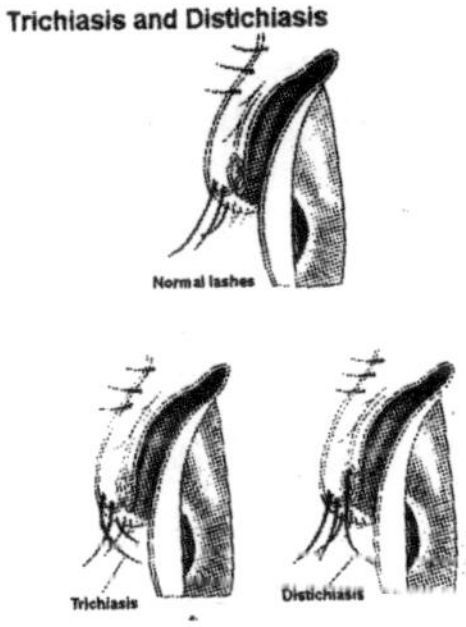

• **diuretic**
agent which increases the secretion of urine, ridding the body of excess fluid.

• **diurnal**
active during the day, oppo-site of nocturnal, which

means active during the night.

- **DJD**
  degenerative joint disease
- **DLH**
  domestic long hair (non-pedigree cat)
- **DM**
  diabetes mellitus
- **DMSO**
  dimethyl sulfoxide, a topical anti-inflammatory.
- **DNA**
  deoxyribonucleicacid, the chemical compound that occurs in cells and is the basic structure for genes.
- **DO**
  days old (following a number)
- **DOA**
  dead on arrival
- **Dogue de Bordeaux**
  the Dogue de Bordeaux, known variously as the French Mastiff and Bordeaux Bulldog, is a truly ancient breed of France said to have descended driectly from the Molossus of Rome. The breed's large brachycephalic skull, deep protective instincts, and overall massive build speak of this direct relationship. A frequent sight on French estates for centuries, the Bordeaux dog is a fearless guardian. Employed as a hunter of pigs, bears, boars and wolves, these formidable titans were never over-esteemed by their twelfth-century French masters. During the Middle Ages, the dogs were used for cattle droving. For many generations, the dogs were employed as both war dogs and flock guardians. Their fearlessness and power are formidable and can be aptly compared to any dog that has ever intimidated the likes of men, wolves, and bears. Frequently used in baiting sports, as well as dogfights, the Bordeaux has proven himself versatile through the ages. With the outlawing of animal baiting, Dogues were pitted against Dogues and provided hours of blood-stirring and -spilling entertainment for the onlooking French peasants and noblemen. Never a dull moment, a full-grown jaguar would be introduced to

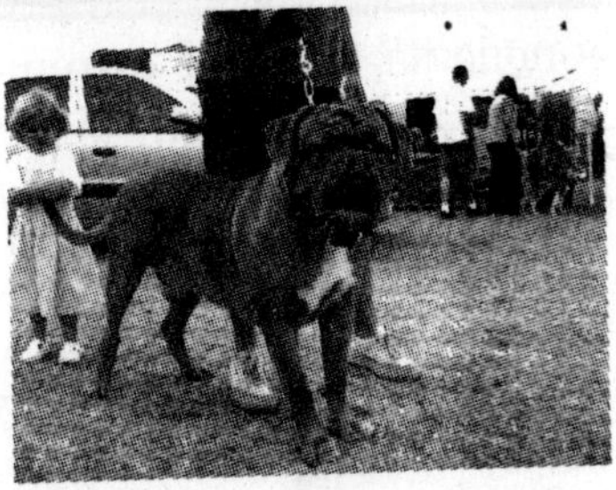

liven up a less than exciting match.

- **domboro's solution**
  aluminum acetate solution. A topical drying agent (astringent).

- **domed skull**
  synonymous with apple skull, the term used in the Chihuahua standard. A domed skull is sloping on all sides, somewhat like one-quarter of a globe. Such a skull has a rounded and smooth appearance.

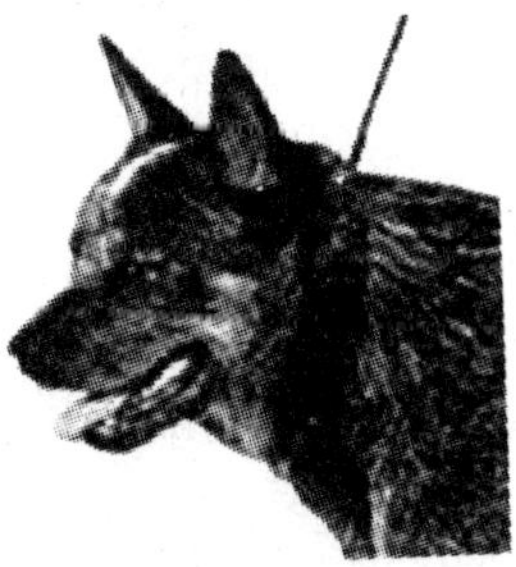

- **domestic animal**
  an animal that has been housed and fed by man for generations and has little fear of man as a result. Some domestic animals learn to depend on human provision so completely that they have little ability to survive if returned to a natural habitat.

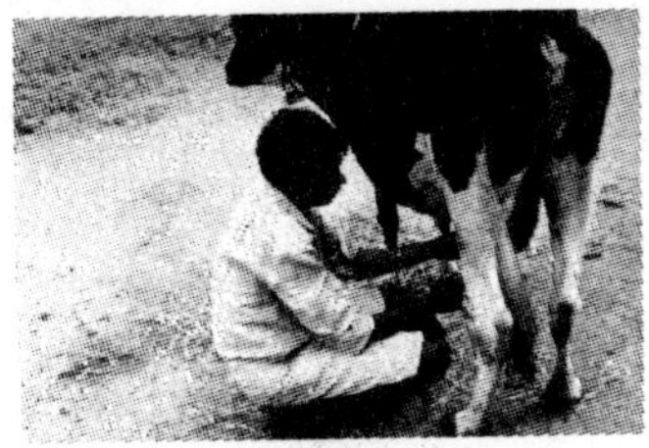

- **domestication**
  a process that tames animals and their offspring, so that they may live in close contact with humans.

- **dominant**
  only one copy of a gene is necessary for a trait to be exhibited. At least one of the parents would also exhibit this same trait.

- **dominant follicle**
  the largest follicle on the ovary that secretes hormones that will suppress the other follicles so that the female will have only one egg and will prevent twinning.

• **dope**
any illegal drug.

• **dors**
dorsal

• **dorsal**
up towards the back or spine. Also used to describe the front of the lower limb below the knee (front) or hock (rear).

• **dorsal displacement of the soft palate**
a condition in which the soft palate, located on the floor of the airway near the larynx, moves up into the airway. A minor displacement causes a gurgling sound during exercise while in more serious cases the palate can block the airway. This is sometimes known as 'choking down, ' but the tongue does not actually block the airway. The base of the tongue is connected to the larynx, of which the epiglottis is a part. When the epiglottis is retracted, the soft palate can move up into the airway (dorsal displacement.) This condition can sometimes be managed with equipment such as a figure eight noseband or a tongue-tie. In more extreme cases, surgery might be required, most commonly a 'myectomy.'

• **dosage**
Although there are actually many 'Dosage theories, ' the one most commonly thought of as Dosage is the one as interpreted by Dr. Steven Roman. A variation of Dr. Franco Varola's work on pedigree analysis, the system identifies patterns of ability in horses based on a list of prepotent sires, each of whom is a chef-de-race. The Dosage system puts these sires into one of five categories brilliant, intermediate, classic, solid and professional, which quantify speed and stamina. Sires can be listed in up to two chef-de-race categories. Each generation of sires is worth 16 points, divided up by the amount of sires, i.e., the immediate sire is worth 16 points while the four sires four generations back are worth four points apiece.

• **dosage index (DI)**
a mathematical reduction of the Dosage profile to a num-

ber reflecting a horse's potential for speed or stamina. The higher the number, the more likely the horse is suited to be a sprinter. The average Dosage index of all horses is about 4.0.

- **dosage profile**
  a listing of Dosage points by category. Used to develop the Dosage index (DI).
- **double coat**
  the dog's usual coat, consisting of an outer coat and an undercoat: two-ply.

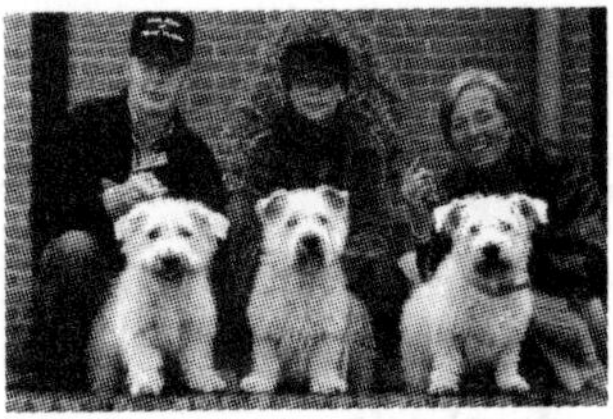

- **doxapram**
  a respiratory stimulant. No longer recommended for use in CPR.
- **DQ**
  abbreviation for disqualified.
- **DR. Lawrence Weed**
  a physician who developed the problem oriented medical record and problem oriented approach to patient care in the 1960's.
- **draft**
  separate sheep into groups.
- **drench**
  liquid administered through mouth.
- **drove/droving (Australian)**
  to move sheep.
- **dry cow therapy**
  antibiotic therapy given at the onset of the non-lactating period of the cow. It is intended to cure and protect against intramammary infection.
- **dry matter**
  feed residue left after all moisture has been removed by drying (i.e., 100% dry matter).
- **dry matter basis**
  an expression of feed nutrient content after the moisture has been removed by drying. Used to compare nutrient composition or animal intake of feeds differing in moisture content.
- **dry period**
  a period of 45-60 days when lactation is halted before the next lactation begins. The dry period is required for rejuvenation of secretory parenchyma.

- **dry eye**
  keratoconjunctivitissicca(KCS) is the technical term for a condition also known as 'dry eye'. It occurs because of inadequate reproduction. Symptoms include a thick, yellowish discharge from the eye.

- **DSH**
  domestic short hair (non-pedigree cat)

- **duodenum**
  the portion of the intestine directly attached to the stomach.

- **duration of immunity**
  length of time an animal is protected from a disease. Vaccines for some diseases provide long durations of immunity (years), while vaccines for other diseases may provide immunity that only lasts for six months.

- **DX**
  diagnosis

- **dysecdysis**
  abnormal shedding of the skin in reptiles.

- **dysfibrinogenemia, Factor I deficiency**
  fibrinogen, or Factor I, is an important component of the 'clotting cascade' which allows your body to stop bleeding. This disease is due to either an abnormally low amount of fibrinogen, or its complete absence, or the presence of a normal amount of an abnormal and less effective fibrinogen. Symptoms include easy or excessive bleeding or no symptoms at all.

- **dysmature cria**
  a cria that has developed too slow inside the uterus. They are born weak and lacking vigour.

- **dysphagia**
  difficulty eating and swallowing.

- **dysphoria**
  agitation or restlessness.

- **dysplasia**
  an abnormal tissue development seen in the bones of dogs.

- **dyspnea**
  difficulty breathing.

- **dystocia**
  difficulty giving birth. Maternal or foetal factors may cause dystocia.

- **dystrophic**
disorder caused by incorrect nutrition.

- **dysuria**
difficult or painful urination.

- **E**
enamel defect

- **E&A**
euthanasia and aftercare

- **E(X)D**
every (x) days

- **E(X)WKS**
every (x) weeks

- **E/D+**
eating and drinking normally

- **E/T**
endo-tracheal

- **EAG**
empty (or express) anal glands

- **ear canal**
the tube that connects the external ear with the ear drum.

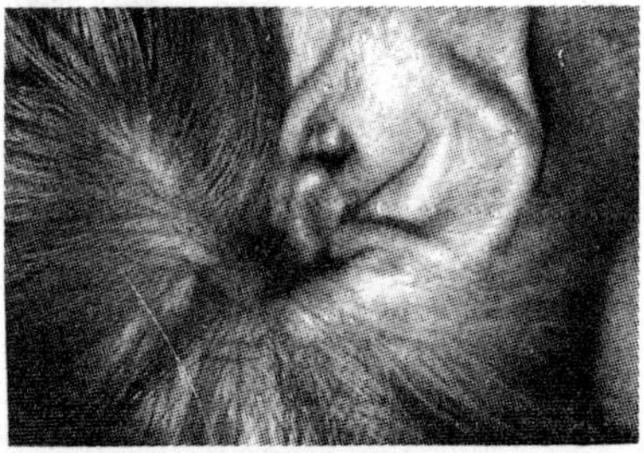

- **ear drum**
the membrane that divides the outer ear from the inner ear where the mechanism of hearing takes place. The membrane prevents infection from reaching the inner ear as well as vibrating to amplify sounds.

- **ear mites**
small parasitic insects that live in the ear canal of an animal, and that are able to survive outside the ear for only very short periods of time.

- **ear muffs**
a piece of equipment that covers a horse's ears to prevent it from hearing distracting sounds.

- **Eastern Equine Encephalitis**
Eastern Equine Encephalitis is a retrovirus. An infected animal either dies, or becomes a chronic carrier, much like a cat with FeLV.

- **EBT**
English Bull Terrier

- **ecdysis**
shedding of the external layers of the skin in reptiles.

- **ECG**
  a printout of an analysis of the electrical activity in the heart.
- **echocardiogram**
  the image produced by performing an ultrasound examination of the heart.
- **echocardiography**
  an ultrasound exam of the heart. Passing sound waves through the heart to see the internal structure of the heart. A plain radiograph (x-ray) only shows the shape of the heart but not its internal structure.
- **eclampsia**
  low blood calcium occurring in female dogs and cats at the end of gestation, or more commonly during early lactation. Small breed dogs are more commonly affected. Low calcium causes signs of muscle tetany.
- **ecp**
  a type of oestrogen sometimes used to mismate.
- **ectoparasite**
  a parasite that lives on the outside surface or skin of another animal. Ectoparasites include fleas, ticks, lice, and mange mites.
- **ectopic**
  nonmalignant tissue growing in an unusual location e.g., an ectopic pregnancy is conception of a normal embryo outside the normal location, which is the uterus.
- **ectopic cilia**
  hairs on the inside of the eyelids causing irritation to the eye.

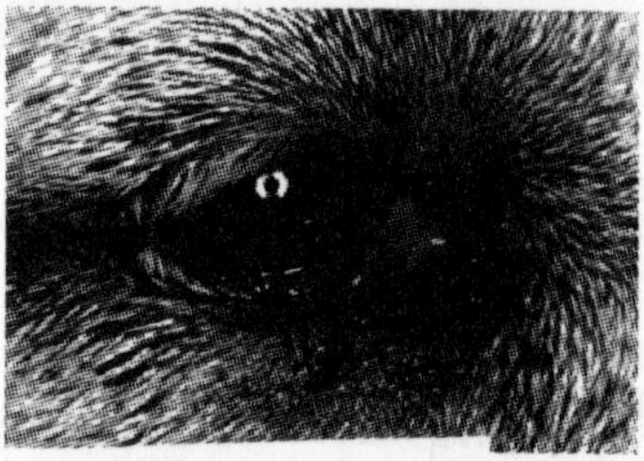

- **ectropion**
  eyelid turns outward. Allows for the accumulation of foreign matter causing eye irritation.
- **edema**
  a condition in which the tissues of the body contain too much fluid. The fluid accumulation may cause swelling in the affected area.

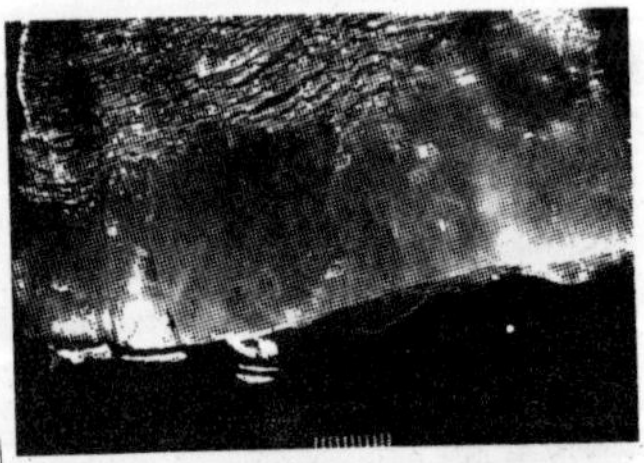

- **edema in pregnant mares**
  ventral edema is fairly common in near-term mares.
- **EDUD**
  eating, drinking, urinating and defaecating
- **EEE (Eastern Equine Encephalomyelitis)**
  one of several different types of encephalomyelitis that are extremely contagious, causing sickness and death in horses by affecting the central nervous system. EEE is spread by mosquitoes and can affect humans. Can be prevented by annual vaccinations.
- **Egistry Berner-Garde**
  bernese Mountain Dog data repository used to track health trends and provide reports about a dog's family on request.
- **Egistry Cerf**
  canine Eye Registry Foundation - closed registry of eye test results.
- **Egistry Closed Registry**
  repository of health test results, but allows access of information only about normal results.
- **Egistry GDC**
  institute for Genetic Disease Control, open registry reporting orthopaedic and ophthalmologic evaluation reports, tumour, epilepsy, heart registry and some other breed specific health information.
- **Egistry ofa**
  orthoapedic Foundation for Animals, closed registry of hip, elbow, heart, thyroid, and other results.
- **Egistry Pennhip**
  Penn Hip Improvement Program - closed registry of hip laxity measurements. Uses a DI (distraction index), a number from 0.0 - 1.00 with the lower the number the better the hip.
- **Egistryopen Registry**
  repository of health test results, allows full access to the information.
- **Enamel Hypoplasia**
  a condition where enamel is thin or absent. Appears as areas of shiny enamel surrounded by opaque areas of dentin. In time, the opaque regions become stained a brownish colour. In dogs, enamel hypoplasia is usu-

ally caused by a febrile disease, occurring before the animal is six months old as the enamel is forming.

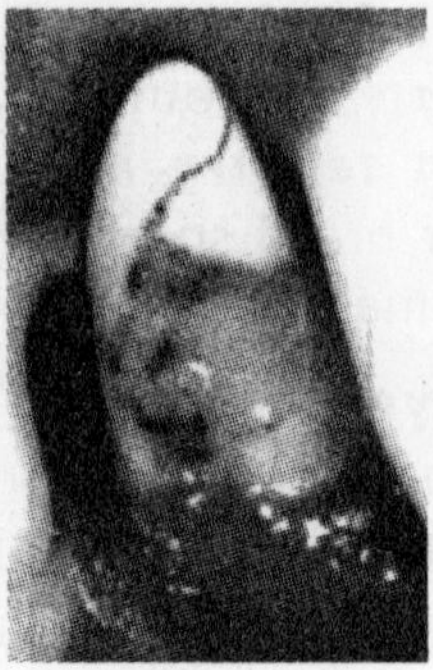

- **EIPH**
  exercise-induced pulmonary haemorrhage.
- **ejaculate**
  the movement of semen through the urethra to outside the penis.
- **ejaculation**
  the ejection of sperm from the penis.
- **ECG**
  a print out of an analysis of the electrical activity in the heart.
- **elbow dysplasia, ED**
  asynchronous growth of the bones of the foreleg causing the joint to meet improperly.
- **electrocardiogram (ECG)**
  a printout of an analysis of the electrical activity in the heart.
- **electrocautery**
  an instrument with a very hot tip, heated by electricity, is applied to a tissue. Electrocautery may be used to make an incision, remove a mass, or to stop bleeding.
- **electroejaculation**
  using an electrical stimulus to cause the male to ejaculate semen.
- **electrolyte**
  an element that when dissolved in water will cause the solution to transmit electricity. This includes certain elements in the blood which are critically important to life including sodium, potassium, chloride, calcium, and phosphorous.

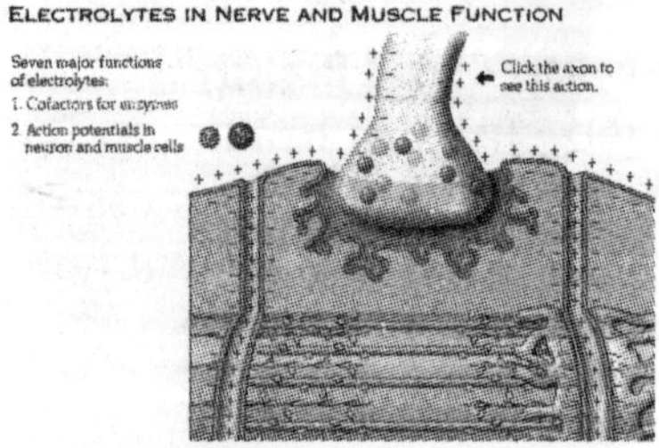

- **electroretinography**
  a diagnostic technique used to evaluate the function of the photoreceptors, specifically used to diagnose retinal degeneration.
- **elizabethan collar**
  a large plastic collar that is placed over the head of a dog or cat. It has a cone shape and is used to keep them from licking or chewing on themselves.
- **emaciation**
  severe weight loss. Extremely thin. Also called cachexia.
- **embryo**
  the early stages of development of a baby in the uterus.
- **embryonic vesicle**
  the sac containing the embryo which later in pregnancy develops into a foetus.
- **emesis**
  a synonym for vomitting.

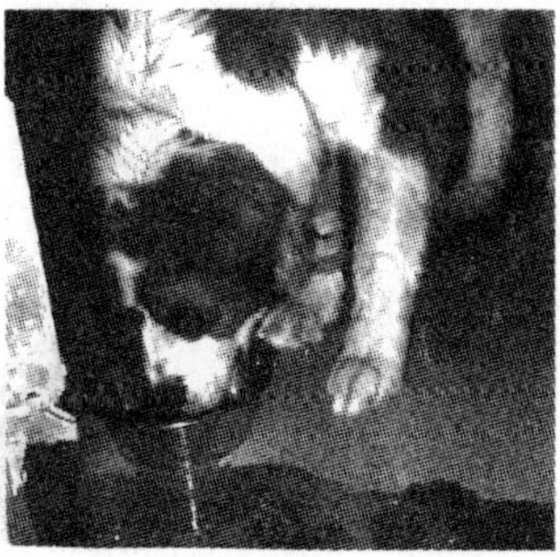

- **emetic**
  agent that decreases or stops vomitting.
- **emollient**
  a softening agent.
- **encephalitis**
  inflammation of the brain.
- **encephalopathy**
  any degenerative disease of the brain. Causes include liver disease resulting in build up of toxic byproducts of metabolism, heavy metal (e.g., lead) poisoning, and loss of blood supply.
- **end stage renal disease (Abrev: ERSD)**
  advanced, irreversible chronic renal disease. Also a non-specific histological finding on renal biopsy that may be the end result of renal disease of any aetiology.
- **endemic disease**
  an infection that is engrained in a particular area.
- **endocrine**
  the body system that produces hormones. Endocrine organs include the pancreas, thyroid gland, parathyroid glands, and adrenal glands. Diseases of the endocrine system may lead

to the production of too much or too little hormone.

- **endogenous**
  produced inside the body. Insulin produced by the pancreas is endogenous insulin.
- **endometritis**
  uterine inflammation or infection due to bacteria or fungi.
- **endoparasites**
  they live within the animal.
- **endorphin**
  a morphine-like peptide that is produced in the brain and which binds to certain receptors to reduce the sensation of pain.
- **endoscope**
  an instrument used for direct visual inspection of a hollow organ or body cavity such as the upper airway or stomach. A 'fibre optic endoscope' is comprised of a long, flexible tube that has a series of lenses and light at the end to allow the veterinarian to view and photograph the respiratory system through the airway. Other internal organs may be viewed through a tiny surgical opening. A 'video endoscope' has a small camera at the tip of the instruments.
- **endoscopy**
  passing an instrument into a cavity to see the insides.
- **endothelial dystrophy**
  an inherited condition seen mainly in older dogs characterised by death of endothelial cells allowing water to enter the stroma resulting in permanent edema.
- **endothelium**
  the epithelial cells lining the inside of a blood vessel.

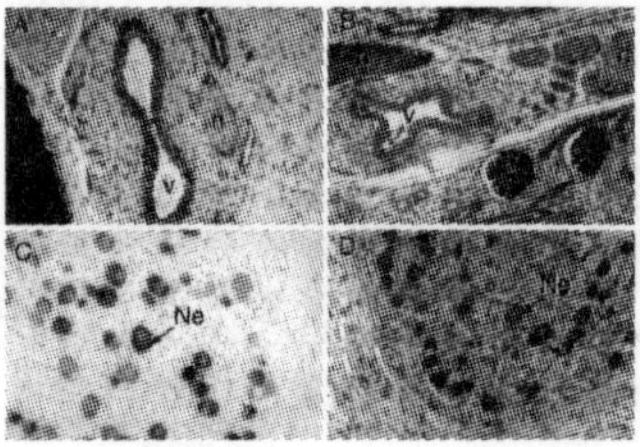

- **endotoxemia**
  a type of shock caused by absorbing endotoxin which is released from some types of bacteria in the intestine when those bacteria die.
- **endotoxin**
  a substance released from some types of bacteria in the intestine that which absorbed into the blood causes fever and shock called endotoxic shock.

- **endotracheal tube**
this tube is placed into the animal's trachea (windpipe) to allow the oxygen and gases to be breathed into the lungs.

- **end-tidal CO2**
monitoring CO2 of exhaled gases provides information about the patient's approximate CO2 levels and is an indirect indicator of cardiac output and blood flow.

- **energy**
a nutrient essential for maintenance, growth, production and reproduction. Energy is required in larger amounts than any other nutrient except water, and is often the limiting factor in livestock production.

- **energy terminology**
Gross Energy (GE) The total combustible energy in a feed, determined by measuring the amount of heat produced when a feed sample is completely burnt in a bomb calorimeter.

- **English Setter**
there is some evidence that the English Setter was in use as a trained bird dog in England about 400 years ago. The development of the modern English Setter began around 1852 when Mr. Edward Laverack obtained a pair of setters from Rev. A. Harrison. Mr. Laverack reportedly continued strict breeding along these lines for the next 50 years. The Laverack setter is the representative of the breed, which one usually finds on the show bench. When the Laverack strain was at its peak of popularity, Mr. R. Ll. Purcell Llewellin purchased a number of Laveracks dogs and crossed them with setters from the north of England. This introduction of new blood resulted in a new strain of setter that proved to be enormously successful at field trials. The Llewellin setter is primarily known as a field dog.

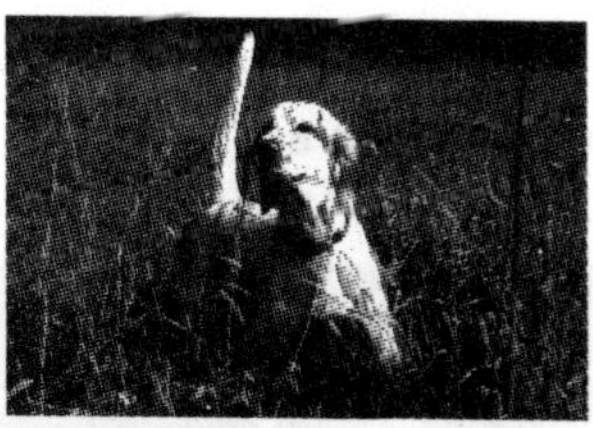

- **enophthalmos**
retraction of globe into the orbit resulting in a sunken eye.

- **enteral**
  delivery of drugs or nutrients to the intestinal tract by deposition in the mouth, stomach or jejunum.

- **enteral feeding**
  a method of feeding an animal in which a tube is placed through the body wall into the gastrointestinal tract and a nutritious liquid is forced through the tube.

- **enteric**
  a pathogen that is related to E. coli.

- **enteritis**
  an inflammation of the intestines.

- **enteropatogenic E. coli**
  specific strains of E. coli that attach very tightly to gut wall and secrete various toxins, causing both excess secretion and malabsorption as well as general systemic effects on the calf.

- **enterotoxemia**
  a highly fatal disease related to the proliferation of Gram-negative organisms in the intestine of susceptible animals.

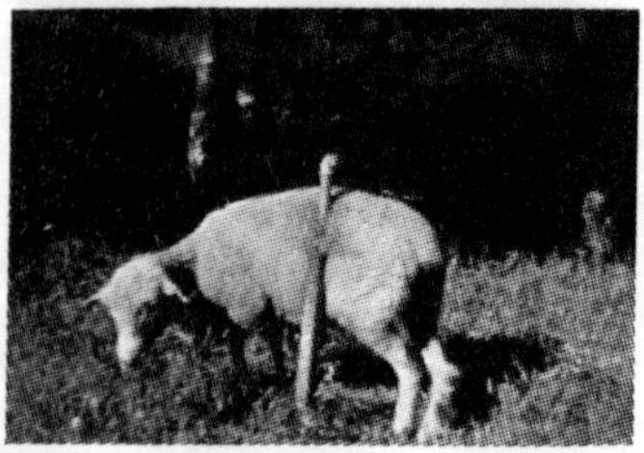

- **enterotoxigenic E. coli**
  a specific strain K99 that attaches to intestinal cells and causes a hypersecretory diarrhoea.

- **entrapped epiglottis**
  a condition in which the thin membrane lying below the epiglottis moves up and covers the epiglottis. The abnormality may obstruct breathing. Usually treated by surgery to cut the membrane if it impairs respiratory function.

- **entropion**
  eyelids turn inward causing hair to irritate the surface of the eye. Normally requires surgical correction, and sometimes requires multiple surgeries.

- **enucleation**
  removing the eye from the orbit: leaves most of the orbital contents behind.

- **envenomation**
  the act of injecting a poisonous material (venom).

- **environmental history**
  this includes a travel history of the animal, a description of the home environment, the percentage of time the patient spends indoors vs outdoors, and the presence of other pets in the household.
- **environmental mastitis**
  mastitis caused by coliforms and environmental *Streptococci.*
- **enzyme**
  a complex protein compound produced in living cells which speeds up chemical reactions without itself being changed or destroyed. It is added to animal feeds to supplement low enzyme production by some young animals or to improve utilisation of feeds.
- **enzyme-linked immunosorbentassay (Abrev: ELISA)**
  an immunological technique for measuring the amount of a substance such as antibody or antigen in blood.
- **EOD**
  every other day
- **eosinophil**
  a type of white blood cell observed in increased numbers in allergies.
- **epulis**
  a periodontal growth classified as either fibromatous, ossifying, or acanthomatous
- **EPI**
  exocrine pancreatic insufficiency
- **epidemiologists**
  scientists that study disease in its natural habitat, rather than in a controlled laboratory environment.
- **epidemiology**
  the study of health and disease in populations of animals.
- **epidermal membrane**
  also called the fourth membrane. A membrane that covers the cria entirely at birth.
- **epidermis**
  the outer-most layer of skin which is made of sequential layers called the stratum corneum, stratum granulosa, stratum spinosum, stratum basalie, and basal lamina.

- **epididymis**
  a structure that is connected to the testicles and stores sperm prior to ejaculation.
- **epididymitis**
  inflammation of the epidiymis often resulting in infertility in rams.
- **epidural anaesthesia**
  injection of an anaesthetic agent into the space outside

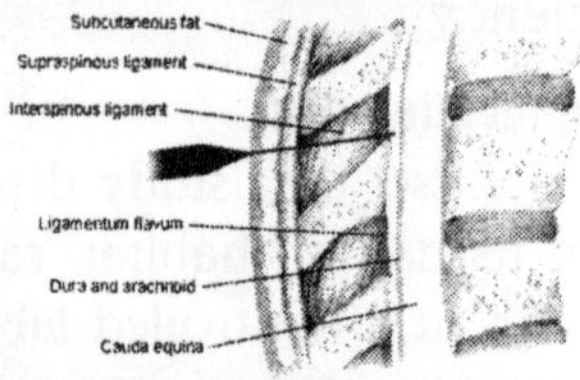

  the dura matter of the spinal cord.
- **epiglottis**
  a triangular-shaped cartilage that lies at the base of the airway just in front of the arytenoid cartilages which cover the airway during swallowing. It is normally located above (dorsal) the soft palate.
- **epilate**
  removing hair.
- **epilepsy**
  abnormal electrical function of the brain causing disturbances of the nervous system.
- **epilepsy acquired**
  acquired due to injury to the brain at birth, tumour, blow to the head, endocrine (hormonal) disorder, etc.
- **epilepsy idiopathic**
  no demonstrable cause, may be genetic.
- **epinephrine**
  a vasopressor drug which via alpha stimulation increases systemic vascular resistance and improves coronary and brain blood flow.
- **epiphora**
  an overflow of tears upon the cheeks due to a blockage or narrowing of the tear ducts.

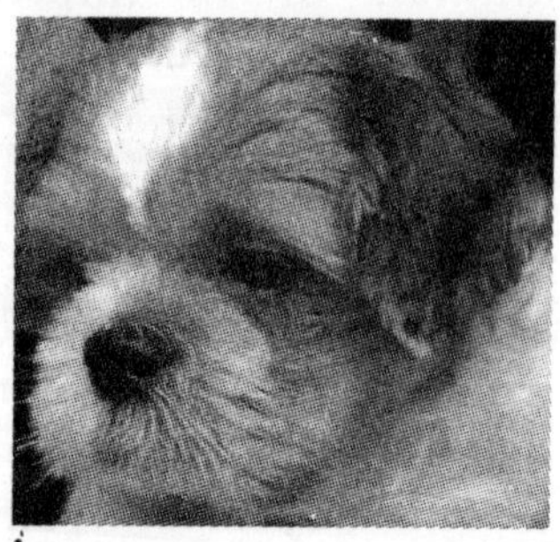

- **epiphysitis**
  an inflammation in the growth plate (physis) at the

ends of the long bones (such as the cannon bone). Symptoms include swelling, tenderness and heat. Although the exact cause is unknown, contributing factors seem to be high caloric intake (either from grain or a heavily lactating mare) and a fast growth rate.

- **epistaxis**
  bleeding from the nose.

- **epithelial cells**
  cells that line the surface of an organ such as the epithelial cells lining the vagina.

- **epitope**
  the site on a bacteria that specific antibody recognises and binds to.

- **Equine Infectious Anaemia**
  the closest thing to HIV in horses is EIA (Equine Infectious Anaemia). It is, as the HIV virus is, a retroviral disease. There is no treatment. Most states require euthanasia or lifelong quarantine for such animals.

- **equitainer**
  a container originally designed for shipping horse semen, also used to maintain temperature control of semen from other species.

- **ER**
  external resorption

- **erosion**
  a shallow defect in the skin. When healed, it will not cause a scar.

- **erythema**
  redness of the skin caused by blood clogging in small blood vessels.

- **Erythema Multiforme (Abrev: EM)**
  an acute, self-limiting eruption of the skin and mucous membranes characterised by distinctive gross lesions and a diagnostic sequence of pathologic changes.

- **Erythrocyte (Abrev: RBC)**
  red blood cell. Contains haemoglobin, which carries oxygen to the tissues.

- **escape rhythm**
  when the SA node is firing at an abnormally slow rate, another location in the heart takes over pacing the heart. This may be the AV node or a ventricular focus.

- **oesophageal reflux**
a condition in which stomach contents move backwards into the oesophagus, i.e., heartburn.

- **oesophagus**
a muscular tube leading from the mouth to the stomach.

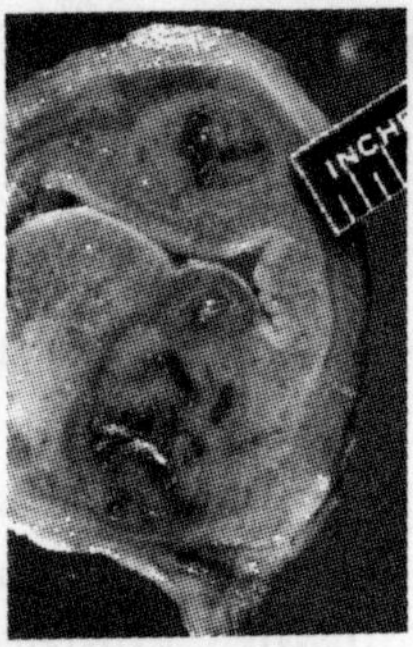

- **essential amino acids**
amino acids that must be supplied in the diet, as the animal either cannot synthesise them or cannot synthesise them in sufficient quantities to meet requirements.

- **essential host**
humans are an essential element of the organisms life cycle. Example: Taeniasis - cysticercosis.

- **essentials of the Australian Cattle Dog**
a strong, compact, and balanced dog of symmetry, strength, and substance. The essential charateristics of the breed are the ability to control and move cattle in all environments and to protect and guard stockmen, herd heads, and property. The Australian Cattle Dog is naturally suspicious of strangers but amenable and easily trainable. The head is balanced with the body and general conformation: skull broad and slightly curved between the ears cheeks muscular but not coarse. The quarters are broad, blending and well developed. The chest is deep and muscular. The outer coat is medium-short and medium textured; the undercoat is short and dense. The coat forms breeches behind the quarters and 'broom' of the tail. Color should be red, blue or blue-mottled, with acceptable markings being black, blue and tan, preferably evenly distributed. Height: 17-20 inches (43-51 cm). Weight: 35-45 pounds (16-20.5 kg).

- **est**
estimate

- **estimated crude protein from non-protein source (Abrev: ECP from NPS)**
  non-protein nitrogen sources such as urea or ammonia. used in ruminant diets in limited amounts to enhance dietary protein levels.

- **estrogen**
  a female hormone produced by the ovaries, which results in the onset of estrus.

- **estrous**
  refers to the entire reproductive cycle compared to estrus which refers to the phase of the cycle that follows proestrus.

- **oestrous cycle**
  describes all parts of the heat cycle whereas oestrus is just the stage of the heat cycle during which the female is receptive to the male.

- **ether extract laboratory test**
  a test to measure the total fat content of a feed.

- **ethyl lactate**
  topical agent that alters follicular environment to reduce bacterial flora.

- **EUA**
  examine under anaesthetic

- **euth**
  euthanase

- **euthanasia**
  a process of killing animals because they are very ill, injured or contribute to pet overpopulation.

- **equine viral arteritis (EVA)**
  a highly contagious disease that is characterised by swelling in the legs of all horses and swelling in the scrotum of stallions. Can cause abortion in mares and can be shed in the semen of stallions for years after infection.

- **ex lap**
  exploratory laparotomy

- **ex or ext**
  external

- **excoriation**
  superficial loss of the epidermis caused by physical damage such as scratching.

- **exogenous**
  supplied to the body from an external source. Insulin injected into the body is exogenous insulin.

• **exophthalmos**
the abnormal outward protrusion (bulging) of the eye.

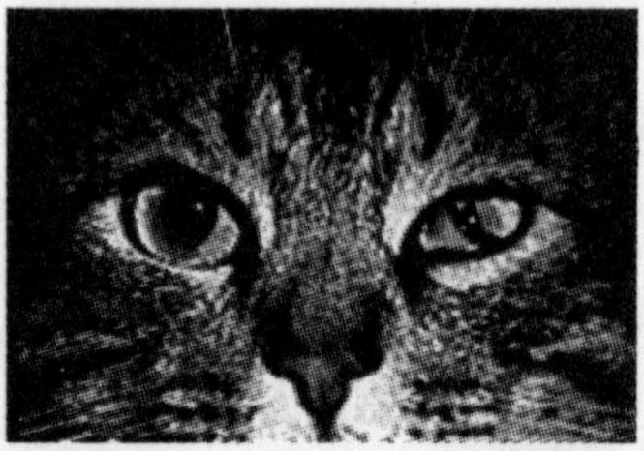

• **exotic**
an animal not native to the geographical area where it is living.

• **exposure**
exposure does not equal poisoning. If you smell ammonia you have been exposed but you have not been poisoned with ammonia gas.

• **extended**
running at top speed.

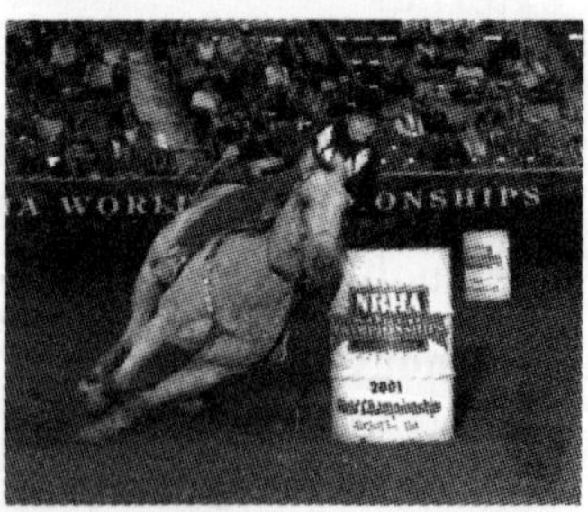

• **extensor tendon**
extends the knee (carpus) joint, ankle joint, pastern and foot and flexes the elbow. The muscles begin above the knee and attach to the coffin and pastern bones.

• **extensor rigidity**
a condition in which muscles contract and tend to straighten the limb, prevent it from relaxing.

• **extra-celluar fluid (Abrev: ECF)**
includes fluid around cells and in the plasma. Comprises 1/3 of total body water.

• **extra-cranial**
originating external to the cranial (brain) cavity.

• **extra-hepatic**
outside of the liver.

• **eyelid agenesis**
born without part of the upper eyelids.

• **F**
furcation exposure

• **F/L or FL**
front legs

• **F1**
Class I (incipient) furcation exposure exists when the tip of a probe can just 1-mm) enter the furcation area.

Bone fills most of the area where the roots meet

- **F1/4**
  forequarters
- **F2**
  Class II (definite) furcation exposure exists when the probe tip extends more than one millimetre horizontally into the area where the roots converge
- **F3**
  Class III (through and through) - alveolar bone has eroded to a point that the explorer probe passes through the defect unobstructed
- **face**
  foreface, that is, the eyes, nose, mouth, cheeks and lips.

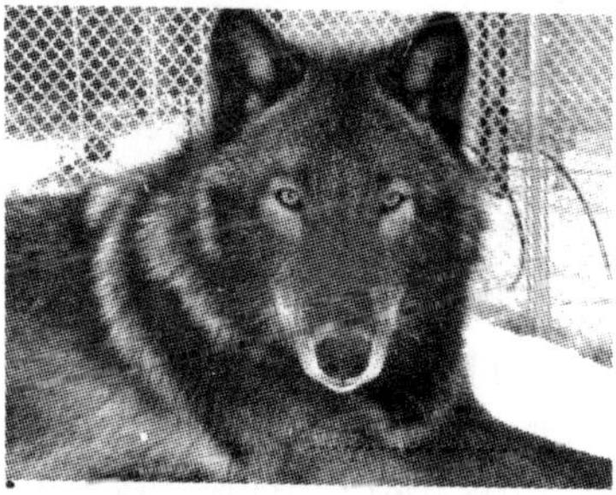

- **facial fold trichiasis**
  seen in brachycephalic breeds that have a large facial fold and the hair from the facial fold touches the medial aspect of the cornea.
- **Fad**
  flea allergic dermatitis
- **fading puppy syndrome**
  an apparently normal puppy gradually weakens and dies within a week or two of birth. Not a specific disorder, but generally applied to infectious causes.
- **false positive test result**
  the result of a diagnostic test is positive but the animal actually does not have the condition tested for.
- **fang**
  canine teeth.
- **farrow**
  to give birth.
- **farrowing area**
  where the sow farrows.
- **fat**
  a term used in a general sense to refer to both fats and oils. Fat supply 2.25 times as much energy as carbohydrates. Both fats and oils share the same general structure and chemical properties, but have different physical properties, i.e.,

oils are liquid at room temperature.

- **fat corrected milk**
  adjustment of milking production records to reflect the energy cost of fat production.

- **fat soluble vitamins**
  includes vitamins A, D, E and K. Vitamins A, D and E are supplemented in many livestock rations. Fat-soluble vitamins are stored in body fat reserves.

- **fat++**
  obese

- **FB**
  foreign body

- **FDIU**
  Field Disease Investigative Unit

- **fe**
  female (entire)

- **faecal-oral transmission cycle**
  a cycle of disease spread where the pathogen is shed in the sick animal's faeces and infects other animals when they ingest something contaminated by the infected faeces.

- **faeces**
  body wastes excreted through the anus from the large intestine; also called stool.

- **feed additives**
  products added to basic feed mixes to improve the rate and/or efficiency of gain, prevent certain diseases, or preserve feeds.

- **feed efficiency**
  a ratio describing the amount of feed required per unit of production (grain, milk, eggs).

- **feed grade**
  term to describe the quality of feedstuffs suitable for animal, but not human consumption.

- **feed processing**
  physical or chemical changes in feedstuffs which influence their nutritional value.

- **feedstuff**
  an edible material that contributes nutrients to animals' diets.

- **feline**
  pertaining to cats.

- **Feline Immunodeficiency Virus (Abrev: FIV)**
  a virus that chronically suppresses the immune system of cats resulting in secondary infectons.

- **Feline Leukaemia**
  a group of diseases that often cause cancer and death.
- **Felv**
  feline leukaemia virus
- **feminisation**
  a male showing signs of being under the influence of the female hormone, estrogen.
- **fen**
  fenestration - a round or oval defect or opening in the alveolar cortical plate of bone over the root surface
- **fenoxycarb**
  an insect growth regularor withdrawn from the market.
- **fentanyl patches**
  a sticky patch impregnated with the narcotic fentanyl which is applied topically for sustained release and absorption of the drug.
- **fenthion**
  A 'pour-on' organophosphate preparation.
- **Feral Cat**
  an untamed domestic cat that was born, or has reverted to living in the wild.
- **fertility**
  capable of conceiving and bearing offspring.
- **fertilisation**
  the process of sperm combining with eggs.
- **fertilisation rate**
  the percentage of females bred that get pregnant. A 90% fertilization rate means that 9 out of 10 females bred get pregnant.
- **foetal**
  pertaining to an unborn animal, or foetus.
- **fetlock (joint)**
  joint located between the cannon bone and the long pastern bone, also referred to as the 'ankle.'
- **foetotomy**
  cutting a dead foetus into parts to allow removal of the pieces from the dam.
- **foetus**
  The later stages of development of a baby before birth.

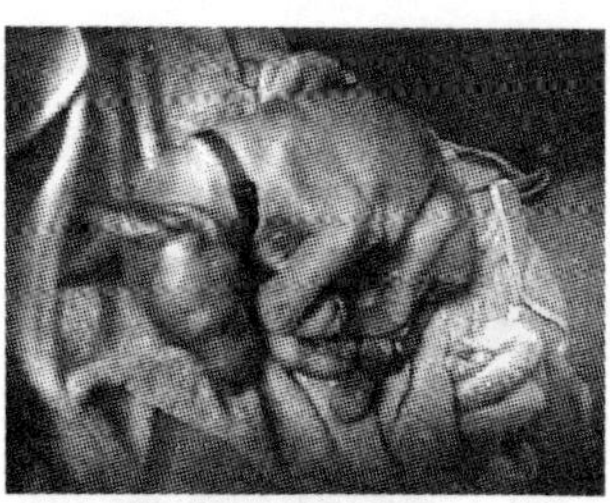

- **FGG**
  free gingival graft - transplanting attached gingiva

from one area of the mouth to another

- **FIA**
feline infectious anaemia (Haemobartonellosis)

- **fibrosarcoma**
a malignant tumour arising from collagen-producing fibroblasts (an immature fibre-producing cell of connective tissue).

- **fibrosis**
scarring.

- **fibro-vascular membranes (Abrev: PIFMS)**
cats with uveitis form fibrovascular membranes due to chronic inflammation. Chronic uveitis that smolders for a long time causes these membranes to form on the iris and they eventually block the drainage angle causing glaucoma.

- **filly**
female horse four-years-old or younger.

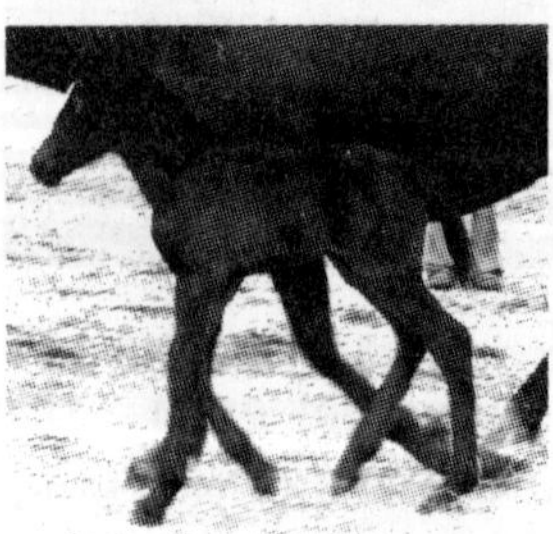

- **FIN**
finish this treatment

- **finasteride**
proscar is a 5 alpha-reductase inhibitor that prevents the conversion of testosterone to dihydrotestosterone.

- **fine needle aspirate**
suction is applied to a hollow needle which has been inserted into tissue and a core of the tissue is withdrawn to culture and/or examine microscopically.

- **FIP**
feline infectious peritonitis

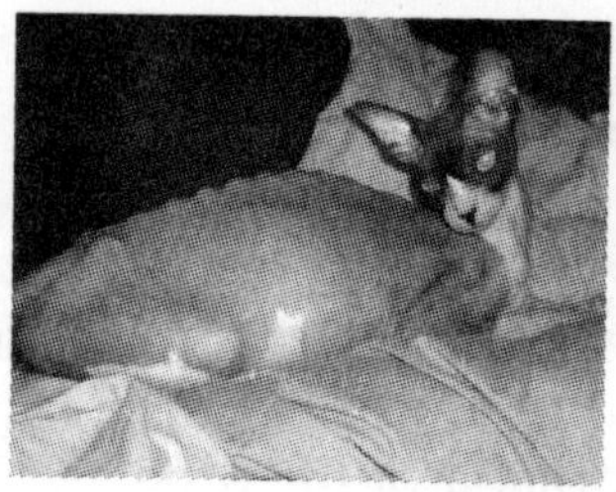

- **fipronil**
phenylpyrazole insecticide, which acts as a neurotoxin.

- **first generation drugs**
a description of medications developed from an earlier form of the medication. First generation medications were developed from the original form of the drug. Second generation medications

are adaptations of first generation drugs. Third generation drugs are adaptations of second generation drugs.

- **fissure**
splitting of the skin surface.

- **fissure (fracture)**
longitudinal crack through only one surface of a bone.

- **FIV**
feline immunosuppressive virus

- **flatten out**
a very tired horse that slows considerably, dropping its head on a straight line with its body.

- **flatulence**
passing gas from the intestinal tract. May be a sign of disease of the small intestine.

- **flea dip**
a solution made to kill fleas applied to an animal and not rinsed off to allow it to have residual action.

- **fleas**
wingless, jumping parasites that feed on blood.

- **flehmen**
a curling of the upper lip or open mouth behaviour, which is a normal mating behaviour in the male alpaca and llama.

- **flehmening**
the grimace a cat makes when it draws air over the Jacobsen's Organ in its mouth.

- **float**
an equine dental procedure in which sharp points on the teeth are filed down.

- **flow sheets**
records of patient data over time. These may include a tabular summary of laboratory test results, vital signs or drugs administered.

- **fluid therapy**
fluid therapy is broadly defined to include the administration of many types of fluids including crystalloids and colloids. Fluid therapy may be given to prevent or correct fluid deficits or electrolyte abnormalities, correct water imbalance from excessive fluid loss or inadequate intake. Haemorrhage Vomitting Diarrhoea Polyuria expand blood volume, correct electrolyte imbalance(s) correct acid-base imbalance supply blood components supply

calories and nutrients, promote renal blood flow.

- **fluorescein stain**
  a stain applied to the cornea to assess for corneal and conjunctival epithelial defects or to assess the patency of the nasolacrimal ducts.

- **fluoroscopy**
  a type of radiograph (x-ray) in which motion can be seen.

- **flushing**
  increasing the feed amount and/or quality (energy intake) prior to mating to increase the ovulation rate.

- **flutd**
  feline lower urinary tract disease. A collection of signs in cats resulting in blood in the urine, straining to urinate, and urinating in abnormal locations. The older term is feline urologic syndrome (FUS).

- **fly strike**
  cutaneous myiasis. A result of cutaneous parasitism by larvae of flesh flies, blow flies and/or the screwworm flies.

- **fly-snapping**
  repeated snapping at non-existent flying object has been associated in BMDs with partial seizures, in some cases with ear infections, and in a few cases with food allergies. Some forms may be alleviated by seizure medications. A few have been alleviated with behavioural modification techniques, which may indicate that some forms are simply behavioural problems often caused by boredom.

- **FMD**
  feline miliary dermatitis

- **FN**
  female (neutered)

- **FNA**
  fine needle aspirate

- **FNAB**
  fine needle aspirate biopsy

- **foal heat/diarrhoea**
  foal heat is a term used to describe the first heat cycle of the mare after she's had her foal. It usually comes on 5-7 days after birth. Some believe foals get diarrhoea due to a slight change of the milk. Foal diarrhoea probably has nothing to do with the milk, as the phenomenon is also observed in orphan foals at the same age.

More likely related to a changing of gut microflora, just coincidental with the mare's heat.

- **foal(ed)**

  1. a horse of either sex in its first year of life.
  2. as a verb, to give birth. Also known as 'dropped.'
  3. can also denote the offspring of either a male or female parent.

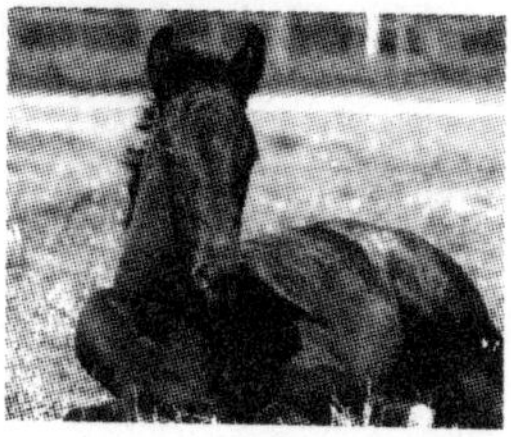

- **follicle**

  1. structures on the ovary that contain the eggs.
  2. the group of cells in the skin in which hair develops.

Anatomy of the Ovary and Follicle

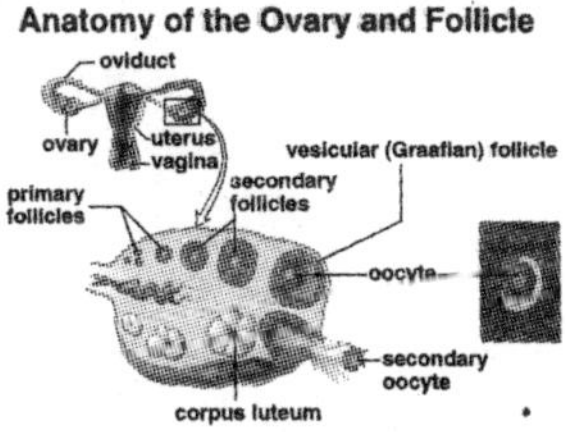

- **follicle stimulating hormone (Abrev: FSH)**

  its primary responsibility is promoting growth of follicles on the ovaries.

- **follicular cycle**

  the series of events that occur when the ovary produces a follicle (an egg) and the follicle goes through a series of changes.

- **folliculitis**

  superficial bacterial dermatitis associated with the hair follicle.

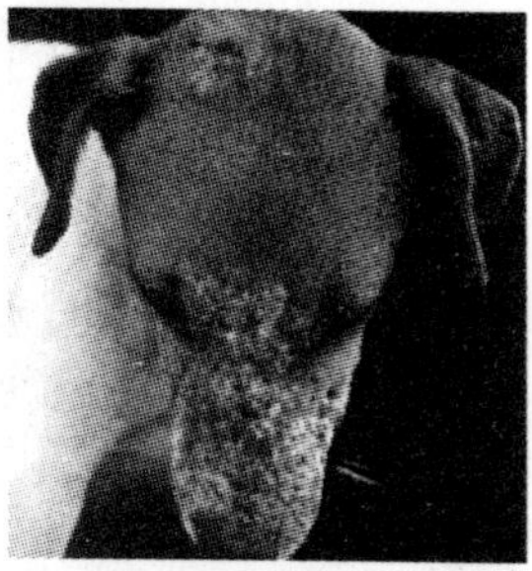

- **fomite**

  a vector of disease transmission that has no part in the pathogen's life cycle. A contaminated milking towel that spreads disease from cow to cow with each subsequent use is a fomite.

- **food hypersensitivity**

  an allergy. An adverse reaction to food with a proven immunologic basis.

- **food intolerance**

  an adverse reaction to food that does not have a proven immunologic basis.

- **food poisoning**
an adverse reaction to a food caused by a direct effect of a toxin.

- **forage**
plants or plant parts fed to, or grazed by, domestic animals. Forage may be fresh, dry or ensiled (i.e., pasture, green chop, hay, haylage). Often used interchangeably with roughage.

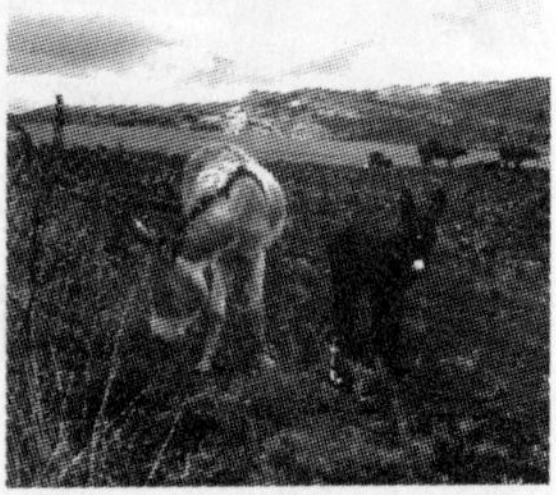

- **foreign body**
any abnormal substance within the body. Examples include wood slivers, cloth, balls, glass, etc.

- **fracture**
a break in the bone generally caused by trauma, twisting, or weakened bone structure due to disease.

- **fragmented coronoid process, FCP**
the coronoid process fragments forming a loose body in the elbow joint, called a joint mouse.

- **free mating**
free mating is also called paddock mating. A single male is introduced with a band of females.

- **free radical**
atom which carries an unpaired electron. Free radicals can potentially injure cells and may be responsible for numerous age related diseases.

- **free stall barn**
housing for cattle where cows can freely enter unoccupied stalls.

- **free-feed**
a feeding process that gives a cat open access to a food bowl all day.

- **free radical**
atom which carries an unpaired electron; free radicals can potentially injure cells and may be responsible for numerous age-related diseases.

- **frenulum**
a piece of tissue that maintains adhesion between the penis and prepuce.

- **fresh frozen plasma**
  plasma that has been separated from the RBC shortly after blood collection and then frozen. Coagulation factors are preserved in this blood product.
- **freshening**
  parturition, calving.
- **frog**
  the V-shaped, pliable support structure on the bottom of the foot.
- **front limbs**
  the front limbs of the horse have no bony connection whatsoever with the spine. They are attached by a muscular sling. Quite different from the human animal.

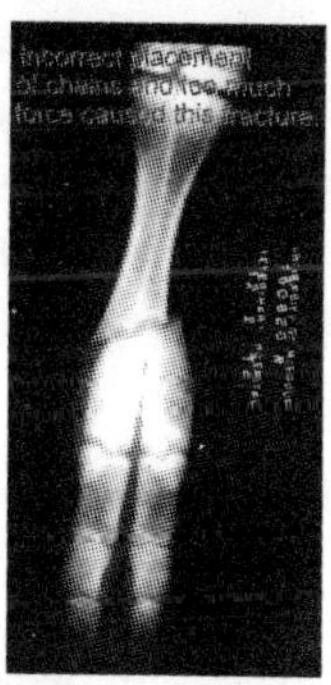

- **frozen plasma**
  plasma that has been separated from RBC after blood collection but not with the intent of preserving the labile coagulation factors. Used primarily to provide plasma protein in hypoproteiemic patients.
- **fu**
  fusion - union of two teeth buds. The root canals may be separate or joined. Clinically there is one less tooth in the arch. Radiographically there will be two roots with one crown
- **full-brother, full-sister**
  horses that share the same sire and dam.
- **fungicide**
  a drug that kills fungi.
- **FUO**
  fever of unknown origin
- **furosemide**
  a medication used in the treatment of bleeders, which acts as a diuretic, reducing pressure on the capillaries.
- **furuncle**
  a painful, nodular adcess in the skin.

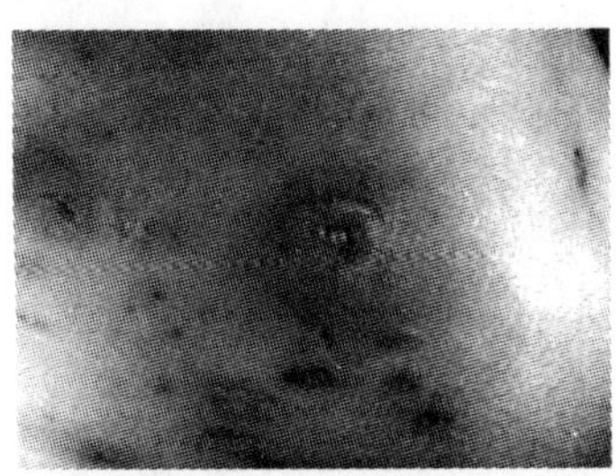

- **FUS**
  feline urologic syndrome. A collection of signs in cats resulting in blood in the urine, straining to urinate, and urinating in abnormal locations. The more current term is feline lower urinary tract disease (FLUTD).
- **FWS**
  freeway space - the space between the maxillary and mandibular premolar opposing teeth cusp tips when the mouth is closed
- **FX**
  fractured tooth
- **GA**
  general anaesthetic
- **gait**
  1. the appearance of the animal as it is moving. The gait is evaluated for lameness, noncoordination, dragging toenails, etc.

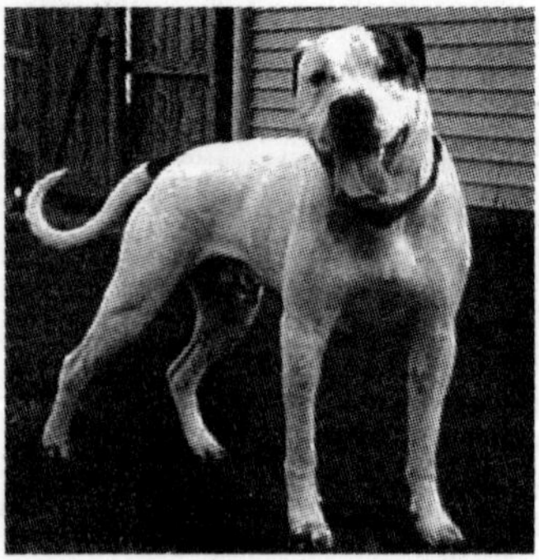

2. the characteristic footfall pattern of a horse in motion. Thoroughbreds have four natural gaits-walk, trot, canter and gallop. Thoroughbreds compete at a gallop.

- **gastric**
  relating to the stomach.

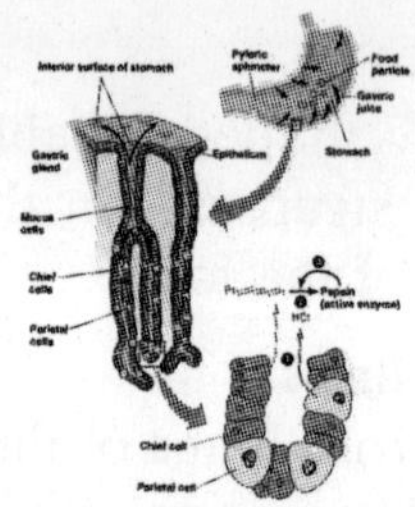

- **gastric dilatation-volvulus, bloat**
  gastric dilatation means stomach distension or enlargement, caused by expanding gas. This may or may not be accompanied by volvulus, or torsion, or twisting of the stomach on its long axis.
- **gastric ulcers**
  ulceration of a animal's stomach. Often causes symptoms

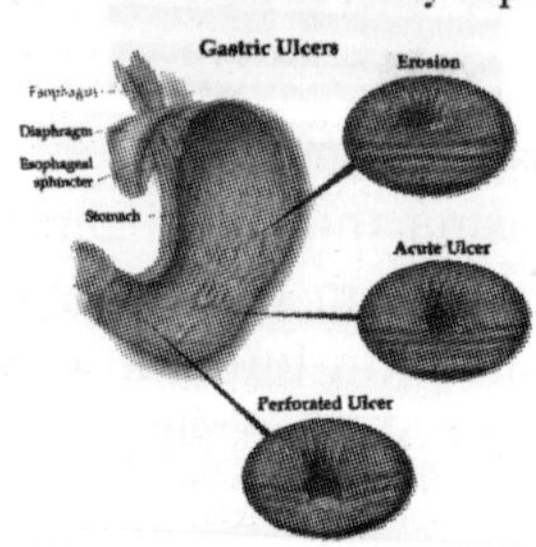

of abdominal distress (colic) and general unthriftiness.

- **gastriclavage**
  to flush out the stomach.

- **gastritis**
  an inflammation of the mucous membrane surrounding the stomach.

- **gastrointestinal tract**
  pertaining to the stomach and intestines. The term 'digestive system' includes the mouth, gastrointestinal tract, anus, pancreas, and liver.

- **gemination**
  the division of a single tooth at the time of development resulting in incomplete formation of two teeth. On radiographs, there will be one root with a split crown. Clinically there will be an extra tooth in the arch

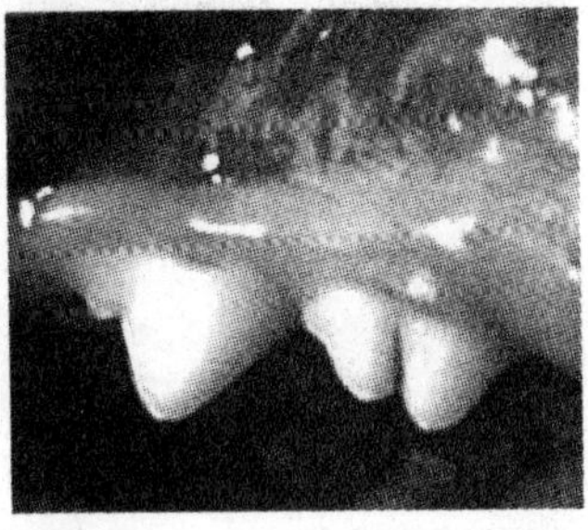

- **gelding**
  a male animal of any age that has been neutered by having both testicles removed ('gelded').

- **genetic**
  inherited.

- **genome**
  the total gene complement of a set of chromosomes.

- **germs**
  microscopic organisms that can cause disease. May include bacteria and viruses.

- **gestation**
  the duration of pregnancy.

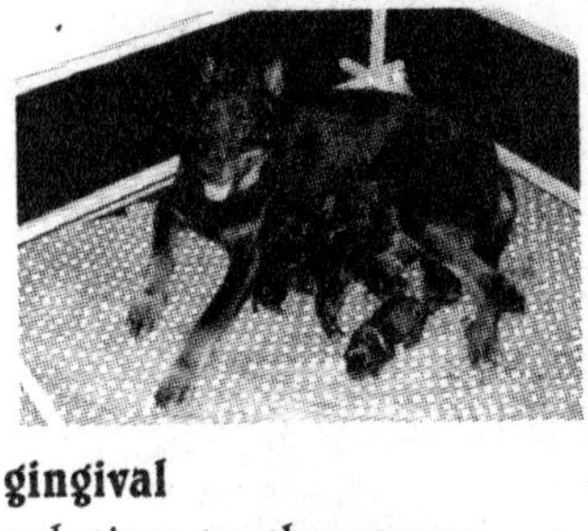

- **gingival**
  relating to the gums.

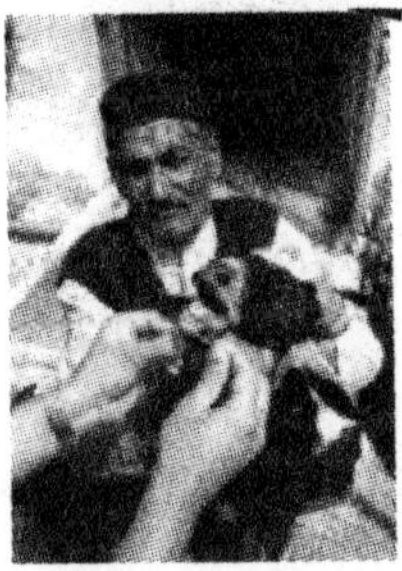

- **gingivitis**
  inflammation and swelling of the gums surrounding

the teeth. The gingiva is normally pink and becomes red when inflamed.

- **girth**
an elastic and leather band, sometimes covered with sheepskin, that passes under a horse's belly and is connected to both sides of the saddle.

- **glabrous**
hairless areas of skin.

- **glaucoma**
increased fluid accumulation in the eye causing increased pressure, pain and leading to blindness if untreated.

- **glipizide**
an oral medication that can be used to control blood glucose levels in some diabetic cats who still have some insulin production.

- **glomerular filtration rate(Abrev: GFR)**
the rate at which the glomeruli form filtrate from blood in glomerular capillaries. GFR correlates with renal function and to renal blood flow. Kidney disease and dehydration both result in a decrease in GFR.

- **glomerulonephritis**
inflammatory disease of the glomerulus, part of the kidney which filters toxic waste from the blood. Tests of the urine can show a variety of abnormalities. Complete loss of kidney function can occur.

- **glomerulonephropathy (Abrev: GN)**
disease that begins in the glomerulus

- **glomerulus**
the microscopic functional unit of the kidney. Disease of the glomeruli causes protein to leak into the urine.

- **glucagon**
a hormone secreted by the alpha cells of the pancreas. Glucagon is responsible for raising blood glucose.

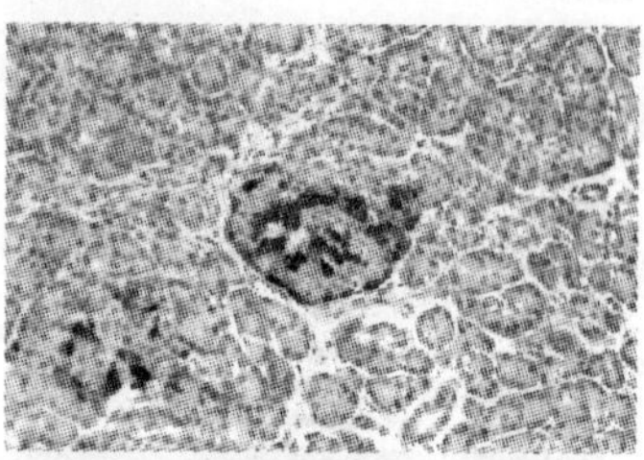

- **glucocorticoid**
hormones produced by the adrenal gland which regulate protein, carbohydrate and fat

metabolism, and are important to almost every function of cells and organs. They also stabilise cell membranes, which is an important part of their function in treating allergic reactions. Also called glucocortico steroids.

- **glucosamine**
  one of the building blocks the body uses to make new cartilage.

- **glucose**
  a molecule (single unit) of sugar. Glucose is one of the main sugars used by the body's cells for energy.

- **glucosuria**
  glucose in the urine. Also called glycosuria.

- **glycogen**
  a storage form of glucose in the body.

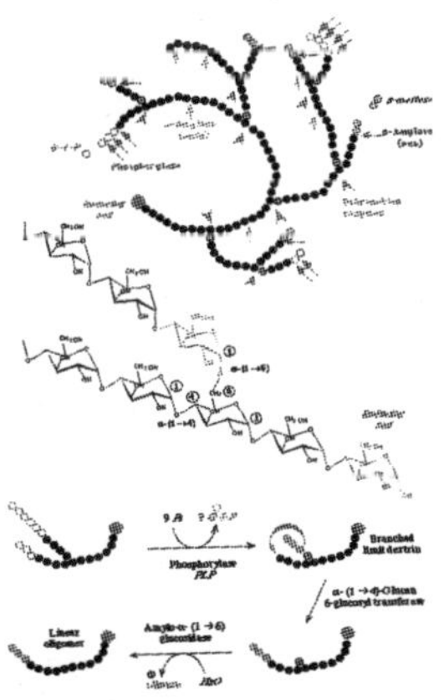

- **glycosaminoglycans**
  compounds which serve as the building blocks of cartilage, which covers the ends of bones within a joint. Glucosamine and chondroitin are necessary for the body to make glycosaminoglycans.

- **goldenseal**
  goldenseal hydrastis cnadensis contains several active constituents—berberine, hydrastine, and canadine, concentrated in the rhizome. Hydrastine is the chief active ingredient. As well as dyeing things yellow, it has an astringent effect on inflamed mucous membranes, and has been used to treat oral ulcers, digestive upset, and hemorrhoids. It also has a laxative effect. In the form of snuff, it has been used to treat the nasal passages, and a solution of the extract is sometimes employed as eyewash.

- **gonadotropin-releasing hormone (Abrev: GnRH)**
  a hormone released from the hypothalamus that stimulates the release of follicle stimulating hormone

(FSH) and luteinising hormone (LH).

• **gonioscopy**
a technique used to evaluate the iridocorneal angle to help judge the risk of glaucoma in an eye.

• **Gordon Setter**
Gordons are a sturdily built dog with a long black coat and tan markings. They were developed for hunting upland game birds, such as pheasant and quail. George Blunt and Daniel Webster imported the breed to America in 1842.

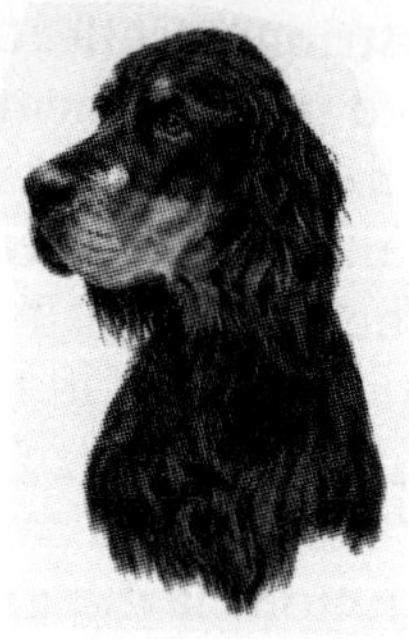

• **gingival recession**
areas where the gingival margin exists apical to the cemento enamel junction (CEJ)

• **grab a quarter**
injury to the back of the hoof or foot caused by a horse stepping on itself (usually affects the front foot). Being stepped on from behind in the same manner, usually affects the back foot. A very common injury during racing. Generally, the injury is minor.

• **grade cow**
a cow that is not registered.

• **gram**
a measure of weight. 28 grams = 1 ounce, 454 grams = 1 pound.

• **Gram negative bacteria**
a classification of bacteria based upon their lack of retention of a certain stain in the laboratory. The staining quality is based on the structure of the cell wall surrounding the bacteria. This structure of the cell wall influences which antibiotics will kill the bacteria. This laboratory staining method was developed by Hans Gram in 1884.

• **Gram positive bacteria**
a classification of bacteria based upon their uptake of a certain stain in the laboratory. The staining quality is based on the structure of the cell wall surrounding the

bacteria. This structure of the cell wall influences which antibiotics will kill the bacteria. This laboratory staining method was developed by Hans Gram in 1884.

- **grandsire**
  the grandfather of a horse father ('sire') of the horse's dam or sire.

- **granuloma**
  the formation of a nodule as a result of inflammation.

- **gravel**
  infection of the hoof resulting from a crack in the white line (the border between the insensitive and sensitive laminae). An abscess usually forms in the sensitive structures and eventually breaks at the coronet as the result of the infection.

- **greasy wool**
  the wool as it comes off the sheep. It contains yolk (wool grease lanolin) suint (sweat) and dirt and vegetable fibre.

- **green osselet**
  an inflammation and swelling in the fetlock joint of young horses, particularly on the front of the joints where the cannon and long pastern bones meet.

- **griseofulvin**
  oral treatment for dermatophytes.

- **grooming kit**
  a collection of materials needed for the care of a cat's coat, including brush, comb and feline shampoo.

- **GSD**
  german shepherd dog.

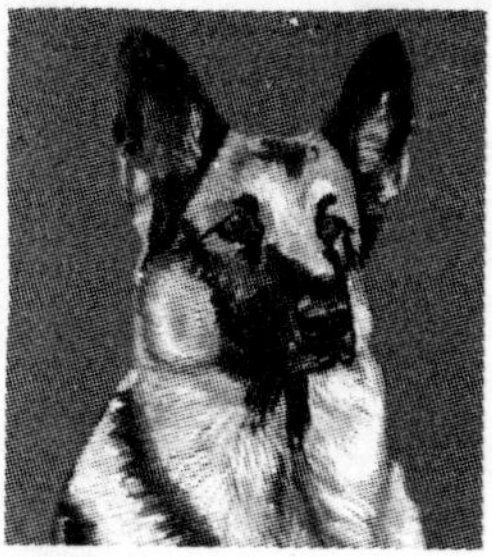

- **guard hair**
  long, course hairs that make up the cat's top coat. These carry the pattern of the fur.

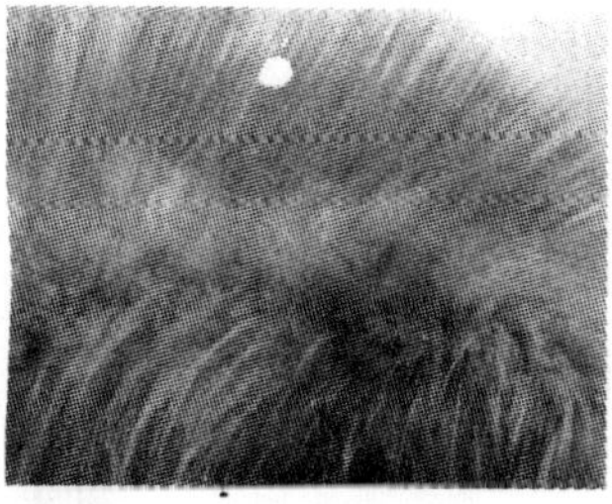

- **gulps**
  exaggerated swallowing movements.

- **guttural pouch**
  a sac in the side of the head that may become infected. The sac is a pouch that is part of the eustachian tube, a passage between the pharynx and the inner ear and is unique to the horse.

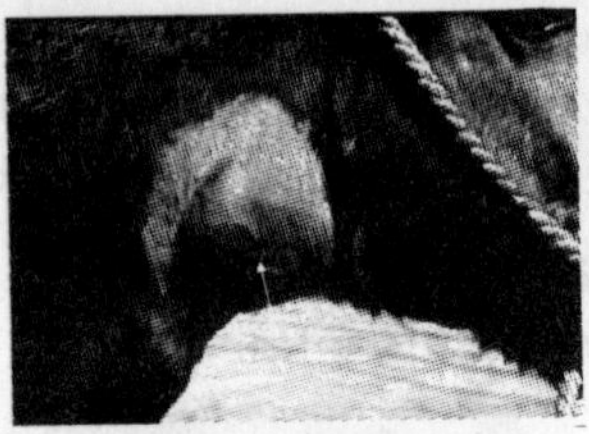

- **GV**
  gingivectomy.
- **gingival hyperplasia**
  proliferation of attached gingiva coronal to the cemento enamel junction (CEJ)

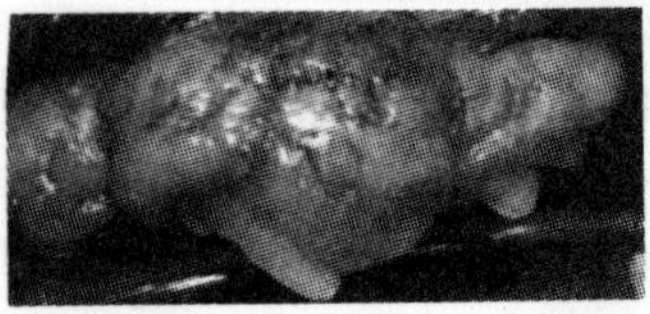

- **H/L or HL**
  hind legs
- **H+**
  history
- **H1/4**
  hindquarters
- **H2 Antagonist**
  a compound, which binds to the areas on cells where histamine also binds. By binding at the same sites, H2 antagonists block histamine from binding and therefore prevent histamine from producing effects such as the production of stomach acid.
- **habit**
  a fixed or constant practice established by frequent repetition, an acquired mode of behaviour that has become nearly or completely involuntary.
- **HAC**
  hyper adreno corticism
- **half-brother, half-sister**
  Horses out of the same dam but by different sires.
- **half-life**
  the time required for the level of a substance in the body (e.g., adrugortoxin) to be reduced by half.
- **halter**
  like a bridle, but lacking a bit. Used in handling horses

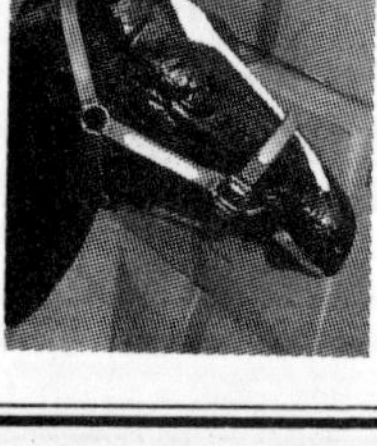

around the stable and when they are not being ridden.

- **hand**
four inches. A horse's height is measured in hands and inches from the top of the shoulder (withers) to the ground, e.g., 15.2 hands is 15 hands, 2 inches. Thoroughbreds typically range from 15 to 17 hands.

- **hand breeding**
also called hand mating. The females are completely supervised during the mating process and the male is led to the female and controlled during the breeding process.

- **hand ride**
urging a horse with the hands and not using the whip.

- **hand-feed**
a feeding process that offers a cat food periodically during the day and for a limited time (usually twice a day, for about 20 minutes).

- **hapten**
a substance that becomes antigenic when it complexes with proteins.

- **hard-pad disease**
crusty, dry footpads that may occur as a consequence of canine distemper infection.

- **harrow**
implement or unit with pulling teeth or tines used to rake and loosen the upper surface of a track.

- **haw eyes**
eyes with a large amount of conjunctival membrane visible, a result of pouching lower eyelid due to looseness.

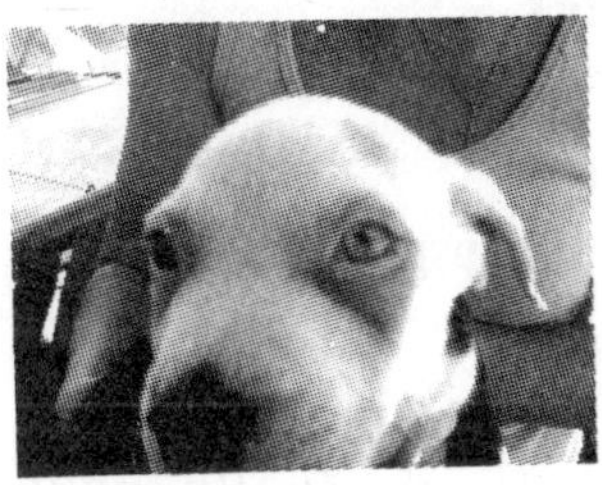

- **hay**
a forage that has been dried.

- **hay additives**
organic acids or acid-forming compounds designed to allow hay to be harvested at higher than normal moisture contents by preventing the microbial activity responsible for spoilage.

- **hazard**
the likelihood or the probability that a substance, i.e., the poison, will induce a disease state under conditions of use.

- **HBB**
hit by bullet

- **HBC**
hit by car

- **HBT**
hit by truck

- **HCM**
hypertrophic cardiomyopathy

- **HCT**
haematocrit

- **HD**
hip dysplasia

- **head**
the foremost part of the skeleton usually including all the bony structures associated with the skull.

- **head mange**
common name for notoedric mange.

- **heart block**
a condition in which the electrical impulses of the heart are not properly conducted from the atria (chambers which receive the blood) to the ventricles (chambers which pump the blood).

- **heartworm**
a parasitic worm that lives and reproduces in the hearts of animals. Microscopic immature worms (microfilariae) circulate in animals' blood and are ingested by mosquitoes when they bite. Microfilariae mature in the mouthparts of mosquitoes and are transmitted to susceptible animals bitten by mosquitoes at subsequent feedings.

- **heat**
a period of time when female animals are sexually receptive.

- **heaves**
emphysema.

- **heel crack**
a crack on the heel of the hoof. Also called a 'sand crack.'

- **heifer**
young bovine female starting her first lactation having calved for the first time. Age at first calving should be 2 years.

• **Heinz body anaemia**
a condition in which the red blood cells are destroyed. Called Heinz body anaemia because the red blood cells develop abnormalities called Heinz bodies, which can be seen under the microscope. This anaemia can occur as a reaction to certain medications and also in cats after ingestion of onions.

• **hemangiosarcoma**
a malignant tumour of endothelial cells (the layer of cells that lines the cavities of the heart and of the blood and lymph vessels). (Epithelial cells cover all body surfaces, inside and out.)

• **haematocrit**
a laboratory test to monitor relative number of red blood cells present in the blood. A blood sample is placed in a tiny glass tube and spunina centrifuge. The cells are heavier than the plasma and are compacted at one end of the tube. After the tube is spun, it is examined and the packed cell volume is determined as the percentage of the red cellular portion relative to the total amount of blood in the tube (i. e., remainder being the plasma). The normal for dogs is 40-59 and cats are 29-50.

• **haematology**
the study of blood.

• **haematoma**
localised collection of blood, a lump. Dogs can get them in their earflaps from violent and repeated shaking of the head, from such things as ear infections or insect stings.

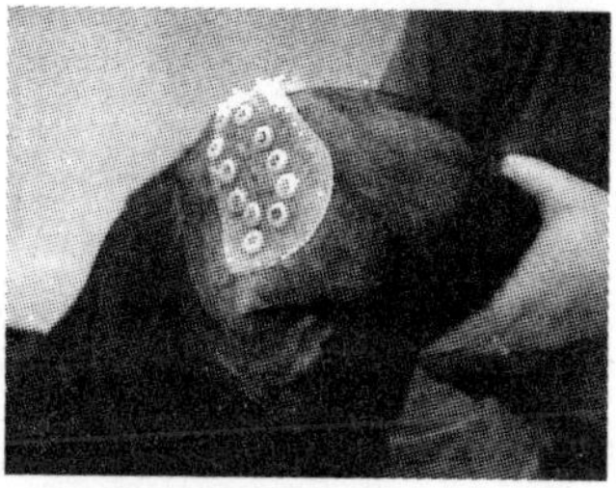

• **haematuria**
red blood cells in the urine.

• **haemocytometer**
a piece of equipment that is used to count white blood cells and can also be used to count sperm.

• **haemodialysis**
a process used to remove waste products from the blood.

• **haemoglobin**
the substance contained in red blood cells that carries oxygen to parts of the body.

• **haemolysis**
the breakdown of red blood cells.

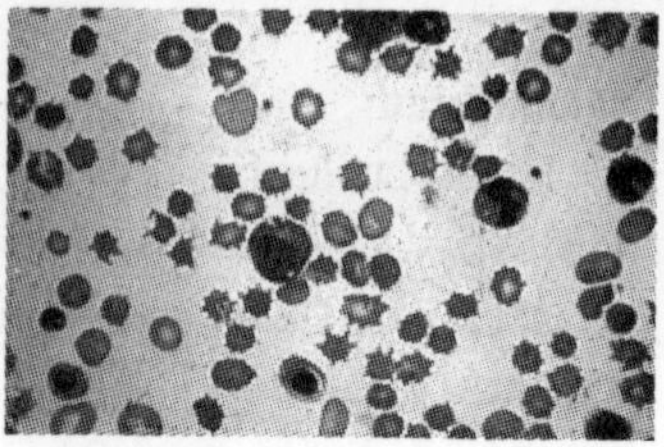

• **haemolytic**
causing the red blood cells to break open.

• **haemophilia**
the blood lacks coagulating factors, causing a strong tendency to bleed, and difficulty in getting the bleeding to stop.

• **haemoptysis**
blood in the sputum.

• **haemorrhage**
to bleed excessively may be the result of injury or blood clotting abnormalities.

• **haemorrhagic follicle**
also called a corpus haemorrhagicum. A follicle that has been present on the ovary and has not been given the chance to ovulate so it will continue growing and becomes large and cyst-like and bleeds inside.

• **haemospermia**
blood in the ejaculate.

• **haemostat**
a surgical instrument used to pinch small blood vessels to stop bleeding (haemostasis is to stop bleeding). Haemastats may be used in non-surgical procedures, for example to pluck hair from the ear canals.

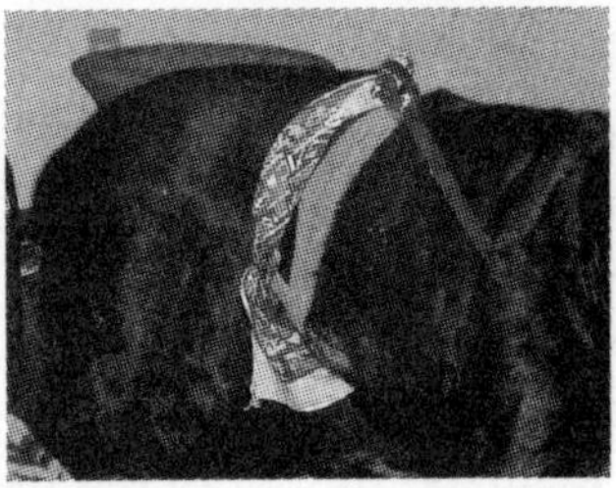

• **hepatic**
pertaining to the liver.

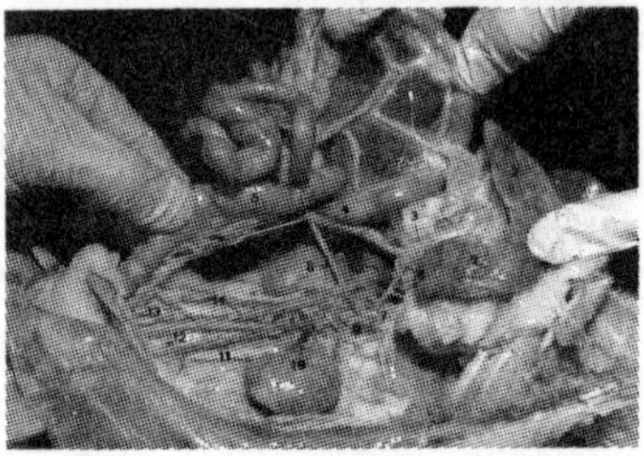

• **hepatic fibrosis**
scarring of the liver.

- **hepatitis**
inflammation of the liver. This can result from a variety of causes including infections (particularly viral), drugs, autoimmunity and genetics. The liver stores and filters blood, secretes bile, converts sugars, processes fat, produces proteins, which help to control blood volume, and produces some of the clotting factors.

- **hepatocerebellar degeneration**
death of liver cells causing poisoning of the white matter of the brain.

- **hepatomegaly**
enlargement of the liver.

- **herbivore**
animal that eats primarily plants and vegetation.

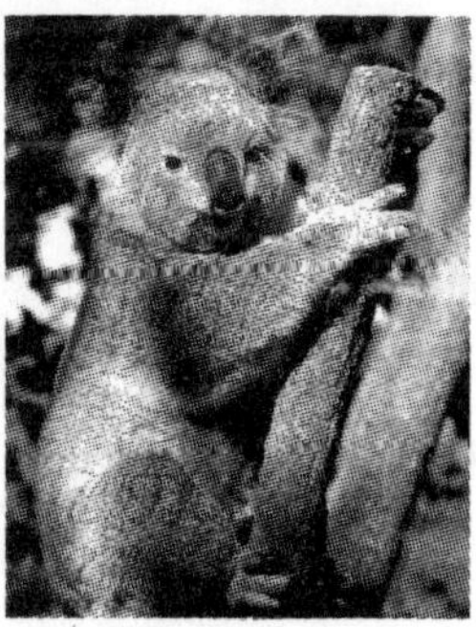

- **herd summary**
summary statistics for herd production, reproduction, health, and demographic factors.

- **hereditary**
derived from ancestry, describing a genetically transmitted or transmittable characteristic, inborn, independent of prior learning.

- **hermaphrodism**
a condition where reproductive structures of both the male and the female are in one body.

- **hernia**
abnormal protrusion of organs through a weak spot or abnormal opening, usually in the abdominal or groin areas.

- **hetastarch**
a colloid solution of hydrolysed amylopectin containing a range of particle sizes, from 10, 000 daltons to over 3 million daltons.

- **heterologous**
derived from an animal of a different species.

- **HGE**
haemorrhagic gastro-enteritis

- **high titer vaccine**
  a modified live vaccine that contains a higher number of virus particles than the average vaccine. High titer vaccines can generally elicit an immune system response in young animals who have a maternal antibody level that would prevent them from responding to an average vaccine.

- **high/low string**
  High/low producing cows are split into feeding groups to optimise ration inputs for milk output.

- **hip dysplasia, chd, hd**
  improper development of the hip joint, typically, the acetabulum (socket) is not deep enough for the femoral head (ball) to fit fully into place.

- **hippomanes**
  normal formations in the cavity of the placenta where the foetus was located.

- **histamine receptor antagonist**
  a compound which binds to the areas on cells where histamine also binds. By binding at the same sites, the antagonist blocks histamine from binding and prevents histamine from producing effects such as the production of stomach acid.

- **histiocytomas**
  a small wart-like skin growth that will eventually disappear.

- **histiocytosis**
  abnormal appearance of histiocytes in the blood. (Histiocytes are produced by the bone marrow and are normally immobile until stimulated by inflammation. They are a type of antigen presenting cell.)

- **hob**
  a male ferret.

- **hock**
  a large joint just above the shin bone in the rear legs. Corresponds to the level of the knee of the front leg.

- **hogget**
  sheep 12 to 24 months of age.

- **homebred**
  a horse bred by its owner.

- **homologous**
  related or similar in characteristics.

- **honeymoon**
  a period where the diabetic enters a phase of either re-

duced insulin requirement, or requires no exogenous insulin. The 'honeymoon' happens relatively soon after diagnosis (weeks to months) and is temporary. It may be related to irregular functioning of beta cells. 'Honeymoon' occurs in dogs, cats, and humans. The term 'honeymoon' is often used interchangeably with 'transient diabetes' - but they have different meanings.

- **hood**
  a (usually) nylon covering which goes over a horse's head to which blinkers or earmuffs are attached.

- **hoof**
  the projected part of the foot of some animals.

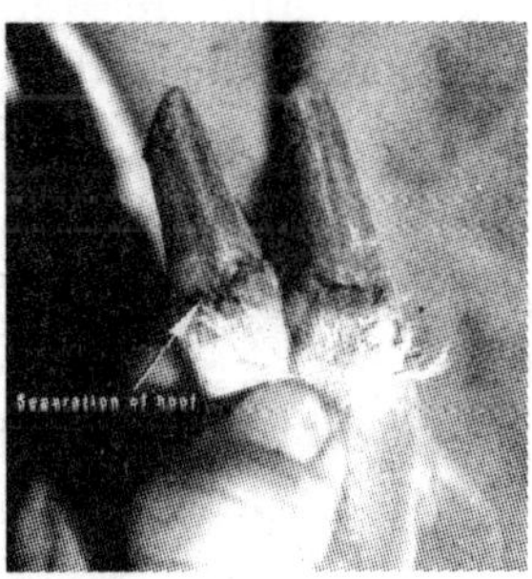

- **hookworm**
  a parasitic worm that thrives in unsanitary conditions.

- **hopped**
  a horse that has been illegally stimulated.

- **horizontal transmission**
  disease transmission from one animal to another.

- **hormone**
  a substance produced by one part of the body that travels throughout the body and controls functions of other cells. Both insulin and glucagon are hormones: they are produced by the pancreas and travel through the body and control glucose metabolism in other cells.

- **horner's syndrome**
  loss of sympathetic innervation resulting in miosis, ptosis and enopthalmos.

- **horse**
  when reference is made to sex, a 'horse' is an ungelded male five-years-old or older.

- **horsing**
  behaviour of a mare in heat (in season).

- **host**
  the organism in or on which a parasite lives. For example, dogs and cats are

hosts for fleas and roundworms.

- **hot nursery**
  a nursery where piglets are raised until they are 4 weeks old and the ambient temperature is very warm.

- **hot spots**
  inflammation of the skin, dermatitis. Frequently caused by fleabites, or a hypersensitivity to an allergen. Can also be caused by bacteria building up in an area that the dog bites or scratches.

- **hotz- Celsus technique**
  a surgical procedure for correction of lower lid entropion.

- **housetraining**
  process of instruction that teaches a cat to eliminate in a litter box.

- **HQ**
  hind quarters

- **HR**
  heart rate

- **HRS**
  high rise syndrome (animal fell off balcony/windowsill)

- **H'S**
  horner's syndrome

- **human albumin**
  a colloidal solution prepared from pooled human plasma and heated to kill many types of blood borne diseases.
  a stimulation test which measures testosterone in response to HCG administration. Used to detect retained testicles.

- **humane societies**
  with the state intention of preventing cruelty towards animals, these organisations are formed. Humane societies typically adopt a code listing the rights that animals are entitled to and state the ways in which these rights can be provided and upheld. Rights may include medical treatment, housing and protection from abuse, and euthanasia.

- **humoral immunity**
  the immunity that is the result of antibody production by B cells. Compare with 'cell-mediated immunity'.

- **HX**
  history

- **hyaluronic acid**
  a normal component of joint fluid. Also can be a

man-made intra-articular medication used to relieve joint inflammation.

- **hybrid**
an animal that has parents of two different species, for instance, a mule's mother is a horse and its father is a donkey.

- **hybridomas**
myeloma cells cultured in the lab survive indefinitely. Myeloma cells can be fused with a normal B cell. The resulting hybridoma produces large quantities of monoclonal antibody.

- **hydrocephalous**
the accumulation of fluid in the ventricles of the brain. The head may appear to be large and dome shaped. Many small breeds of dogs have a degree of hydrocephalous that is normal for the breed. Severe hydrocephalous damages brain tissue.

- **hydrolysed**
breaking a compound into smaller and simpler compounds by a chemical reaction with water.

- **hydroxyzine HCl**
atarax an antihistamine.

- **hymen**
a thin membrane partially occluding the opening to the vagina in a virgin.

- **hyper**
This prefix is used in conjunction with many terms and means an increase, for example, hyperthermia means an increase in temperature.

- **hyperalgesia**
unexpected increased pain intensity from a stimulus. Excessive sensitivity to pain.

- **hypercalcemia**
elevated blood calcium. The most common cause is the production of a bio-chemical substance by tumours, resulting in the retention of calcium. This is called pseudohyperparathyroidism, most commonly occurring in patients with lymphoma or tumours of the apocrine anal sac. Pseudohyperparathyroidism has been reported associated with other tumour types. Primary hyperparathyroidism occurs uncommonly.

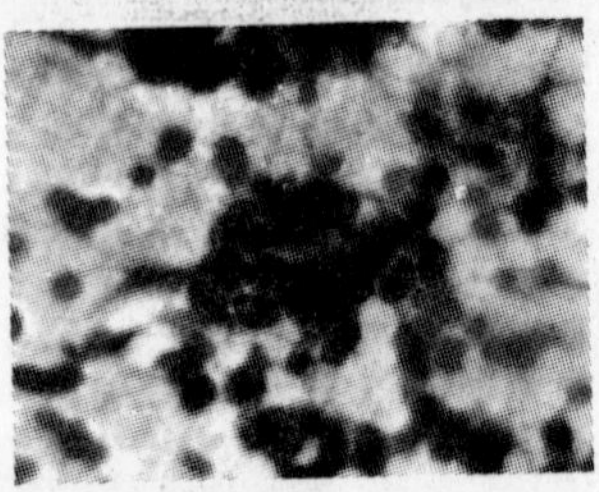

- **hyperchloremia**
elevated blood chloride.

- **hyperesthesia**
increased sensitivity to stimulation. Is most commonly seen with peripheral nerve diseases, such as, tumours and polyradiculoneuritis.

- **hyperglycemia**
elevation of blood glucose. There are numerous causes of hyperglycemia including diabetes mellitus, hyperadrenocorticism, excitement and the administration of glucose or glucocorticoids.

- **hyperkalemia**
increased level of potassium in the blood.

- **hyperkeratosis**
increased thickness of the horny layer of the epidermis.

- **hypermagnesemia**
elevated blood magnesium.

- **hypernatremia**
elevated blood sodium. Hypernatremia is uncommon in dogs and cats and most often is iatrogenic from the repetitive administration of high sodium containing solutions. Animals who have severe hypernatremia in excess of 170 meq/L show signs of depression progressing to coma.

- **hyperosmolarity**
an increase in the osmotic concentration of the blood. Hyperosmolarity of the blood can draw water from RBC's causing lysis or from neurons causing neurologic signs such as coma.

- **hyperosmotic agents**
drugs such as mannitol and glycerine which draw water to themselves. Used to control edema and swelling.

- **hyperphosphatemia**
elevated phosphorus.

- **hyperpigmentation**
an increased dark colour in the skin caused by the pigment melanin.

- **hyperplasia**
an increase of the number of cells within an organ.

- **hyperplastic**
abnormal increase in the amount of tissue, e.g., a hyperplastic ear would have increased numbers of cells in the ear canal, sometimes to the point of closing off the ear canal. In prostatic hyperplasia, the prostate enlarges due to an increased number of normal, not cancerous, cells.

- **hyperreactive**
producing an exaggerated, or greater than normal response to a stimulus.

- **hypersensitive**
a type of allergic condition in which the body overreacts to a certain agent such as a bee sting or medication.

- **hypersensitivity type IV**
an exaggerated reaction of the cellular components of the immune system.

- **hypertension**
blood pressure above normal.

- **hypertensive**
elevation in blood pressure.

- **hypertensive retinopathy**
retinal damage caused by edema or haemorrhages beneath the retina causing it to detach. Systemic hypertension is the cause of the detachment.

- **hyperthermia**
an increase in body temperature above normal.

- **hyperthyroidism**
a condition, more commonly seen in cats, in which the thyroid gland produces too much thyroid hormone.

- **hypertonic**
a fluid that contains a ratio of electrolytes to water that is greater than extra-celluar fluid.

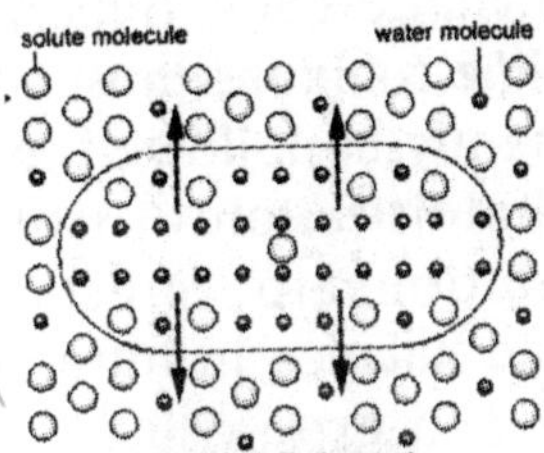

Hypertonic Environment
The water concentration is greater inside the cell; the solute concentration is greater outside. Water flows out of the cell.

- **hypertonic dehydration**
dehydration that develops after a hypotonic fluid is lost from the body. The fluid lost from the body contains a ratio of electrolytes to water that is less than extracelluar fluid. The osmolality of ECF is hypertonic after the electrolyte-poor fluid is lost. This

is a rare form of dehydration in dogs and cats.

- **hypertonic saline**
hypertonic saline has a concentration of sodium and chloride greater than 0.9% and is used in states of hypovolemic shock. A very small volume of hypertonic saline administered to a hypovolemic patient will result in the mobilisation of fluid from the cells into the extra-cellular fluid compartments, causing an expansion of blood volume and maintenance of blood flow to vital organs. Hypertonic saline solutions must subsequently be followed by the administration of isotonic solutions to re-establish fluid balance in intra-cellular and extra-cellular fluid locations.

- **hypertrophic**
a thickening or an enlargement of an organ.

- **hypertrophic osteodystrophy (HOD)**
inflammation of the growth plates, and can be accompanied by depression, weight loss, and fever. The joints may be swollen and feel hot. Mild cases usually resolve with no lasting ill effects. However, in the rare case of severe HOD, permanent damage to the bone joints can result in limb deformities.

- **hypertrophy**
enlargement.

- **hyperventilate**
an increase in the rate and/ or depth of respiration such that the body loses too much carbon dioxide.

- **hyperventilation**
fast breathing. Also called hyperpnea.

- **hyphema**
blood in the anterior chamber.

- **hypo**
this prefix is used in conjunction with many terms and means a decrease, for example, hypothermia means a decrease in temperature.

- **hypoalbuminemia**
low concentration of blood albumin.

- **hypocalcemia**
low blood calcium. Hypocalcemia causes tetany (ri-

gidity of muscles) in dogs and cats but flaccid muscle weakness in cattle.

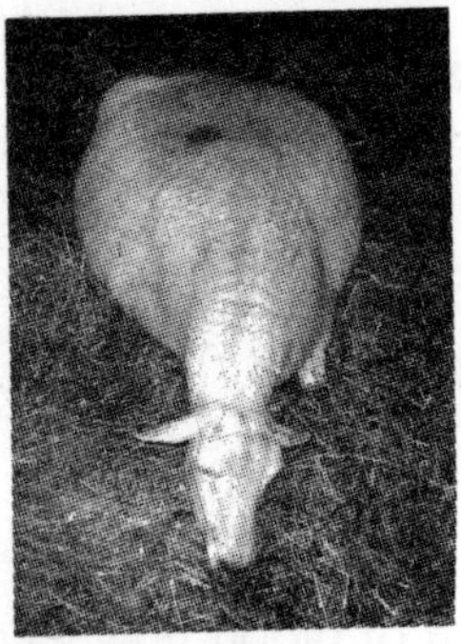

- **hypodermoclysis**
  a synonym for subcutaneous.
- **hypoglycemia**
  abnormally low blood glucose.
- **hypokalemia**
  lower than normal level of potassium in the blood.
- **hypomagnesemia**
  low blood magnesium.
- **hypomyelination, tremblers**
  reduction in the amount of myelin (cover or sheath) on the nerves. The disease has an early onset, In BMDs is considered to be an autosomal recessive trait.
- **hyponatremia**
  Low blood sodium. The most common cause is Addison's disease or iatrogenic from the administration of electrolyte free solution, such as 5% dextrose.
- **hypoplasia**
  inadequate or defective development of tissue.
- **hypopyon**
  pus in the anterior chamber of the eye.

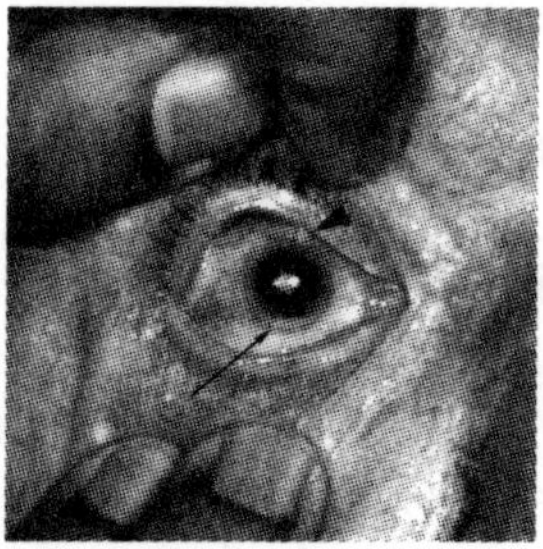

- **hyposensitisation**
  the administration of increasing doses of antigen to reduce sensitisation to the antigen.
- **hypot4**
  hypothyroidism
- **hypotension**
  abnormally low blood pressure.
- **hypothalamus**
  a part of the brain. Some hormones associated with reproduction are produced or stored in the hypothalamus.

a decrease in body temperature below normal.

- **hypothyroid**
  low function of the thyroid gland.
- **hypothyroidism**
  a condition, more common in dogs, in which the thyroid gland does not produce enough thyroid hormone.
- **hypotonic**
  a fluid that contains a ratio of electrolytes to water that is less than extracelluar fluid. A fluid that contains a concentration of electrolytes less than extracellular fluid.
- **hypotonic dehydration**
  dehydration that develops after a hypertonic fluid is lost from the body. The fluid lost from the body contains a ratio of electrolytes to water that is greater than extracelluar fluid. The osmolality of ECF is hypotonic after the electrolyte-rich fluid is lost. The best example of this type of dehydration is hypoadrenocorticism (Addison's Disease).
- **hypotony**
  decreased intraocular pressure.
- **hypovitaminosis A**
  a condition in which the body suffers from a deficiency in vitamin A.
- **hypovolemia**
  reduced circulating blood volume either due to blood or fluid loss or to redistribution of blood flow as occurs during shock.
- **hypoxia**
  low oxygen level in blood and tissues.
- **hysterectomy**
  a sterilisation process that removes a female cat's uterus.
- **hysteropexy**
  a surgical procedure during which the uterus is 'tacked' to prevent prolapse.
- **I**
  incisor (tooth - followed by a number to indicate which one)
- **impacted tooth**
  a tooth that cannot erupt or complete its eruption due to its contact with an obstruction

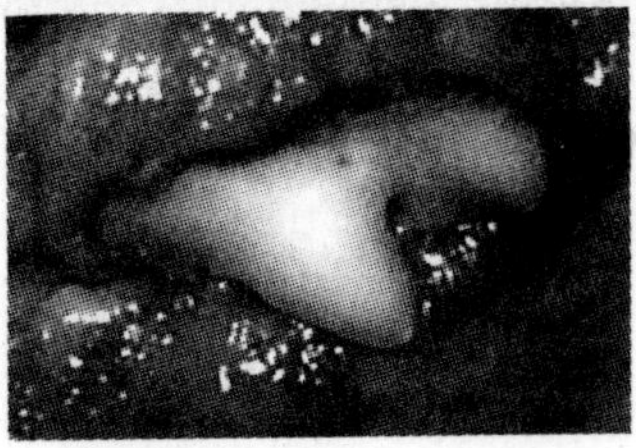

- **I.V.**
  intravenous
- **I/D**
  inter-digital
- **IAAAM**
  International Association of Aquatic Animal Medicine.
- **iatrogenic**
  disease that was caused while trying to diagnose or treat another condition. For example, if a complication such as excessive bleeding arises during a biopsy procedure, the complication is iatrogenic.
- **iatrogenic infection**
  infections that are acquired through human intervention. Also referred to as nosocomial infections.
- **icing**
  1. a physical therapy procedure, properly known as 'cryotherapy.'
  2. when a horse is stood in a tub of ice or ice packs are applied to the legs to reduce inflammation and/or swelling.
- **icterus**
  commonly referred to as jaundice. A yellowing of the tissues, usually as a result of abnormal liver function.

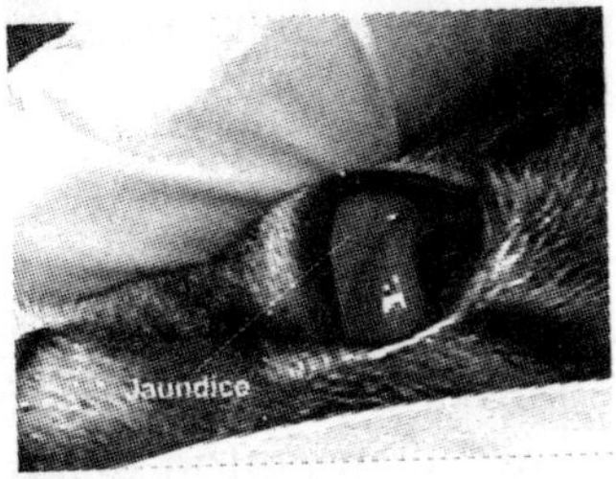

- **ID**
  identification or Identichip
- **IDDM**
  insulin dependent diabetes mellitus (IDDM) : a form of diabetes in which so little insulin is produced that supplemental insulin must be given for the animal to live. Also called Type I diabetes mellitus.
- **idiopathic**
  no known cause
- **idiosyncrasy to food**
  a qualitatively abnormal response to a food or food additive that resembles a hypersensitivity.

- **IID**
once a day
- **ilritis**
inflammation of the iris.
- **ileus**
a condition in which there is an absence of muscular contractions of the intestine which normally move the food through the system can result in an intestinal obstruction.
- **IM**
abbreviation for intra-muscular an injection given in a muscle.
- **IMHA**
immune-mediated haemolytic anaemia
- **imidocloprid**
is a neurotoxin available as a topical 'pour-on' for use in dogs and cats over 4 months of age.
- **immune mediated disease**
immune mediated indicates that the immune system is involved in the genesis of disease. Immune mediated diseases can be due to a foreign antigens (viruses, drugs) acting as haptens, adhering to or altering the surface of cells so that antibodies form against the hapten - cell complex or against cell antigens that become exposed. True autoimmunity indicates that the immune system is damaging unaltered 'self'. Often it is not possible to differentiate between true autoimmunity and immune mediated diseases.
- **immune system**
The body's defence system, which recognises infectious agents and other foreign compounds (such as pollen) and works to destroy them.
- **immune-mediated**
the immune system is supposed to protect against disease by destroying foreign objects such as bacteria. If the immune system attacks normal parts of the body such as red blood cells, the disease is immune-mediated.
- **immune-mediated reaction or disease:**
a condition or disease caused by abnormal activity of the immune system in which the body's immune system either over-reacts (e.g., immune-mediated

contact dermatitis) or starts attacking the body itself (e.g., autoimmune haemolytic anaemia).

- **immunity**
  a condition in which the animal's immune system has been primed and is able to protect the body from a disease-causing agent such as a certain virus or bacteria. An animal could have immunity to one agent, such as parvovirus, but not have immunity to another agent, such as rabies.

- **immunisation**
  the process of rendering an animal protected (immune) against a certain disease. Vaccination is a way to produce immunisation. However, just because an animal has been vaccinated (received a vaccine) does not necessarily mean the animal is immune. If the body did not correctly react to the vaccine or if the vaccine was defective, immunity would not occur. No vaccine produces immunity in 100% of the population to which it was given. 'Vaccination' is not the same as 'immunisation'.

- **immunodeficiency**
  reduced function of the immune system of an animal making it more susceptible to infectious disease. Can be an inherited defect or caused by drugs, radiation, or viruses.

- **immunoglobulins**
  there are several kinds that contribute to immunity overall. IgG is most abundant in serum and colostrum. IgM is 'early' antibody the first one to appear when there is an infection. IgA secreted on mucosal surfaces of respiratory, intestinal and genital tracts. IgE allergic antibody to allergens.

- **immunoprophylaxis**
  administration of vaccines to confer protection against infectious agents.

- **immunostimulant**
  a compound which stimulates the immune system to work more effectively to kill bacteria, viruses or cancer cells.

- **immunosuppression**
  any failure of the immune response usually becomes apparent through increased susceptibility to infection and disease.

- **immunosuppressive**
  something, for instance a drug, hormone or virus, that reduces the function of the immune system of an animal.

- **impaction**
  a type of colic caused by a blockage of the intestines by ingested materials (constipation).

- **impetigo**
  superficial pustular pyoderma seen in dogs less than 9 months of age.

- **impost**
  weight carried or assigned.

- **impr**
  improved: followed by a variable number of +'s to indicate degree of improvement

- **IMTP**
  immune-mediated thrombocytopenia

- **in foal**
  pregnant mare.

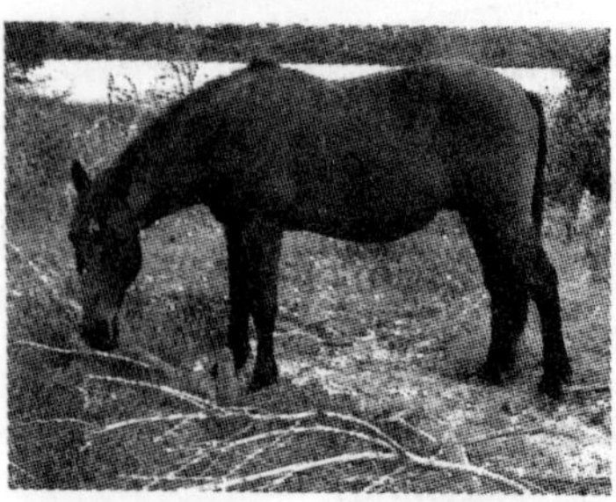

- **in hand**
  running under moderate control, at less than top speed.

- **inactive problems**
  inactive problems are unresolved problems that are not being addressed diagnostically or therapeutically. Usually they are problems of a minor nature.

- **innate**
  inborn, inherited existing or determined by factors present from birth congenital.

- **inbreed**
  to mate together closely related cats, for example brother and sister, or father and daughter.

- **incidence**
  the proportion of sampled animals that develop a condition of interest over a defined period of time. It is the measure of the occurrence of disease over time in a defined group of susceptible animals. Incidence can also be applied to measuring the occurrence of new cases of disease in an ever-changing population over time.

- **incisions**
  a wound made by something sharp like glass fragments or a scalpel blade, that penetrates all layers of the skin.
- **incisors**
  the front teeth.
- **incontinence**
  inability to control urination and/or defecation.
- **incubation period**
  the time between the exposure to a disease, causing agent, and the onset of signs of the disease.
- **index of bone**
  circumference of metacarpals x 100 divided by height
- **index of format**
  oblique length of dog x 100 divided by height at withers
- **index of leg height**
  measure of forearm to elbow x 100 divided by height at withers
- **indirect lifecycle**
  there are multiple hosts and so the parasite is actually required to pass from one host to another host, and sometimes to another host, before it comes back to the original host in this lifecycle.
- **indirect transmission**
  a mode of disease transmission where the environment is somehow part of the transmission cycle, e.g. contaminated water in a water trough spreads the disease.
- **indolent ulcer**
  ulcerative lesions found most frequently on the upper lips, but also seen in the skin elsewhere or in the oral cavity.
- **induced ovulator**
  an animal such as the queen that requires vaginal stimulation in order to ovulate.
- **infection**
  multiplication of organisms such as bacteria in the body usually leading to disease.
- **infectious agents**
  the agents that cause disease. They may be bacteria, viruses, fungi and parasites
- **infectivity/infectiousness**
  capacity of parasite to become established in the animal's tissues – e.g. rotavirus and corona virus in calf scours, are carried in the gastrointestinal tract of calves (> 4 weeks of age)

and older cattle without clinical signs of disease.

- **inferior check ligament**
  a direct continuation of the posterior (back) ligaments of the knee (carpus), located below the knee. Function is to support the deep flexor tendon.
- **infertility**
  inability to conceive and bear offspring.
- **infestation**
  a term used to describe an invasion of parasites.
- **infield**
  area encompassed by the inner rail of the racetrack.
- **inflammation**
  a condition in which tissue reacts to injury and undergoes changes during the healing process. As an example, a toe with a sliver of wood in it would be inflamed and show the signs of inflammation which include redness, increased temperature, pain, swelling and a loss of or disordered function. The toe is swollen, red, hot, painful, and the animal is reluctant to walk on that toe.
- **infusoria**
  microscopic organisms which are cultured as a food for the fry of fresh water fish.
- **inherent**
  implanted by nature intrinsic, innate involved in the constitution or essential character belonging by nature or habit.
- **inherited**
  a trait passed from one generation to the next in the genes from each parent.
- **initial database**
  the initial information collected on a patient when the patient is first seen. The minimum amount of information that will be collected should be defined in advance and may differ for different types of patients.
- **initial problem list**
  a listing of problems identified from history and physical examination. This list becomes more specific as the results of diagnostic tests become available.
- **initiation**
  a stage in the development of acute renal failure de-

fined as the time from renal insult to recognition of decreased GFR, decreased urine output and increased BUN and creatinine. This phase lasts 1-2 days.

- **inj**
  inject or injection
- **inotropic**
  affecting the force of muscle contractions. For example, a positive inotropic drug increases the force of contraction.
- **insensible fluid loss**
  insensible routes of fluid loss are those that are not readily observed and include the loss of fluid through the respiratory tract during respiration and loss of fluid by sweating. Dogs and cats sweat minimally through their footpads so most insensible losses are through the respiratory tract. The fluid lost during breathing is close to pure water and does not contain many solutes (a hypotonic loss). The basal loss of water through breathing is about: 10-15 ml/lb/day. High environmental temperatures, fever and activity result in increased insensible losses.
- **insensitive laminae**
  the layer just under the wall of the hoof; similar to the human fingernail. It is an integral structure that helps to attach the hoof wall to the underlying coffin bone.
- **insoluble carbohydrate**
  also, insoluble fibre. Fibre that resists enzymatic digestion in the small intestine.
- **instinct**
  a propensity that urges an animal to perform actions that are for the most part useful or beneficial, a natural or inherent aptitude that is largely hereditary and usually unalterable.
- **insulin**
  a hormone produced by the pancreas which is necessary for glucose to be able to enter the cells of the body.

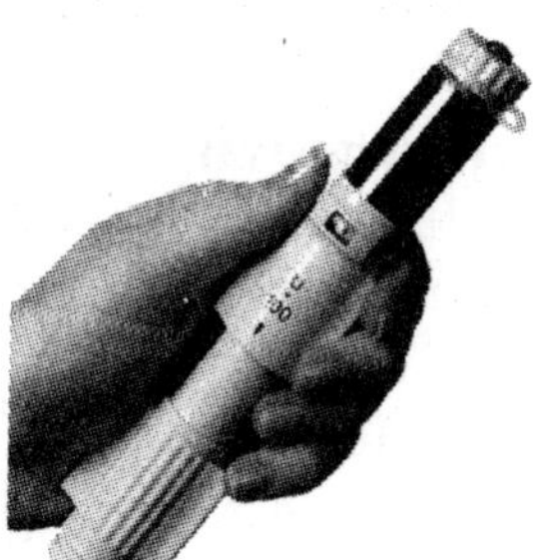

- **insulin abbreviations**
  R regular (fast acting)
  N NPH [a big long name] (intermediate acting)
  L lente (intermediate acting)
  U ultralente (long acting) not to be confused with U as in Units of insulin

- **insulin resistance**
  a condition in which the blood glucose level remains higher than it should at an insulin dosage of 2 units per pound of body weight per day in cats.

- **insulinoma**
  insulin-producing tumour of the pancreas. The increased production of insulin resulting from these tumours can cause low blood sugar (hypoglycemia).

- **int**
  internal

- **interdigital pyoderma**
  bacterial infections between the toes.

- **inter-estrus interval**
  the duration between consecuative estrous cycles, usually about 4 months in the bitch.

- **interferon**
  a glycoprotein produced by macrophages, lymphocytes and epithelial cells in response to viral infection.

- **inter-leukins**
  they are also referred to as cytokines. These are regulatory proteins that are secreted primarily by lymphocytes to help the interaction between the lymphocyte and a macrophage.

- **intermediate host**
  in the life cycle of some parasites, the immature form of the parasite must pass through a different type of host (animal, insect, snail, etc.), called the intermediate host, before it can re-enter and infect the type of animal it came from. An example would be heartworms. The adult worm lives in the dog or cat. The immature form, laid by the adult heartworm, is taken up by the mosquito. The immature form develops within the mosquito, and is then reintroduced into another dog or cat where it develops into the mature adult and the cycle repeats

itself. The intermediate host for heartworms, then, is the mosquito.

- **international unit (Abrev: IU)**
  a standard unit of potency of a biological agent. Example: vitamin, hormone, antibiotic, antitoxin. Also called a USP unit.
- **interposed abdominal compression CPR**
  in CPR, interposed abdominal compressions with chest compressions with an alternating rhythm between the abdomen and the chest.
- **interstitial**
  within the spaces of tissues.
- **interstitial cell tumour**
  a testicular tumour that usually displays benign biological behaviour.
- **interstitial cystitis (Abrev: IC)**
  a condition of the bladder resulting in haematuria and pollakiuria that resembles the condition in humans with the same name.
- **interstitial fluid**
  interstitial fluids are a subset of extra-cellular fluids that surround cells and include fluid in: dense connective tissue, bone, cartilage, cerebrospinal fluid, the gastrointestinal tract, and bile.
- **interstitial space**
  a subset of extra-cellular fluid including fluid surrounding cells, in connective tissue, in bone, in cartilage, cerebrospinal fluid, fluid in the gastrointestinal tract and bile.
- **intertriginous pyoderma**
  skin fold pyoderma occurring in lip folds (spaniels), facial folds (brachycephalic breeds), vulvar folds (obese, spayed females) and corkscrew tails (brachycephalic breeds).
- **inter-trochanteric fossa**
  a depression located between the greater and third trochanters of the femur. This is the site at which a needle penetrates into the femur for intraosseous administration or for collection of bone marrow.
- **inter-vertebral disk disease, IVDD**
  pain and often paralysis resulting from displacement of the centre of a vertebral disk.

- **intestine**
  the gut. A tubular organ that attaches to the stomach. The intestine is responsible for absorbing nutrients and water and eliminating wastes. The first part of the intestine is the duodenum, followed by the small intestine, large intestine, colon and rectum.
- **intra-articular**
  within a joint.
- **intra-cardiac route**
  the administration of drugs directly into the heart through the chest wall.
- **intra-cellular**
  within a cell.

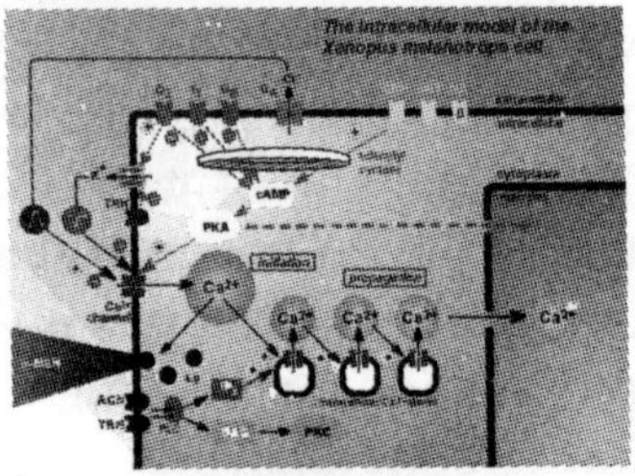

- **intra-cellular fluid (Abrev: ICF)**
  fluid located inside cells. Comprises 2/3 of total body water.
- **intra-cellular parasites**
  parasites that reside within the hosts cells.
- **intra-cranial**
  inside of the head.
- **intra-dermal skin testing (Abrev: IDST)**
  injection of known amounts of allergens intra-dermally and comparing the reaction to a positive (histamine) and negative control (saline).
- **intra-lipid**
  a solution of lipids available in 10 or 20% solution that can be administered.
- **intra-mammary antibiotics**
  antibiotics instilled directly into the mammary gland.
- **intra-muscular (IM)**
  into the muscle.
- **intra-nasal (IN)**
  into the nose.
- **intra-ocular pressure (Abrev: IOP)**
  the pressure within the globe. IOP is increased in glaucoma.
- **intra-tracheal route**
  the administration of drugs into the trachea usually using a catheter placed near the tracheal bifurcation.
- **intra-vascular space**
  the vascular space. Space located in the blood vessels.

- **intra-vascular (Abrev: IV)**
given directly into the blood stream.
- **intra-venous (IV)**
into the blood via a vein.
- **intromission**
the act of placing the penis in to the vagina.
- **intussusception**
a telescoping of a part of the intestinal tract into another part of the intestine.
- **IOL**
intra-ocular lens
- **ionofores**
one of the most common feed additives that we give cows to increase production, to increase efficiency, and increase rate of gain.
- **ionophore**
a carboxylic polyether antibiotic that affects the transport of ions across cellular membranes and inhibits the growth of some Gram positive bacteria. It is used in growing cattle to enhance feed efficiency and stimulate growth. Examples: Bovatec, Rumensin.
- **IP or I/P**
intra-peritoneal
- **iridencleisis**
treatment for glaucoma in which a window is made in the sclera and the iris pulled through and sutured under the conjunctiva.
- **iris**
the coloured portion of the eye. As with humans, dogs' iris colours vary. In the centre of the iris is the black opening called the pupil. This opening can be made larger or smaller by muscles called ciliary bodies that attach to the coloured iris causing it to expand or contract.
- **iris bombe**
posterior synechiae that occur all the way around the pupil and aqueous cannot flow through.
- **iris hypoplasia**
in blue-eyed animals one may see iris hypoplasia where the iris fails to develop properly and the irises of these young animals are almost transparent.
- **iris prolapse**
prolapse of the iris through a defect (ulcer) in the cornea.

- **irritable bowel syndrome**
soft or watery faeces, often with mucus. Associated with stress. Also called colitis.

- **ischemia**
deficiency of blood supply, which may be temporary or permanent. Caused by the shutting down of the blood vessels.

- **isoflavone**
an oestrogen-like substance produced by pasture plants a type of phytoestrogen.

- **iso-ionic**
iso-ionic refers to a similar concentration of a particular electrolyte in a solution compared to extra-cellular fluid. Therefore solutions which are iso-ionic with regard to sodium will have sodium concentrations comparable to the sodium concentration of extra-cellular fluid and plasma, which is approximately 145 mq/l in the dog and cat.

- **isolation barn**
a facility used to separate sick horses from healthy ones.

- **isomer**
different spacial configurations of a drug or chemical compound.

- **isosthenuria**
urine with the same specific gravity as glomerular filtrate indicating that the renal tubules have performed no work to either concentrate or dilute glomerular filtrate. There are also nonrenal causes of isosthenuria.

- **isothermaliser**
part of the Equitainer semen container system.

- **isotonic**
isotonic or iso-osmotic fluids have the same tonicity or osmolality as extra cellular fluid, which in the dog and cat is approximately 280-310 mOsm/l.

- **isotonic dehydration**
dehydration characterised by the loss of water and electrolytes in a ratio similar to extra-cellular water. Dogs and cats most often have isotonic dehydration as water and electrolytes are lost.

- **isotretinoin**
accutane-Roache. A retinoids, which is a synthetic derivative of vitamin A.

- **itraconazole**
  sporanox-Janssen. An oral treatment for dermatophytes.
- **ITW**
  Intertrack wagering.
- **IV or I/V**
  intravenous
- **ivermectin**
  ivermectin works on gamma amino butyric acid, which mammals most assuredly have. The trick with ivermectin is that it doesn't cross the blood/brain barrier in any appreciable quantity, so it doesn't affect GABA in mammals except in very high doses.
- **IVSA**
  International Veterinary Student Association
- **jacobsen's organ**
  an organ in the roof of a cat's mouth that is linked with the sense of smell and taste.
- **jaundice**
  the condition in which there is a build up of waste products in the body called bilirubin. Bilirubin is yellow in colour therefore an animal with jaundice will have yellow gums, skin (often seen on the inside flap of the ear), and a yellowish cast to the 'whites' of the eyes. It can occur if a large number of red blood cells are destroyed, the liver is not functioning normally, or the bile ducts are blocked.
- **jejunum**
  the longest part of the small intestinal tract.
- **jen chung**
  an acupunture technique also referred to as governing vessel 26 which causes sympathetic stimulation.
- **jill**
  a female ferret.
- **joining**
  putting the rams and ewes together for mating. Tupping is the same thing.
- **joint capsule**
  the structure that comprises the boundary to the joint space.

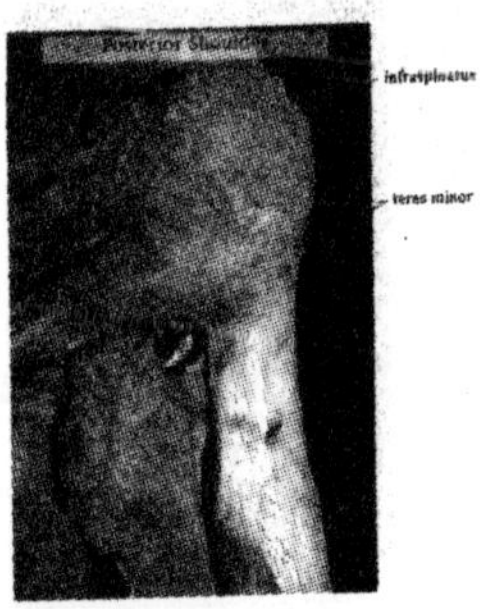

- **joule (Abrev: J)**
  a unit adopted by Systeme International (SI) for expressing energy. The Joule is more commonly used in Europe than in North America (4.184J = 1 calorie).
- **jowls**
  loose flesh around the neck and throat.

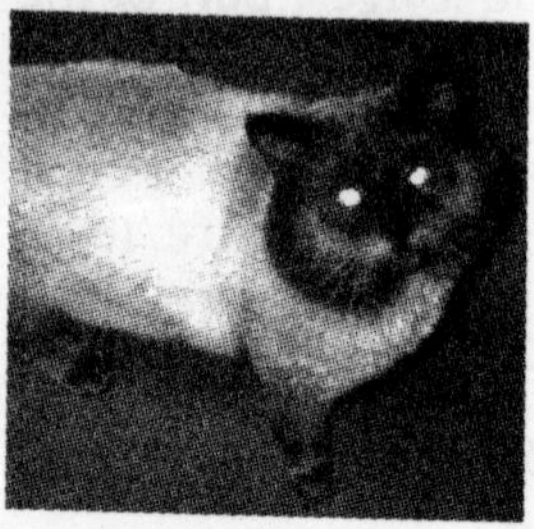

- **jt**
  joint
- **jugular**
  a large vein on the bottom surface of the neck that may be used to collect blood samples or to place catheters.
- **jumper**
  steeple chase or hurdle horse.
- **juvenile**
  two-year-old horse.
- **juvenile cellulitis**
  an inflammatory disease of young (less than 4 months) puppies, characterized by inflammation and severe edema of the face, muzzle, periocular skin, and ears.
- **KC**
  kennel cough (infectious tracheobronchitis)
- **KCS**
  Keratoconjunctivitis sicca. Dry eye.
- **kemp**
  non-wool hair fibres in the fleece.

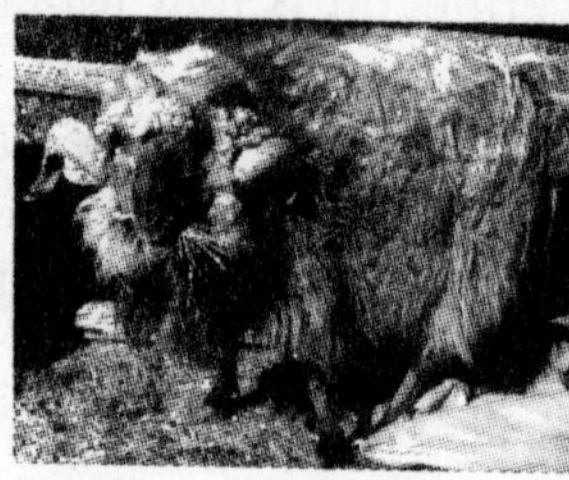

- **keratic precipitates**
  clusters of inflammatory cells on the back (endothelial surface) of the cornea.
- **keratin**
  a cystine rich protein produced by the epithelial cells.

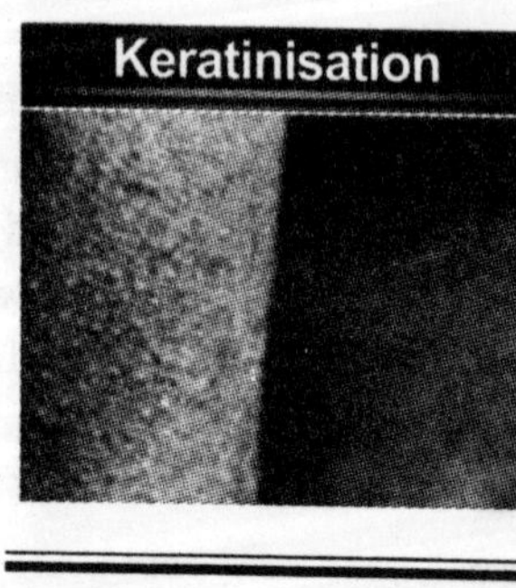

- **keratinisation disorders**
cutaneous disorders characterised by scaling.

- **keratitis**
inflammation of the clear part of the eye, the cornea.

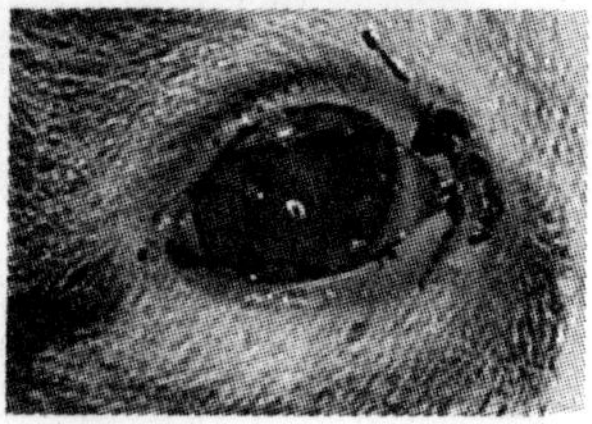

- **keratolytic**
softens and loosens crusts and scales on the skin.

- **keratotomy**
removal of part of the thickness of the cornea.

- **ketoacidosis(Abrev: DKA)**
a form of diabetes mellitus in which the pet has increased amounts of acids in the blood and is very sick.

- **ketoconazole**
nizoral-Janssen. An oral treatment for dermatophytes.·

- **ketone**
waste product produced when the body is using fat as an energy source. Ketones are acids, and can cause damage or death to cells. Excess ketones accumulate in the blood and are excreted in the urine. Acetone is a ketone which can be eliminated through the lungs. Ketoacidotic animals often have a chemical smell to their breath (Some nail polish removers contain acetone - it is a similar smell).

- **ketonuria**
ketones in the urine. Occurs when the diabetes is uncontrolled and the body is producing ketones.

- **ketoprofen**
another of the nonsteroidal anti-inflammatories.

- **killed vaccine**
vaccines which are made by taking the real, disease-causing viruses (or bacteria), killing them, and putting them into a liquid base.

- **kinetic skull**
having mobile joints between various parts of the skull, e.g., being able to unhinge the jaws. This allows the mouth of the animal, e.g., snake, to open wider so that it can eat large prey.

- **kink**
a twist, curl, bend or bump in the tail bone.

- **kit**
  a baby ferret.
- **kittens**
  offspring of a female cat.

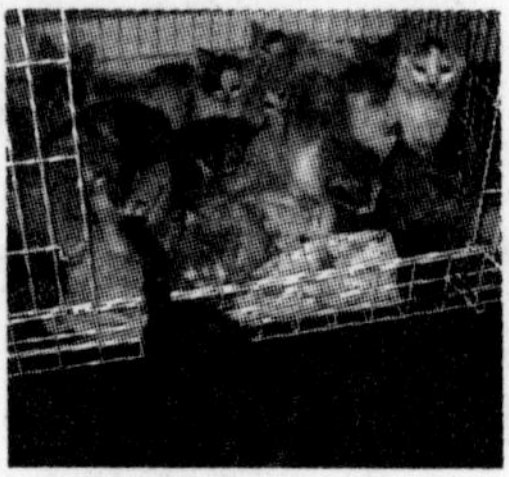

- **koch's postulates**
  used in infectious diseases to determine if the parasite will cause disease. The traditional criteria used are as follows: the organism must be regularly isolated from cases of the disease. The organism must be grown in pure culture or free of the animal host. Such a pure culture should cause disease upon innoculation into susceptible animal. The same organisms must be re-isolated from the experimentally induced disease.
- **l**
  lumbar (vertebra - usually followed by a number to denote which one)
- **LA**
  left atrium
- **LA**
  local anaesthetic
- **laces**
  white markings on the legs.

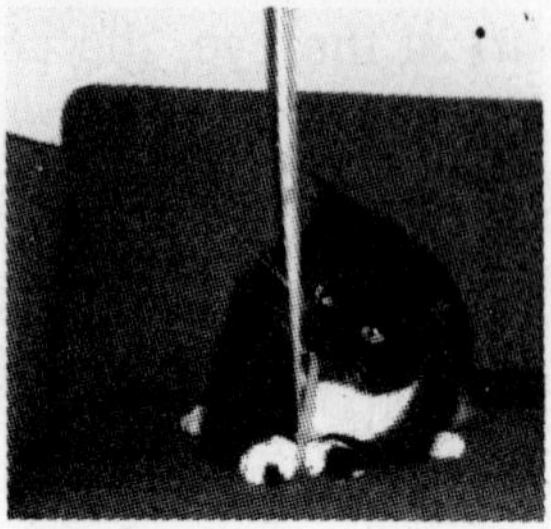

- **lacrimal system**
  consists of 2 glands that produce the aqueous tear film component, one in the dorsolateral orbit and one on the bulbar surface of the nictitans. Tears flow through the nasolacrimal duct to the nose
- **lactate**
  to produce milk.
- **lactated ringer's solution**
  lactated ringer's solution is one of the most common crystalloid solutions used in a small animal practice. It has an osmolality comparable to extracellular fluid, so it is considered an isotonic solution. Most lactated Ringer's solution that are commercially available are marketed for people, there-

fore the actual osmolality of lactated Ringer's solution is slightly less than the osmolality of canine and feline extracellular fluid/plasma. The sodium, potassium, and chloride concentrations of lactated Ringer's solution are comparable to extracellular fluid, although the sodium concentration is iso ionic to human extracellular fluid/plasma and is slightly lower than the sodium concentration of canine and feline extracellular fluid/plasma. Lactated Ringer's solution contains lactate, which is converted by the liver to bicarbonate.

- **lactating**
  producing milk.

- **lactation**
  the time a cow is producing milk.

- **lactation curve**
  a graphic plot of days in milk vs. pounds of milk produced.

- **lactic acid**
  organic acid normally present in muscle tissue, produced by anaerobic muscle metabolism as a by-product of exercise. An increase in lactic acid causes muscle fatigue, inflammation and pain.

- **lactogenic immunity**
  a form of local immunity in milk (post colostrums) that bathes the intestinal tract and prevents colonisation by virulent bacteria and neutralised viruses passing through the gut.

- **lae**
  left atrial enlargement

- **lagophthalmos**
  inability to fully close the eyelids over the eyeball.

- **lamb bed**
  uterus.

- **lame**
  a deviation from a normal gait due to pain in a limb or its supporting structures.

- **laminae**
  a part of the hoof.

- **laminitis**
  an inflammation of the sensitive laminae of the foot. There are many factors involved, including changes in the blood flow through the capillaries of the foot. Many events can cause laminitis, including ingest-

ing toxic levels of grain, eating lush grass, systemic disease problems, high temperature, toxemia, retained placenta, excessive weight-bearing as occurs when the opposite limb is injured, and the administration of some drugs. Laminitis usually manifests itself in the front feet, develops rapidly, and is life-threatening. In mild cases, however, a horse can resume a certain amount of athletic activity. Laminitis is the disease that caused the death of Secretariat. Also known as 'founder.'

- **laminitis - nerving**
in laminitis (there) is an arteriovenous shunting upstream from the laminae, resulting in hypoxic damage. If a similar phenomenon is taking place post nerving, that would certainly be a Bad Thing.

- **laparotomy**
a surgical procedure to open the abdominal (belly) cavity.

- **large intestine**
the lower part of the intestinal tract usually made up of the colon, cecum, and rectum.

- **larva**
the worm-like offspring of an insect (plural larvae).

- **Laryngitis**
an inflammation of the larynx, often temporarily making speech difficult.

- **larynx**
the voice box. The larynx closes during swallowing to keep food out of the airways.

- **lat**
lateral

- **late double**
a second daily double offered during the latter part of the programme.

- **latency**
a virus which remains hidden and does not cause disease but which may reactivate and cause clinical signs of disease at a later time.

- **latent**
a dormant stage of disease. The patient is infected with an organism, but is not yet ill.

- **lateral**
towards the side and farther from the centre. Pertains to a side.

- **lateral recumbant**
  laying down on the side.
- **lateral torsion**
  twisted or rotated out.
- **level bite**
  where the maxillary and mandibular incisors meet at the incisal edges.

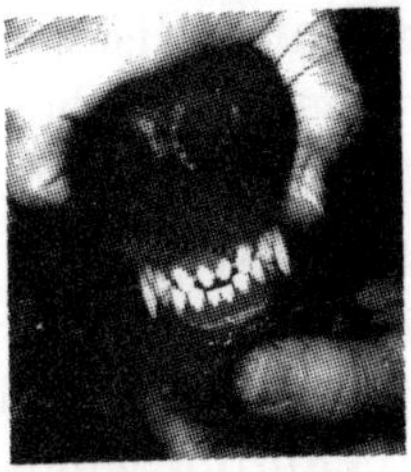

- **leash**
  a set of three animals, such as hounds.
- **lecithin**
  phospholipids found widely in animals and plants, (e.g., egg yolk) that have emulsifying, wetting, and antioxidant properties.
- **lens**
  structure in the eye which functions to transmit and focus incoming light rays directly on the retina. This is facilitated by accommodation - the subtle change in lens shape brought about by contraction and relaxation of the ciliary body the accommodative ability of the lens is limited in domestic species.
- **lens capsule**
  a clear elastic membrane surrounding the lens body.
- **lens luxation**
  primary or secondary displacement of the lens either anterior into pupil or anterior chamber or posterior into the vitreous chamber.
- **lethargy**
  malaise or inactivity.
- **leukemia**
  a cancerous proliferation of one of the subsets of White Blood Cells.
- **leukocytosis**
  high white blood cell count.
- **leukopenia**
  a condition in which the number of white blood cells in the blood is lower than normal.

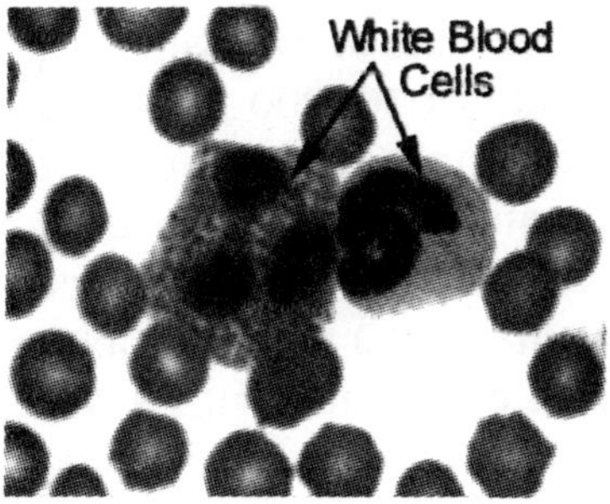

- **leukotriene**
  substances derived from arachidonic acid in cell membranes that mediate allergic responses.
- **levator palpebrae superioris**
  muscle in the upper lid that elevates the upper eyelid. It is innervated by cranial nerve 3, the oculomotor nerve.
- **IF**
  left fore
- **LH**
  left hind
- **Lhasa Apso**
  the Lhasa Apso is a small Oriental canine, with a 2, 000 year history in his homeland of Tibet. This little dog from the roof of the world is 'gay and assertive, but chary of strangers', reflecting the isolation of his Tibetian background, where strangers were few and far between. Originating in the Himalyan Mountains at an average altitude of 16, 000 feet, in an extreme variation of temperature, he is tough, sturdy and free from general genetic faults. He is rather stubbon and deliberate, with a regal attitude that loves admiration and praise. Playful and clownish, but never foolish or fawning. Slow to mature at two or three years of age, he keeps a youthful appearance well into his teens. At a general size of fourteen to eighteen pounds, the Lhasa Apso is large enough to withstand trauma and disease, and never toyish or delicate. His profuse 'coat of many colours is long, heavy and of rather harsh texture — never soft, silky or whispy, and luxuriously beautiful when clean and brushed. All colours are allowed, as long as pigmentation is black. Weekly brushing and bathing is necessary to care for this coat, but many owners keep their Lhasa Apso trimmed in various little 'shaggy dog' clips to avoid the extra work. Intelligent and loyal to their owners, Lhasas do not change homes easily. Their suspicion of strangers make them excellent watch dogs, and they are generally very clean with no body odour. They are never pests clamouring for attention, but rather content to lie at your feet or in a doorway where they can

watch you and their surroundings. Extremely adaptable, they are nevertheless creatures of comfort and habit, preferring the sofa or your bed to a crate or dog bed. All in all, a big dog in a small package, the Lhasa Apso is beautiful to look at, but much more than just another pretty face!

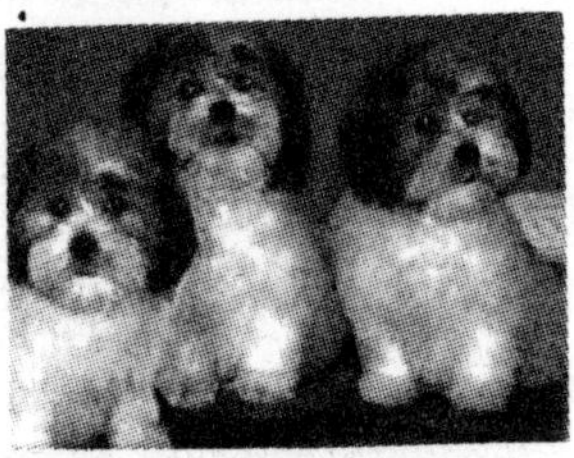

- **LHD**
  long haired domestic (non-pedigree cat)
- **LI**
  large intestine
- **libido**
  sexual desire
- **lichenification**
  thickening, hardening and often hyper-pigmentation of the skin.

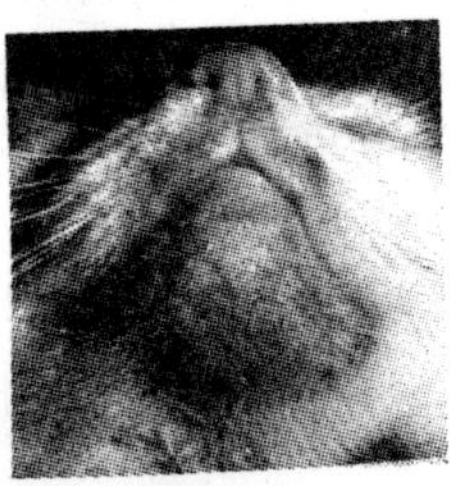

- **lidocaine**
  a drug used as a local anaesthetic and as an antiarrhythmic agent in treatment of certain cardiac arrhythmias such as ventricular fibrillation.
- **ligament**
  a band of fibrous tissues connecting bones, which serves to support and strengthen joints and to limit the range of motion. There are also ligaments that support certain organs.
- **limbic system**
  a group of brain structures which exert an important influence on the endocrine and autonomic motor system and which influence (emotion) mood states.
- **limbus**
  junction between conjunctiva and cornea.
- **linear immunoglobulin A dermatosis**
  clinically present as sub-corneal pustules, epidermal collarettes, etc. Generally truncal in distribution. Most often seen in the dachshund.

- **linebreed**
  to mate together cats that have some of the same ancestors. For example, two cats that have the same grandfather.
- **lipase**
  digestive enzyme, produced by the pancreas, which breaks down fat.
- **lipids**
  substances found in plant and animal tissues that are insoluble in water, but soluble in benzene or ether. Includes fats, oils, glycolipids, phosphoglycerides, waxes and steroids.
- **lipoxygenase (Abrev: 5-LOX)**
  5 lipoxygenase breaks down arachidonic acid to form the leukotrienes. The leukotrienes mediate activation and margination of neutrophils, altered vascular permeability, and promotion of gastric ulceration or degenerative joint disease.
- **liquid protein supplement (Abrev: LPS)**
  a protein product usually containing molasses, urea, added vitamins and trace minerals; particularly useful in pasture feeding.
- **lithe**
  a cat body type that is lean, narrow and small-boned.
- **litter**
  all the kittens born to a mother in a single birth.
- **litter Box**
  a lined container filled with kitty litter, used as a sanitary place for cats to eliminate.
- **LIU**
  lens induced uveitis
- **liver**
  the largest organ in the abdomen, responsible for producing enzymes required for digestion of food, and bile that helps to digest fat. The liver also detoxifies the blood and may be damaged in the process.
- **LL**
  left lower (eg. eyelid, lip)
- **LN**
  lymph node/s
- **loafing area**
  area of farm, often associated with free stalls and milking barn where animals are free to exercise and move voluntarily.

- **lochia**
  the vaginal discharge that appears post-delivery and in the bitch is green coloured.

- **lochia**
  green coloured post-partum discharge. The appearance of lochia before delivery indicates placental separation and impaired blood flow to the foetuses.

- **locket**
  solid white marking on the neck.

- **longhair**
  a cat with relatively long fur, often varying in length over different parts of the cat. Some longhairs have shortish fur on the body, but all longhairs have long fur on the tail, forming a 'plume' or 'brush, ' and most have long fur around the neck forming a 'ruff.'

- **low passage vaccine**
  a low passage vaccine contains virus particles which have been attenuated (or weakened) less so than those in the average vaccine. Low passage vaccines can generally elicit an immune system response in young animals who have a maternal antibody level that would prevent them from responding to an average vaccine.

- **LTF**
  learning to fly (animal fell off balcony or similar)

- **LU**
  left upper (eg. eyelid, lip)

- **lufeneron**
  a benzoyl-phenylurea compound that inhibits chitin development. An insect growth regular.

- **lunge**
  1. horse rearing and plunging.
  2. a method of exercising a horse on a tether ('lunge line').

- **luteinising hormone (Abrev: LH)**
  LH causes ovulation of ovarian follicles. LH is also believed to be involved in testicular descent into the scrotum.

- **luxating tarsus**
  dislocation of the 'ankle'

- **LV**
  left ventricle

- **LVE**
  left ventricular enlargement

- **lymph nodes**
part of the immune system. Lymph nodes contain white blood cells called lymphocytes. Blood from nearby areas is filtered through the lymph nodes allowing foreign or infectious material to be recognised and destroyed.

- **lymphocytes**
the class of cells in the body which are responsible for mounting an immune response. Two main types are B cells and T cells

- **lymphoid organs**
organs that regulate the production and differentiation of lymphocytes. The main lymphoid organs are the salivary glands, the thymus, the spleen, and the bone marrow.

- **lymphokines**
chemicals produced by T lymphocytes. Some lymphokines signal macrophages and other phagocytes to destroy foreign invaders.

- **lymphoma, lymphosarcoma**
malignant tumour that arises from cells of the lymphoreticular system. Commonly present with swollen lymph nodes, masses, enlarged liver or spleen, fevers, weight loss.

- **lyophilised**
freeze dried

- **M**
1. molar (tooth - followed by a number to indicate which one)
2. male (see also Me and Mn)

- **mobile tooth**
an important diagnostic sign that results from a decrease in root attachment or changes in the periodontal ligament. Mobility is noted as M1, M2, M3, based on severity

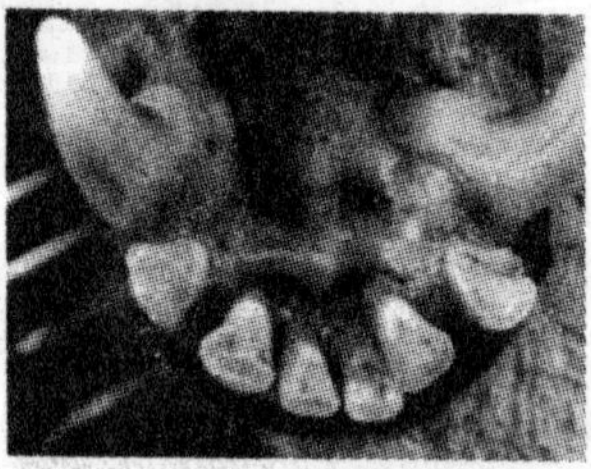

- **M/C**
metacarpal

- **M/T**
metatarsal

- **MacKenzie Brush technique**
this technique employs a sterile toothbrush to comb the hair coat of an animal

suspected to be a carrier of dermatophytes. The bristles of the brush are then embedded or shaken over agar for culture.

- **mackerel**
  a type of tabby pattern where the colours of the coat appear striped.

- **macro minerals**
  minerals required in relatively large amounts by livestock. Includes calcium (Ca), phosphorus (P) magnesium (Mg), potassium (K) chlorine (Cl), sulfur (S) and sodium (Na).

- **macrophage**
  a type of phagocyte (cell in the body which 'eats' damaged cells and foreign substances such as virus and bacteria).

- **macule**
  a circumscribed, flat (not raised or depressed) change in the colour of the skin. Large macules are patches.

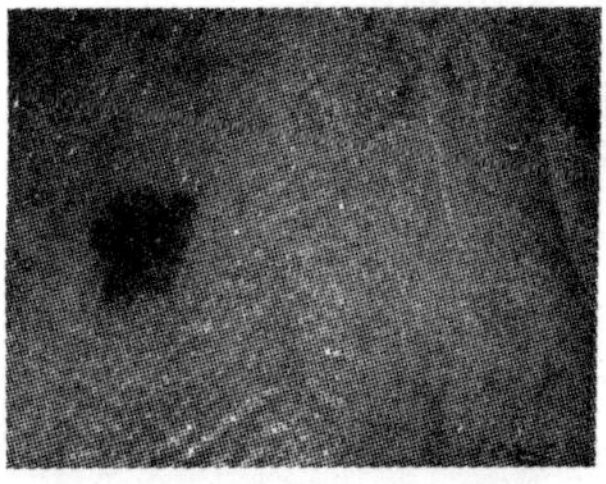

- **magnetic resonance imaging (Abrev: MRI)**
  a very strong magnet is used to produce a 3 dimensional picture of a structure in the body. MRI is a good method to look inside the skull to see the brain.

- **magnetic therapy**
  physical therapy technique using magnetic fields. The low-energy electrical field created by the magnetic field causes dilation of the blood vessels (vasodilation) and tissue stimulation. Magnetic therapy may be used on soft tissue to treat such injuries as tendinitis or bony (skeletal) injuries such as bucked shins.

- **maiden**
  a female that has never been bred.

- **maiden ewe**
  an ewe lambing for the first time.

- **maintenance phase**
  a phase of acute renal failure following initiation during which oliguria persists. Whether an ARF patient is oliguric or polyuric reflects the severity of insult, which caused ARF. The majority of

ARF dogs and cats become oliguric although some ARF patients are never oliguric. In those patients which can repair the renal damage, the oliguric phase lasts 1-2 weeks. Many animals die or are euthanised during the oliguric phase because of the poor prognosis. The most life-threatening consequences of the oliguric phase include hyperkalemia and overzealous fluid therapy resulting in overhydration.

- **maintenance solutions**
  maintenance solutions are hypotonic compared to extra-cellular fluid. They have more potassium than extra-cellular fluid and less sodium than extra-cellular fluid. Maintenance solutions can be purchased or 'created' from other cystalloid solutions.

- **malabsorption/maldigestion syndrome**
  a condition involving the intestine in which food may not be properly digested or the nutrients not absorbed.

- **malassezia pachydermatis**
  a budding yeast considered part of the normal flora of the external ear canal. May become pathologic in certain situations. Formerly called Pityrosporum canis.

- **malignancy**
  cancer.

- **malignant**
  a rapidly invasive proliferation of neoplastic (new growth) histiocytes. No known treatment, always fatal.

- **malnutrition**
  ill health due to dietary deficiency or imbalance.

- **mammary**
  pertaining to the breast.

- **mammary gland**
  the udder or breast.

- **mandible**
  lower jaw.

- **mange**
  any of several skin and ear conditions caused by a variety of mites.

- **manip**
  manipulation

- **MAOIS**
  Mono amine oxidase inhibitors. Substances that inactivate the enzyme monoamine oxidase, which regulates certain transmitter chemi-

cals between nerves. These compounds include certain types of antidepressants and also insecticides containing amitraz.

- **mare**
  female horse five-years-old or older.

- **marsupial**
  an order of mammals including kangaroos, opossums, and sugar gliders in which the female has a pouch on the abdomen which holds the young.

- **mash**
  soft, moist mixture, hot or cold, of grain and other feed that is easily digested by horses.

- **mask**
  the darker shadings on the face.

- **massage**
  rubbing of various parts of the anatomy to stimulate healing.

- **mast cell tumour**
  a nodular growth, usually on the skin, comprised of mast cells (which contain large amounts of histamine). All mast cell tumours in dogs should be considered potentially malignant.

- **master problem list (Abrev: MPL)**
  a list of all the problems shown by a patient. The master problem list is dynamic and may expand over time.

- **masticate**
  chew.

- **mastiff**
  there is no doubt that the Mastiff descends from ancient lines. Dogs of similar type inhabited Europe and Asia deep into B.C. times. These massive canines were employed in the hunting of wild horses and lions, as well as in protecting the homes of Babylonians. The burying of terracotta Mastiff figures under the thresholds of houses was a custom of Assyrian peoples. It was practised to invoke the canine spirits to ward off evil

spirits. Mastiff prototypes, such as the Molossus of Epirus and Babylonian Mastiff, were used as flock guards against wolves and other predators. Romans found the Mastiff in England when they first arrived - how the dogs got to England escapes our knowledge - and took them back to Rome to perform in the arenas. One early writer claims that the Roman government set up a 'Procurator Cynegii' at Winchester, England, to purchase promising canines for use by the army and in the arena. These dogs are believed by many to be the ancestors of the modern Mastiff. Yet, with all the documented evidence of 'giant' dogs, which resemble in general type the Mastiff of today, the origin and development of the breed continue to be speculated on by historians.

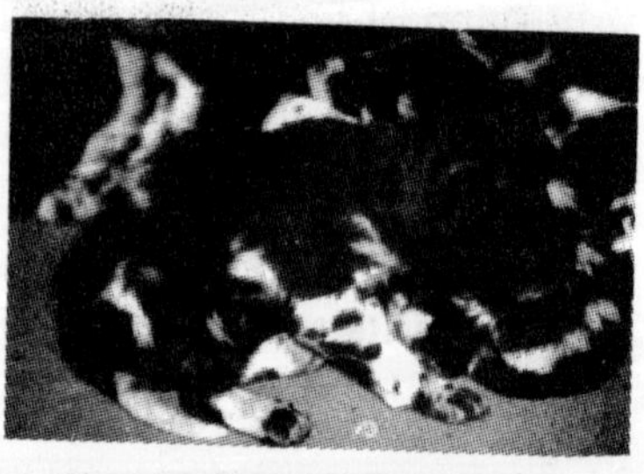

- **mastitis**
  inflammation of the mammary gland, usually due to bacterial infection.

- **mastocytoma**
  a growth of mast cells (cells in the dermis which is directly beneath the outer skin layer, which release histamine to counter allergens). These tumours may become malignant.

- **maternal antibody**
  antibody in a newborn animal which the newborn acquired through the placenta or colostrums (the first milk).

- **mature equivalent**
  a cow reaches maturity at 7 years of age (5th lactation) and thus records can be adjusted for what her production is expected to be at maturity. Allows comparison among herd mates at different ages.

- **mature follicle**
  a large follicle on the ovary that secretes oestrogen that makes the female receptive and she will be able to respond to mating by ovulating.

- **MD**
  myocardial disease

- **ME**
  male (entire)
- **meal**
  when referring to food ingredients, means a ground-up preparation. Chicken meal is ground up chicken, which might include bones and feathers. Meat meal means ground up muscle meat.
- **meconium**
  the first stool or faeces passed by the newborn.
- **med**
  medial
- **medial**
  pertaining to the middle in anatomy, nearer the medial plane (the horizontal plane that bisects the centre).
- **median survival time**
  time at which 50% of the animals had died.
- **medication administration record (Abrev: MAR)**
  a flow sheet charting medications given to a patient over time.
- **medication list**
  a list kept by the track veterinarian and published by the track and Daily Racing Form (when provided by track officials) showing which horses have been treated with legally prescribed medications.
- **megacolon**
  a condition in which the colon enlarges and dilates, which results in faeces accumulating in the colon. Constipation then occurs. This condition is more common in cats than dogs.
- **megaoesophagus**
  overly enlarged oesophagus causing buildup of food and saliva and regurgitation. Associated with aspirative pneumonia from an early age.
- **megestrol acetate**
  a progestin marketed for estrus control in the dog and commonly used for managemnet of severe pruritus in the cat.
- **meibomian gland adenoma**
  a benign tumour of the Meibomian glands.
- **meibomian glands**
  glands located at the eyelid margins that secrete the lipid part of the tear film.

- **melangestrol acetate (Abrev: MGA)**
  a hormone added to diets to suppress estrus cycle and improve feed efficiency and growth rate in feedlot heifers.

- **melanomas in grey horses**
  melanomas in grey horses are, as a rule, non-malignant. They can occur on any part of the body, but do often occur around the anus.

- **melena**
  darkening of the stool due to the presence of digested blood, which indicates bleeding is occurring in the stomach and/or beginning of the small intestine. The faeces generally look black and tarry.

- **memory**
  when an animal mounts an immune response against a foreign substance, some cells are created to 'remember' the antigens on that substance. If the animal is again exposed to the substance, these cells will help the body respond much faster and to a higher degree.

- **menace reflex**
  used to assess vision and the ability to close the eyelids.

- **meningitis**
  not a disease, but a symptom, the inflammation of the membranes covering the brain and spinal cord, the meninges. This can be caused by bacteria, virus, fungi, or chemical toxins.

- **meningitis aseptic**
  is inflammation of the meninges for which no identifiable infectious agent can be cultured or tested for, and is probably genetic.

- **metabolic acidosis**
  a condition in which the blood is too acidic.

- **metabolic reactions to food**
  an adverse reaction due to an effect of a substance upon the metabolism of the host, or as a result of defective metabolism of a nutrient by the host.

- **metabolism**
  the chemical processes in cells that are involved in using energy and building substances the cells need. Glucose metabolism relates to how cells use or store

glucose. Anabolism refers to the building up processes, catabolism refers to the breaking down processes.

- **metabolisable energy (Abrev: ME)**
  a measure of the useful energy in a feed. It represents that portion of the feed gross energy not lost in the faeces, urine and belched gas.

- **metabolise**
  to have molecules transformed within the body tissue through chemical processes.

- **metabolise energy(me)**
  the net energy available to an animal from a certain food.

- **metacarpal (fracture)**
  usually refers to a fracture of the cannon bone, located between the knee and the fetlock joint in the front leg. Also may refer to a fracture of the splint bone.

- **metastatis**
  spread of a tumour from its original location to a remote one, by tumour cells that are carried in the blood.

- **metatarsus**
  the part of the rear limb between the tarsus and the phalanges (toes).

- **methaeamoglobin**
  an altered haemoglobin which does not carry oxygen.

- **methaemoglobinemia**
  a condition of the blood in which there are large amounts of methaeamoglobin which is an altered haemoglobin which does not carry oxygen.

- **methoprene**
  an insect growth regulator. Present in rinses, sprays, collars, and household sprays/foggers. Recently added to a topical pour-on product containing fipronil.

- **metritis**
  infection of the uterus. If the infection follows delivery, it is a postpartum metritis.

- **micro-minerals**
  minor mineral elements required in very small amounts in the ration of animals. Includes manganese (Mn), copper (Cu), zinc (Zn), selenium (Se) iron (Fe),

cobalt (Co), iodine (I) and fluorine (Fl).

- **microencapsulation**
a process whereby an insecticide is packaged into small microspheres (polyurea, nylon, etc). This process increases the LD50 and decreases biodegradation (extends duration of action). Currently, microencapsulated products include pyrethrins, diazinon, and chlorpyrifos.

- **microfilaremia**
the presence of microfilariae in the blood.

- **microfilaria**
the larval form of some parasitic worms, for example heartworms. These worms do not lay eggs, they produce microfilariae instead.

- **microfilaricide**
compound which kills microfilaria, the immature forms of heartworms which circulate in the blood.

- **micro-nutrient**
any ingredient, such as minerals, vitamins or drugs, added in very small amounts to a ration.

- **micro-organism**
a single-celled life form that is invisible to the naked eye and that may cause disease in man or animals.

- **micro-phthalmos**
a small eye that has failed to develop properly.

- **micturition**
a synonym for urination.

- **mid-body (fracture)**
see sesamoids.

- **milbemycin oxime**
a systemic treatment for demodectic mange.

- **miliary**
small, resembling a seed.

- **miliary dermatitis**
a cutaneous reaction pattern characterised by the formation of multiple, circumscribed crusted papules.

- **milk fat test**
the percentage of fat in the milk. To be legal, whole milk must contain at least 3.25% fat.

- **milk replacer**
a substitute for feeding whole milk to calves, generally consisting of milk byproducts and/or plant products and is mixed with wa-

ter. The higher quality replacers have more milk products.

- **milking parlour**
barn where cows are milked. Two prevalent types: Herringbone and Parallel Parlours.

- **min**
minutes

- **mineral supplement**
a rich source of one or more mineral elements.

- **mineralisation**
the process in which minerals are laid down within tissue in an abnormal pattern causing a hardening of the tissue.

- **mineralocorticoids**
hormones produced by the adrenal gland which regulate the amounts of sodium, potassium and chloride in the blood.

- **miniature pinscher**
not a dwarf of the Doberman Pinscher as some believe, the Miniature Pinscher is an ancient breed whose origins can be traced for over 350 years. Its resemblance to the Doberman is an ex post facto coincidence namely, the doing of Herr Dobermann, who greatly admired the sleek Miniature Pinscher. The MinPin was derived from large smooth-coated German Pinschers and was employed to keep down the rat population in the stables that it frequented. The breed was developed in the German Rhineland, where it was known as the Reh Pinscher, allegedly due to its similar appearance, structurally and gait-wise, to the reh deer, a small roe deer.

- **minimum database**
a minimum database is the minimum amount of information collected for a medical record and includes: the chief complaint(s), history, patient signalment and physical examination.

- **miosis**
small pupil.

- **mismate**
a drug given in attempt to prevent pregnancy.

- **missing tooth**
adult dogs normally have 42 teeth, cats 30. Missing teeth occur for various reasons: Congenital absence, Impac-

tion of an unerupted tooth. Previous trauma causing exfoliation or fracture. Previous dental care. To evaluate the cause of missing teeth, radiography will show if there is an impacted tooth, retained, or fractured root, or no root

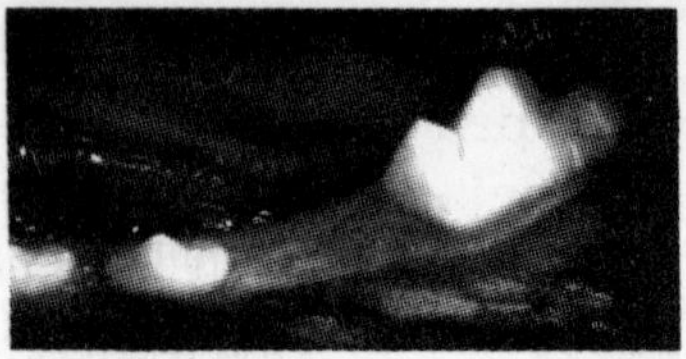

- **mites**
  very small arachnids that cause and carry a variety of diseases.
- **miticide**
  an agent that kills mites.
- **mitochondria**
  parts of the cell which are responsible for providing the cell with energy.
- **mitral valve defect**
  a defect in the heart valve that separates the left atrium and the left ventricle.
- **mixed breed**
  a cat of unknown or mixed parentage. Mixed breed cats can be shown in the household pet (HHP) competitive class.
- **mL**
  short for millilitre. A liquid measure, the same volume as a cc. 28 mL = 1 liquid oz.
- **MLK**
  a multimodal analgesic administration technique combining lidocaine, ketamine and morphine in IV fluids such as LRS.
- **MM or MMB**
  mucous membranes
- **MN**
  male (neutered)
- **MO**
  months old (following a number)
- **modified live vaccine**
  vaccines which are made by altering (attenuating) viruses so that they become incapable of causing disease but are still capable of stimulating an immune response. Compare with killed vaccines and recombinant vaccines.
- **modified live virus (Abrev: MLV)**
  a vaccine which contains a living virus that has been modified to attenuate its virulence.

- **moggy**
  the UK term for mixed breed.

- **monoamine oxidase inhibitor (MAOI)**
  substances that inactivate the enzyme monoamine oxidase which regulates certain transmitter chemicals between nerves. These compounds include certain types of antidepressants and also insecticides containing amitraz.

- **monoclonal**
  originating from a single precursor cell.

- **monoclonal antibody**
  the term used to describe a homologous Ig produced by a clone of B cells. This occurs naturally in neoplasia of B cells resulting in myeloma.

- **monogastric**
  an animal having a single or simple stomach system. Example: swine.

- **monorchid**
  1. a male horse of any age that has only one testicle in his scrotum-the other testicle was either removed or is undescended.
  2. an adult male cat which has only one descended testicle.

- **monovalent vaccine**
  a vaccine that is manufactured to stimulate the body to produce protection against only one disease, e.g., rabies vaccine.

- **morning glory**
  horse that performs well in morning workouts but fails to reproduce that form in races.

- **morphology**
  the structure or appearance of something.

- **motility**
  Movement. Intestinal motility is the muscular contractions of the intestines, which move food from the stomach to the anus.

- **motivational-affective dimension of pain**
  this is the disruption of the feeling of well-being that results in suffering to the degree that it triggers an active response from the animal to pain.

- **movement extension**
  increasing a joint's angle

- **movement flexion**
  decreasing a joint's angle
- **MT**
  mammary tumour
- **mucolytic**
  breaks down mucous.
- **mucopolysaccharide**
  a carbohydrate which also contains a hexosamine molecule and is a component of mucous.
- **muco-purulent**
  a discharge that is a combination of pus and mucus.
- **mucosa, mucous membranes**
  specialised membrane which covers various passages and cavities exposed to the air such as the mouth, nose, inner portion of the eyelids, vagina. Examination of the mucous membranes can provide important information: if they are dry the animal is likely to be dehydrated, pale, and the animal may be anaemic or in shock, yellow, and the animal is said to be jaundiced due to accumulation of waste products which should be eliminated by the liver.

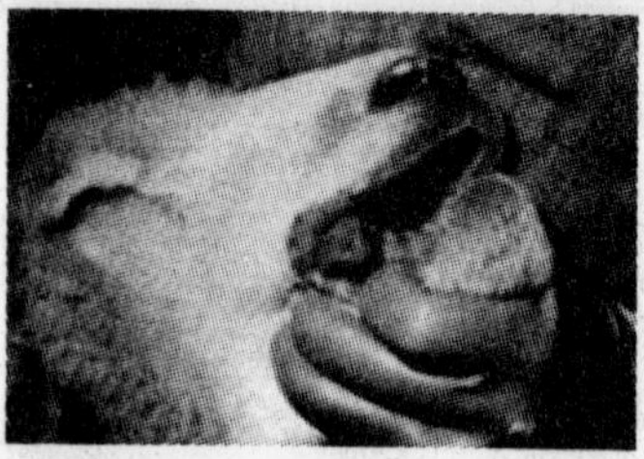

- **mucosal immunity**
  a form of local immunity on the body surfaces of the respiratory, intestinal and genital tracts.
- **mudder**
  horse that races well on muddy tracks.
- **mueller cells**
  cells responsible for support and nutrition of the retina.
- **muller's muscle**
  smooth muscle in the eyelids which provides tone to the lids. Innervated by sympathetic fibres.
- **multi-modal**
  using more than one method.
- **multi-valent vaccine**
  a vaccine that combines two or more components to stimulate the body to produce protection against all the components. Most distemper vaccines for puppies are of the multi-valent type

and commonly include distemper, parvovirus, adenovirus, hepatitis, and parainfluenza.

- **mupriocin**
  topical antibacterial ointment effective against staphylococci.

- **murmur**
  an abnormal heart sound associated with the opening or closing of a heart valve. This may indicate a structural or functional abnormality.

- **musculoskeletal system**
  consisting of the bones, muscles, ligaments, tendons and joints of the head, vertebral column and limbs, together with the associated muscles, tendons, ligaments and joints.

- **music**
  the sounds of hounds at bay.

- **mutualistic**
  a relationship where both participants or parties benefit.

- **muzzle**
  consisting of the forward sections of the jaws, upper and lower, the muzzle is the portion of the skull in front of the brain case. Depending on the skull development, muzzle types vary greatly. Comparing the short or stubby muzzle of the brachycephalic (short-faced) breeds (e.g., Pug, Bulldog) with the long wedge-shaped, tapering muzzle of the dolichocephalic (long-headed) breeds (e.g., Saluki, Greyhound), the differences in type, size and depth are rather apparent. Many terms have been employed to describe the muzzle types: Blunt muzzle: Square muzzle, Pinched muzzle, Snipy muzzle, Pointed muzzle, Short muzzle, stubby muzzle, Tapering muzzle, Wedge-shaped muzzle. Dog muzzles can be made or purchased at a pet shop. A bandage or necktie can provide a workable makeshift muzzle should the need arise. The muzzle is wrapped around the dog's mouth twice and tied above and below the chin and then around the back of the head behind the ears. Most manufactured muzzles are made of leather or some kind of wire. Muzzles chiefly

intend to prevent the dog from biting, injuring, or fighting. In case of an accident where the dog is hurt and in shock, the makeshift muzzle may help to keep the dog under control. In some cities, owners are required to muzzle their dog when walking on pedestrian thoroughfares. This law is aimed at large dogs or potentially vicious dogs.

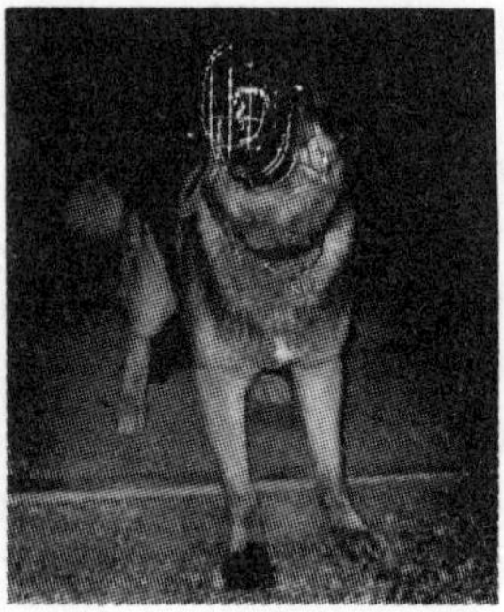

- **MVA**
motor vehicle accident

- **myasthenia gravis**
myasthenia gravis is a neuromuscular disease in which there is a failure of the nerves' ability to stimulate and control the actions of certain muscles.

- **mycobacteriosis**
feline leprosy caused by Mycobacterium lepraemurium.

- **mycoplasma**
these are a group of bacteria that have lost their cell walls.

- **mycosis**
disease caused by a fungus such as blastomycosis, histoplasmosis and ringworm.

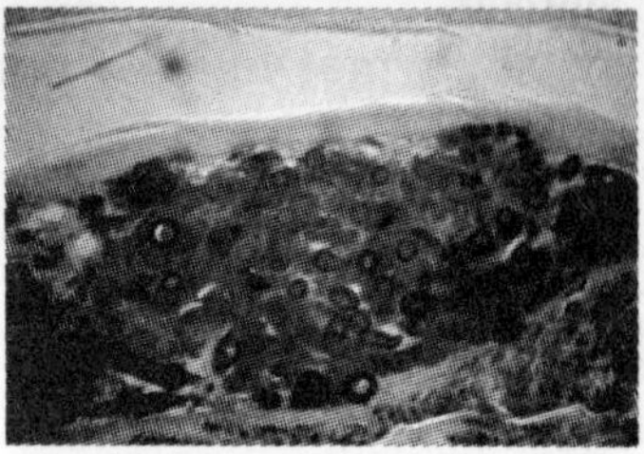

- **mycotoxin**
a substance produced by fungi and toxic to animals, e.g., vomitoxin, zearalenone and aflatoxin.

- **mydriasis**
small pupil size.

- **myelitis**
inflammation or infection of the spinal cord.

- **myelogram**
radiograph (x-ray) of the spinal cord taken after a contrasting dye has been injected into the space around the spinal cord.

- **myelosuppression**
a suppression of the bone marrow so that it does not

produce normal numbers of red blood cells, white blood cells and platelets.

- **myocardium**
  the middle layer of heart muscle.
- **myopathy**
  inflammation of muscle.
- **N**
  1. normal
  2. neck lesion (feline oral resorptive lesion)
  3. Class I - enamel loss only
  4. Class II - enamel and dentin exposure
  5. Class III - pulpal exposure
  6. Class IV - partial crown loss
  7. Class V - full crown loss

  NDEF nerve deficit
- **N/S**
  next step
- **NAD**
  no abnormality detected (or detectable)
- **nadir**
  the lowest point. Refers to the lowest blood glucose concentration on a BG curve.
- **NAF**
  no abnormal findings
- **naloxone**
  an antagonist of morphine and other opiods.
- **nasal**
  a synonym for the cavity behind the nose.
- **nasogastric tube**
  a long tube that is capable of reaching from the nose to the stomach.
- **nasolacrimal system**
  the route of drainage of tears from the eye to the nose.
- **nauplii**
  newly hatched brine shrimp.
- **navicular bone**
  a small, flat bone within the confines of the hoof that helps-along with the short pastern bone and the coffin bone-to make up the coffin joint.
- **navicular disease**
  a degenerative disease that affects the navicular bone (small bone in the back of the foot), navicular bursa and deep flexor tendon. Generally considered a disease of the front feet. Both front feet are often affected, but one will usually be more noticeable than the other.

- **NBG**
  treatment not working
- **NE**
  near exposure
  fractured tooth with near pulpal exposure
- **near side**
  left side of a horse. Side on which a horse is mounted.
- **nebulise**
  convert into a fine spray form.
- **neck**
  unit of measurement. About the length of a horse's neck a little less than a quarter of a metre.

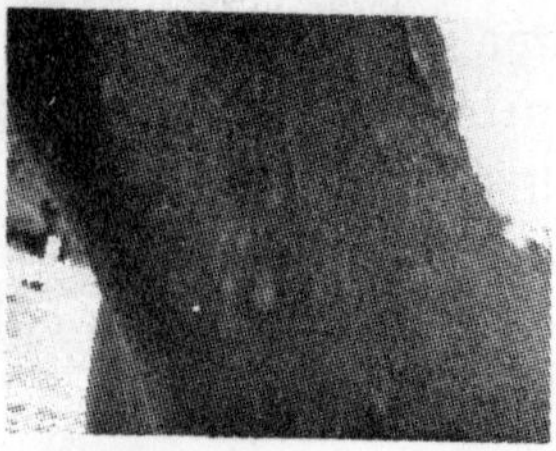

- **necklace**
  bandings of colour across the lower neck and chest area, as if the cat is wearing a necklace.

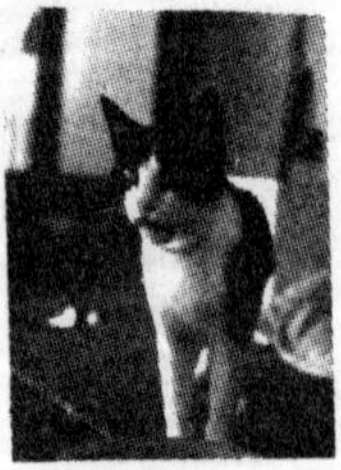

- **necropsy**
  post mortem examination.
- **necrosis**
  the death and breakdown of cells.
- **nematodes**
  a common name for any round worm of the phylum Nematoda.
- **neonatal heart murmur**
  a heart murmur in a neonatal equine is quite common, and not necessarily indicative of any defect.
- **neonate**
  refers to a young puppy or kitten shortly after birth.
- **neoplasia**
  abnormal growth and accumulation of cells. Neoplasia may be benign or malignant.

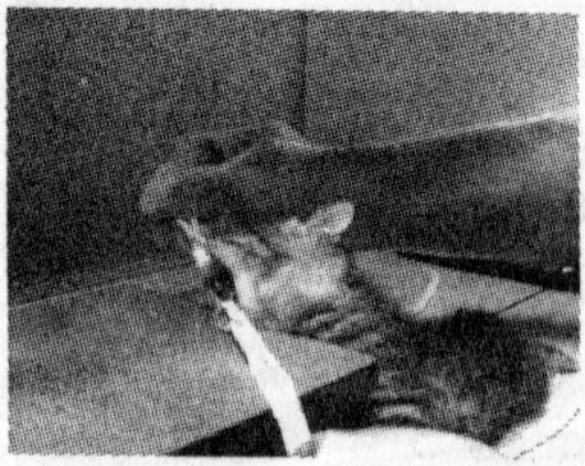

- **neoplasm**
  a lump or cancer. The word means 'new growth'.
- **nephropathy**
  abnormal functioning of the kidney.

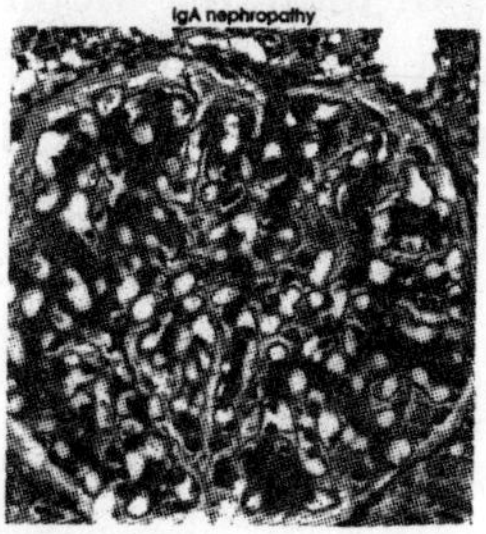

- **nephrotoxic**
a drug or chemical that causes damage to the cells of the kidneys.

- **nerve root signature**
lameness due to nerve root involvement.

- **nerving**
see neurectomy.

- **net energy (Abrev: NE)**
the amount of feed energy actually available for animal maintenance and production. It represents the energy fraction in a feed left after faecal, urinary, gas and heat losses are deducted from the gross energy value of a feed.

- **neuralgia**
pain along the distribution of nerves.

- **neurectomy**
a surgical procedure in which the nerve supply to the navicular area is removed. The toe and remainder of the foot have feeling. Also referred to as 'posterior digital neurectomy' or 'heel nerve.'

- **neuroleptanalgesic**
a combination of a tranquilliser and an opiate which provides a synergistic effect for sedation and analgesia.

- **neuropathic pain**
pain originating in peripheal nerves and nerve roots.

- **neuropathy**
abnormal functioning of nerves.

- **neurotransmitter**
a substance released from a neuron of the central or peripheral nervous system which excites or inhibits the target cell. Examples include: acetylcholine, norepinephrine, epinephrine, dopamine, substance P, enkephalins, endorphins and serotonin.

- **neuter**
sterilisation by surgical removal of the testicles of a male animal.

- **neutral detergent fibre (Abrev: NDF)**
  the insoluble fraction containing all plant cell wall components left after boiling a feed sample in a neutral detergent solution. NDF is of low digestibility, but can be broken down somewhat by the digestive tract micro organisms. NDF value is used to predict ruminant feed intake.

- **neutralise**
  to change from acidic alkaline to a neutral pH.

- **neutralising antibody**
  a type of antibody that specifically blocks virus receptor sites on the virus preventing attachment to target cells in the body.

- **neutrophil**
  the most common type of white blood cell observed in the blood stream.

- **nictitans**
  the third eyelid which is a fold of tissue covered by conjunctiva and containing a lacrimal gland on the inner (bulbar) surface.

- **NIDDM**
  non-insulin dependent diabetes mellitus(NIDDM): A type of diabetes mellitus in which although the blood glucose levels are higher than normal, they are not immediately life-threatening, and the animal can survive without supplemental in sulin. Also called Type II diabetes.

- **nigropallidal encephalomalacia**
  a specific brain lesion seen in horses with yellow star thistle poisoning. The clinical sign is an inability to swallow.

- **Nikolsky sign**
  the epidermis may be rubbed off with slight trauma. Named after a Russian dermatologist.

- **NMDA receptor**
  glutamate dependent N-methyl-D-aspartate (NMDA)receptors. This type of receptor develops in the central nervous system in response to sustained pain and appears to be responsible for amplifying pain, and causing opioid tolerance.

- **NNTSA**
  no need to see again

- **NOC/S/V/D**
  no coughing, sneezing, vomitting or diarrhoea

- **NOAD**
  no other abnormality diagnosed

- **NOAF**
  no other abnormal findings

- **nociception**
  the detection of noxious stimuli by the nervous system.

- **nociceptors**
  peripheral receptors for pain which sense painful stimuli and transmit signals to the central nervous system where the sensation of pain is perceived.

- **nocturnal or crepuscular**
  animals that are active during the night and sleep during the day.

- **nod**
  lowering of head.

- **nodule**
  a circumscribed, solid, raised lesion that involves the deeper layers of the skin.

- **non-steroidal anti-inflammatory drug (Abrev: NSAID)**
  a drug such as aspirin that has anti-inflammatory properties but that is not a corticosteroid.

- **non-contagious disease**
  a disease that cannot be spread between animals by direct contact.

- **non-core vaccine**
  vaccine which should only be given to animals increased risk of exposure to a disease. Example, leptospirosis in dogs or feline leukaemia in cats

- **non-essential amino acids**
  amino acids that can be synthesised by the animal.

- **non-insulin dependent diabetes mellitus (NIDDM)**
  a type of diabetes mellitus in which although the blood glucose levels are higher than normal, they are not immediately life-threatening, and the animal can survive without supplemental insulin. Also called Type II diabetes.

- **non-pathogenic**
  not causing disease. Some bacteria, such as those that normally live in an animal's intestines, are non-pathogenic.

- **non-protein nitrogen (Abrev: NPN)**
  nitrogen not derived from true protein, but can be used by rumen microbes to build microbial protein.

- **non-ruminant herbivore**
  animals with simple stomachs able to digest roughages and other fibrous feeds because of the microbial population in their hindgut. Examples: horse, rabbit.

- **non-septic**
  a condition not caused by an infection. For example, septic arthritis is caused by an infection with bacteria, yeast or other agent a case of non-septic arthritis may be caused by injury or cancer

- **non-structural carbohydrates (Abrev: NSC)**
  simple carbohydrates, such as starches and sugars, stored inside the cell which serve as a cellular energy source. Non-structural carbohydrates are rapidly and easily digested by the animal.

- **non-terrestrial rabies**
  rabies in mammals that do not walk on the ground: bats.

- **normal saline**
  0.9% sodium chloride. It is isotonic. It contains only sodium and chloride. Sodium chloride is used when blood sodium is decreased; such as in Addison's disease because it has a higher concentration of sodium than does lactated Ringer's. It may be used in lieu of lactated Ringer's for rehydration in patients with lymphoma. It is used as a rehydration solution when a patient has an increased potassium or calcium, and the administration of additional calcium or potassium are contraindicated.

- **norwegian catheter**
  A catheter used to deposit semen during artificial insemination.

- **NOS**
  no other symptoms

- **nose band**
  a leather strap that goes over the bridge of a horse's nose to help secure the bridle. A 'figure eight' nose band goes over the bridge of the nose and under the rings of the bit to help keep the horse's mouth closed. This keeps the

tongue from sliding up over the bit and is used on horses that do not like having a tongue tie used.

- **nosocomial**
  an infection contracted in the hospital.
- **nosodes**
  products prepared from infected tissues, infected discharges, or a pathogenic organism, which are processed and administered orally in attempt to 'vaccinate' against an infectious agent.
- **not for breeding**
  a cat that has been designated by the breeder as not to be used for breeding. Such a cat cannot have registered offspring.
- **notobiotic environment**
  an environment with no germs whatsoever.
- **novel protein**
  a diet that contain proteins to which an animal has not previously been exposed(fed).
- **noxious stimulus**
  a stimulus that is potentially or actually damaging to tissue. A stimulus that is of adequate intensity to trigger a nociceptive reaction in an animal (the feeling of pain).
- **NPO**
  nothing per os/nil per os
- **NSAID**
  non-steroidal anti-inflammatory drug
- **NSF**
  no significant finding
- **nuclear sclerosis**
  compression of older lens fibres in the nucleus of the lens which results in light-scattering that clinically appears as a gray, homogeneous, perfectly round area in the centre of the lens which is bilaterally symmetrical. A normal ageing change that does not interfere with vision.
- **nucleatederythrocytes**
  immature form of red blood cells.
- **nuclei (nucleus)**
  a structure located within a cell. Contains amongst other substances the genetic information of the cell.
- **number-averaged molecular weight**
  the mean of the molecular weight of all the polymers in

a solution. The number-averaged molecular weight tells you how quickly a fluid will exert an effect. The smaller the number-averaged molecular weight, the quicker the initial oncotic response.

- **nutraceutical**
  a very broad term describing certain components in food (plant or animal) or nutritional supplements, which contain substances normally present in the body that aid in the proper functioning of body systems.
- **nutrient**
  compounds in foods which are essential for life. Nutrients include protein, fats, vitamins, and minerals.
- **nutrient allowances**
  recommendations of nutrient amounts necessary for maintenance, growth, gestation, lactation or performance that include a safety margin to account for variability in feeds and animals (e.g., environment, health, storage losses).
- **nutrient requirements**
  the minimal amounts of nutrients (energy, protein, minerals and vitamins) necessary to meet an animal's minimal needs for maintenance, growth, reproduction, lactation or work.
- **nutritional value of beet pulp**
  2.56 Mcal/kg on a 100% DM basis digestible energy (for comparison, oats are 3.20)
- **NYD**
  not yet diagnosed
- **nystagmus**
  constant involuntary movement of the eye, often from side to side
- **O**
  owner
- **O/F**
  off food
- **oa**
  osteo-arthritis
- **open bite**
  an area of open space when the jaw is closed, which normally should be occupied by occluding teeth.

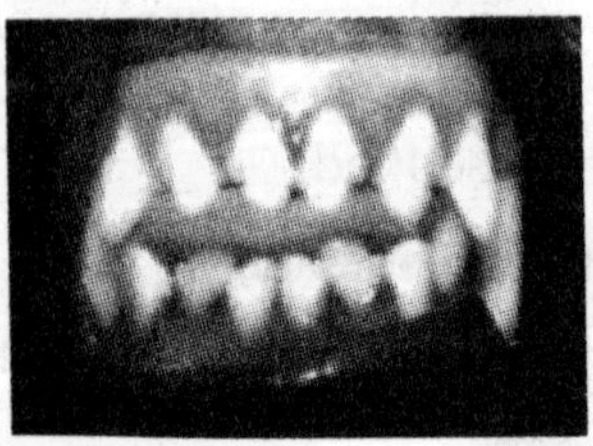

- **obesity**
  overweight.

- **objective information**
  any information that can be quantified such as the size of a mass, a laboratory value or the grade of a heart murmur.

- **obligate carnivore**
  an animal that requires in its diet nutrients that are found in sufficient quantities only in meat or other animal products.

- **obligate pathogen**
  parasite that generally will cause disease – e.g. *Brucella abortus* (Brucellosis); *Yersinia pestis* (Plague); and *Mycobacterium bovis* (Tuberculosis).

- **oblique (fracture)**
  fracture at an angle.

- **obsessive compulsive**
  a behavioural condition in which a pet repeatedly performs an action out of context. It is thought that the behaviour is an expression of stress, frustration, and/or conflict. Certain breeds are more prone to these behaviours. These behaviours include tail chasing, excessive barking, continual licking, and biting the air as if snapping at invisible flies.

- **occiput**
  upper back point of the skull, a feature that varies in prominence from breed to breed. Often referred to as the peak, apex, and occipital bone. The occiput's function is to serve as a point for muscles to attach themselves.

- **occult**
  indicating a disease or condition that is clinically not apparent.

- **OCD**
  osteochondritis dissecans

- **OCD lesion**
  a cartilaginous or bony lesion that is the result of a failure in development.

- **OCNE**
  off colour, not eating

- **ocular**
  relating to the eye.

- **odontoplasty**
  area of reshaped tooth by dental bur.

- **odd-eyed**
  a cat with one blue eye and one green, gold, or copper eye.

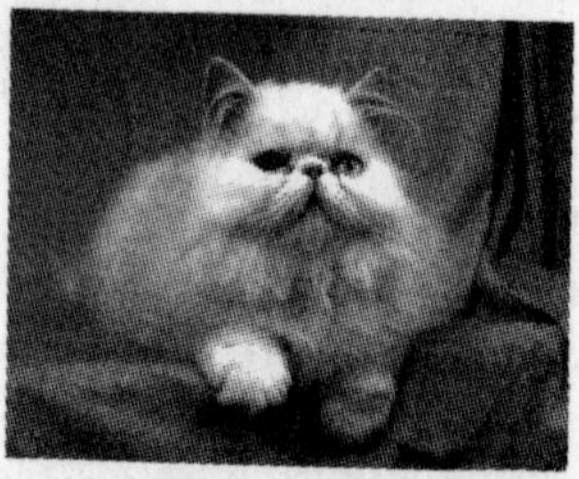

- **OES**
  old English Sheepdog.

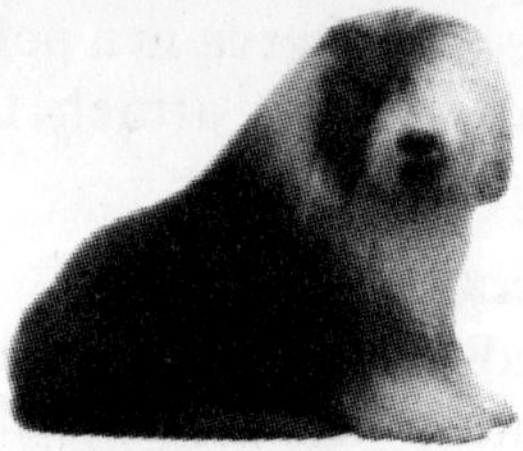

- **off label**
  term used to describe the use of a medication for a condition for which it was not approved. A large number of medications used in veterinary medicine are used off label. If veterinarians only used approved medications, options for treatments of certain conditions would be severely limited or nonexistent.
- **off side**
  right side of horse.
- **offal**
  animal organs rejected at slaughter as unfit for human consumption, e.g. spleen, intestine, brain, lungs.
- **oliguria**
  small volume of urine production. In adult dogs and cats oliguria is defined as urine production of less than 0.5 ml/lb/hr (1 ml/kg/hr).
- **OM**
  oral mass
- **omentum**
  a thin lace-like layer of tissue in the abdomen that partially covers the organs.
- **omnivore**
  animal that eats both flesh and plants.
- **on the body caudal, or posterior**
  toward the south wall or butt.
- **on the body cranial, or anterior**
  toward the north wall or head.
- **on the body dorsal**
  toward the ceiling or back
- **on the body lateral**
  toward the east or west wall or side
- **on the body medial**
  toward the midline, away from the east or west walls.

• **on the body ventral**
toward the floor or belly.

• **on the limbs distal**
away from the body.

• **on the limbs palmar**
the front foot pads.

• **on the limbs plantar**
the rear foot pads.

• **on the limbs proximal**
toward the body.

• **on the muscle**
denotes a fit horse.

• **oncology**
the study of cancer.

• **oncotic**
the pressure or pull of fluids created by colloids in solution. In blood, the oncotic pressure created by particles such as plasma proteins offsets the hydrostatic pressure created by the pumping of the heart that acts to drive fluid out of vessels into the extra vascular space. The oncotic pressure of the plasma proteins holds fluid in the blood vessels.

• **oronasal fistula**
an abnormal communication between the mouth and nasal cavity

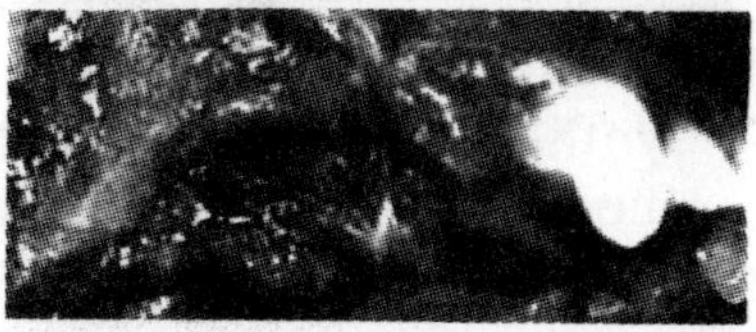

• **onychectomy (Declawing)**
a surgical process that permanently removes the nails on an animal (British vets have unilaterally banned it by deciding they won't ever declaw except in cases of medical necessity, not to be encouraged elsewhere).

• **onychomycosis**
fungal infection of the nail bed.

• **oocyte**
egg, ova.

• **OOH**
out of hours

• **op**
operate or operation

• **open knee**
a condition of young horses in which the physis of the knee has not closed an immature knee. Often used to describe the status of the physis immediately above the knee and is an indicator of long bone growth in two-year-olds.

- **opioid**
  synthetic compounds with effects like opium but which are not derived from opium.
- **opportunist**
  a bacteria that causes clinical disease in animals that are somehow weakened and can not fight off the infection.
- **opportunistic pathogen**
  parasites that are usually harmless commensals in their normal habitat, but can cause disease when they gain access to other body sites – e.g. *Pasteurella haemolytica* (pneumonia) and *Staphylococcus aureus* (mastitis). Impairment of animal's immune defence is the principle factor leading to opportunistic infections.
- **opsinising antibody**
  a type of antibody that coats particles, such as bacteria to promote phagocytosis.
- **optic nerve**
  formed by axons of the ganglion cells of the retina.
- **optic nerve hypoplasia**
  incomplete development of the optic nerve.
- **optic neuritis**
  inflammation of the optic nerve. It can be unilateral or bilateral.
- **oral**
  Giving something by mouth or referring to the mouth.
- **oral cavity**
  the mouth.
- **oral hypoglycemic agent**
  a medication, given by mouth, which lowers the level of glucose in the blood. Example: glipizide
- **oral transmission**
  common route of animal-to-animal exposure due to contact with infected placenta, foetal fluids, milk.
- **orbicularis oculi**
  muscle which is responsible for eyelid closure and is innervated by cranial nerve 7.
- **orbital fascia**
  the connective tissue sheath that lines the orbit and envelopes all the structures within the orbit.
- **orbital rim technique**
  a surgical technique that is no longer recommended for correction of prolapse of the gland of the third eye-

lid. This technique fixed the gland so it could no longer sweep across the eye spreading tears.

- **orbitotomy**
surgical procedure to access the back of the globe for a biopsy.

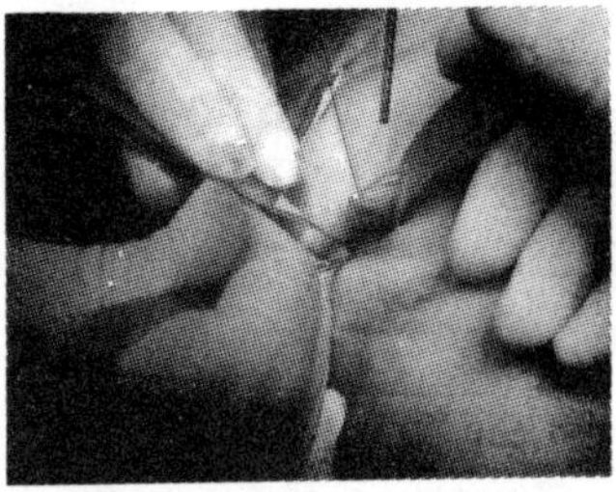

- **orchitis**
inflammation of the testicles.

- **organ system**
a group of organs that function together. For example the digestive system includes the oesophagus, intestinal tract, liver and pancreas because they all function to absorb and digest food.

- **os penis**
a bone in the penis of a dog. This is a structure unique to the dog.

- **osmolality**
a property of fluids determined by the number and size of particles in the fluid. Fluids with large numbers of small particles have a high osmolality.

- **osmolarity**
the concentration of osmotically active particles in solution expressed in as osmoles of solute per litre of solution.

- **osmotic diuretic**
a compound that increases the amount of urine formed and rids the body of excess fluid.

- **osteo-arthritis**
a permanent form of arthritis with progressive loss of the articular cartilage in a joint.

- **osteo-chondritis dessicans, OCD**
a piece of cartilage tears away forming a flap. The flap may reattach to the bone on its own, or it may tear away, becoming a joint mouse in the joint cavity. Symptoms include pain and limping. Often requires surgery.

- **osteo-chondrosis**
exercise causes as much of a growth spurt as does a big

feed intake. If inflamed joints are not backed off, you then risk osteo-chondrosis at stress points. Cartilage dies late and becomes encapsulated in normal bone nearby, leaving a hole that can fracture later on

- **osteo-myelitis**
  an infectious disease of bone that is often of bacterial origin.
- **otic**
  pertaining to the ear.
- **otitis externa**
  inflammation of the external ear canal.

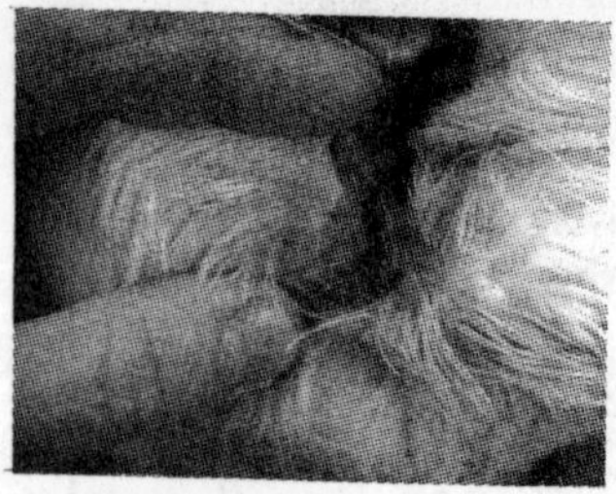

- **otoacariasis**
  ear mites.
- **otobius megnini**
  the spinous ear tick may induce otitis in dogs and occasionally cats.
- **ototoxic**
  destructive to the structures of the ear.
- **outside tie**
  when the male ejaculates with the bulbus glandis engorgement outside of the vagina. Females bred with an 'outside tie' usually don't get pregnant.
- **outcross**
  the mating of cats that have no common ancestors within several generations.
- **ova**
  eggs
- **ovarian bursa**
  a structure that surrounds the ovaries and collects eggs released from the ovary and channels those eggs to the uterus.
- **ovariectomies**
  lots of mares which have had ovariectomies for granulosa cell tumours go on to produce with one ovary.
- **ovariohysterectomy (Abrev: OVH)**
  the removal of the female reproductive organs.
- **ovary**
  the part of the female reproductive tract that produces eggs (ova) and female hormones.

- **over at the knee**
  a leg that looks like it has a forward arc with its centre at the knee when viewed from the side.

- **over the counter (Abrev: OTC)**
  can be purchased without a prescription, like aspirin and vitamins.

- **ovine progressive pneumonia (Abrev: OPP)**
  a chronic inflammatory disease of the lung leading to eventual suffocation.

- **ovulate**
  the release of an egg from the ovary of the female.

- **ovulation**
  the process of releasing eggs (ova) from the ovary.

- **oxidise**
  to combine with oxygen.

- **oxyglobin**
  a red blood cell substitute made from polymerised bovine haemoglobin.

- **oxytocin**
  a hormone that stimulates milk flow in lactating mammals (females nursing their young), and contractions of the muscles of the reproductive tract in many species.

- **P**
  pulse

- **P3**
  The third phalanx, or the third bone in a digit.

- **packed cell volume (PCV, haematocrit):**
  a laboratory test to monitor relative number of red blood cells present in the blood. A blood sample is placed in a tiny glass tube and spun in a centrifuge. The cells are heavier than the plasma and are compacted at one end of the tube. After the tube is spun, it is examined and the packed cell volume is determined as the percentage of the red cellular portion relative to the total amount of blood in the tube (i.e. remainder being the plasma). The normal for dogs is 40-59 and cats is 29-50

- **pain**
  an unpleasant sensory and emotional experience which may cause tissue damage.

- **paint**
  counter-irritant used to increase blood supply, blood flow and to promote heal-

ing in the leg. A mild form of blistering.

- **palatability**
the appeal and acceptability of feedstuffs. Affected by the taste, odour, texture and temperature of the feed.

- **palatable**
tasty; refers to food that is readily accepted.

- **palliative treatment**
palliative treatment is given to patients with untreatable diseases in order to make them more comfortable. Includes a combination of supportive and symptomatic treatments.

- **palmer**
back of the front limb from the knee down.

- **palp**
palpate or palpation

- **palpation**
to examine with the hands or fingers.

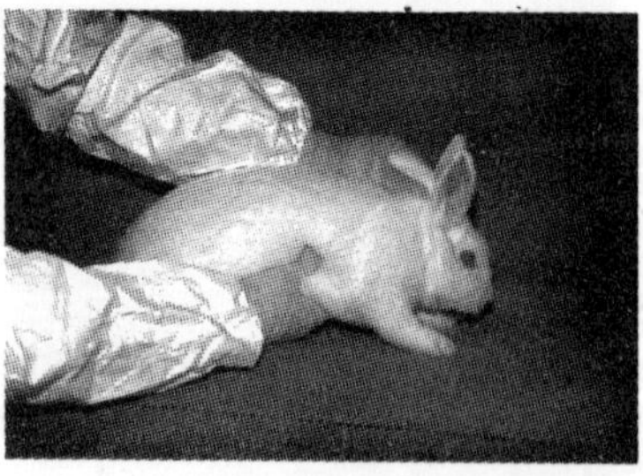

- **palpebral**
pertaining to the eyelids.

- **palpebral fissure**
the opening between the eyelids.

- **palpebral or blink reflex**
used to assess sensation and the ability to close the eyelids.

- **PAN**
peri-arteritis nodosa

- **pancreatitis**
inflammation of the pancreas due to a variety of causes such as infections and drugs. The pancreas produces enzymes and bicarbonate important in digestion and absorption of nutrients as well as insulin. Chronic, severe pancreatitis can result in malabsorption and diarrhoea as well as diabetes mellitus.

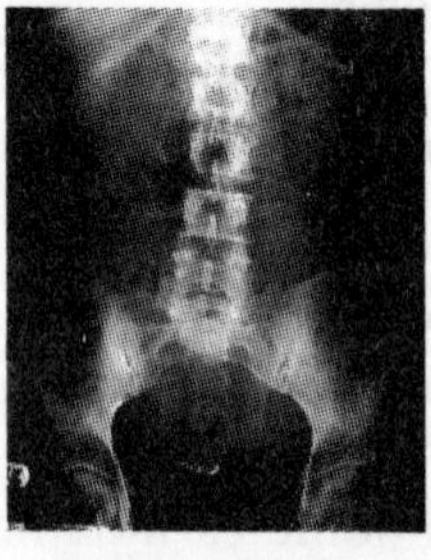

- **panleukopenia**
viral infection that attacks the bones and intestinal walls.

• **panniculitis**
inflammation of sub-cutaneous fat.

• **pannus**
a chronic condition of the eye in which blood vessels grow across the cornea (the clear surface of the eye). The cornea looks hazy and sometimes reddened and may eventually take on a dark pigment. This condition is also called chronic superficial keratitis.

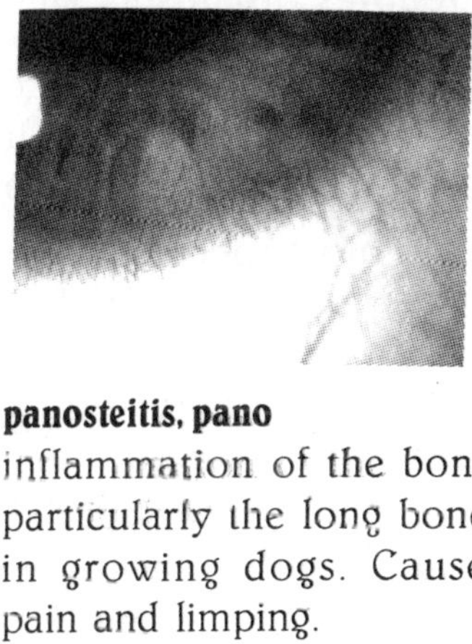

• **panosteitis, pano**
inflammation of the bone, particularly the long bones in growing dogs. Causes pain and limping.

• **PAO_2**
the concentration of oxygen in the blood.

• **papillae**
the tiny, pointed hooks on a cat's tongue that give the tongue its rough surface.

papillae

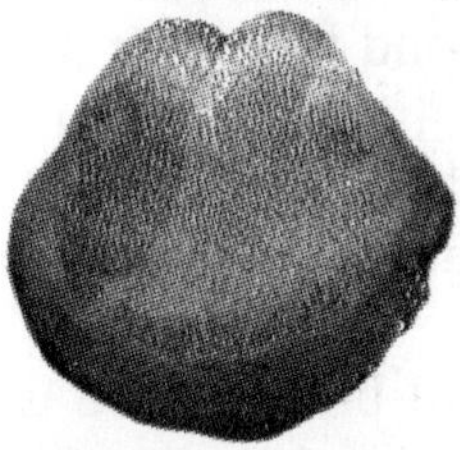

dorsal surface of cat's tongue

• **papule**
a small solid elevation of the skin. Larger lesions are called nodules or tumours and if flat, a plaque.

• **parabasal cell**
epithelial cells exfoliated from the vagina during proestrus. The cells are small and round with large and distinct nuclei. The total area of the cytoplasm of the parabasal cell is smaller than the nucleus.

• **paradoxical CSF acidosis**
paradoxical CSF acidosis is a condition caused by the administration of a large amount of bicarbonate to an acidotic patient, which will result in neurologic dysfunction. When one gives bicarbonate, the equation is shifted towards the left of the screen, towards the generation of CO_2. CO_2 is very diffusible, and will diffuse

across the blood brain barrier and then shift the equation in the cerebral spinal fluid towards the right with a generation of hydrogen ions. Even though additional bicarbonate is being generated in the CNS, the neurons perceive the increase in hydrogen ions and malfunction. The bicarbonate that was administered IV cannot cross the blood brain barrier.

- **parakeratosis**
  abnormal process of cornification.

- **paralysis**
  the loss of movement and/ or sensation on the body.

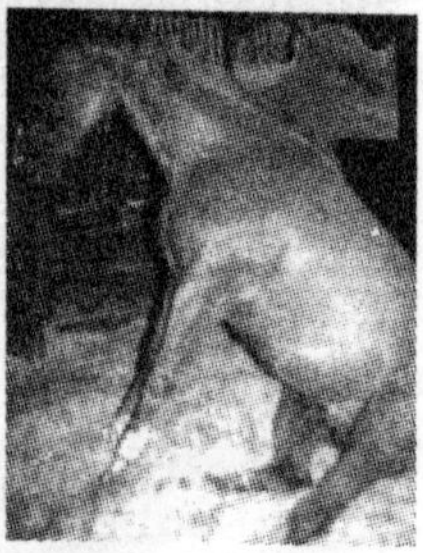

- **paraphimosis**
  paraphimosis is when the penis is extruded from the prepuce and cannot be returned to its normal position. This may occur following breeding or sexual excitement such as being kennelled next to a bitch in heat, or by a traumatic fracture of the dog's penis.

- **parasite**
  an organism that lives in or on another organism and often survives by draining nutrients from its host.

- **parasiticide**
  a substance that kills parasites.

- **parasitism**
  denotes organisms which survive and persist on or within another living organism. The parasite usually does not harm the animal. The most successful parasites achieve a balance whereby both the parasite and host animal survive. Among the parasites found on or within animals are bacteria, protozoans, fungi, mycoplasmas, rickettsia, and viruses.

- **parasympathetic nervous system**
  the portion of the nervous system which stimulates the pancreas to produce digestive enzymes and stimulates many of the smooth muscles in the body includ-

ing those of the stomach and intestine. It also tends to slow the heart rate.

- **parasympathomimetic effects**
  a drug that produces effects similar to the effects produced by stimulation of parasympathetic nerves.

- **parenterally**
  a term used to describe the administration of a drug by means other than by mouth.

- **paresis**
  slight or incomplete paralysis.

- **paronychia**
  inflammation of the nail fold.

- **paroxysmal**
  the sudden onset of a symptom that recurs. For example paroxysmal seizures begin suddenly and occur more than once.

- **parrot mouth**
  a horse with an extreme overbite.

- **partial parenteral nutrition**
  Abrev: PPN
  providing energy and nutritional supplementation to a patient at 50 to 70% of the patient's nutritional needs.

- **particle size**
  measure of the diameter of granular feed materials and/or the length of roughage fragments. Particle size can affect mixing of feed ingredients and digestion rate.

- **particolour**
  a coat pattern consisting of two or more colours in distinct patches.

- **parturition**
  the process of giving birth.

- **passive immunity**
  immunity produced by providing an animal with antibodies or immunologic cells from another source such as colostrums.

- **passive transfer**
  the transfer of antibodies from colostrums into the cria's blood.

- **pastern (bones)**
  denotes the area between the fetlock joint and the hoof. The joint between the long and short pastern bones is called the 'pastern joint.' Can also be used to describe the area of the limb or to describe a specific

bone long pastern bone. Technically known as the P1 (long) and P2 (short).

- **patellar luxation**
  dislocation of the 'knee' cap, causing mild to severe, continuous or intermittent pain.

- **patent ductus arteriosus, PDA**
  the normal opening between the aorta and pulmonary artery, which allows blood to bypass the unoxygenated lung in utero, fails to close after birth.

- **patent period**
  the parasites are producing eggs within the host.

- **pathogen**
  organisms that generally will cause disease

- **pathogenicity**
  capacity of parasite to produce disease.

- **pathogenic**
  causing disease.

- **pathologist**
  a specialist in veterinary medicine who examines the changes in body tissues and organs caused by disease.

- **pavletic**
  a surgical technique used to repair lid defects using skin from the lip.

- **PBT**
  pit bull terrier.

- **PCB (posterior cross bite)**
  a malocclusion where one or more of the mandibular premolar teeth occlude bucally with the maxillary teeth

- **PCV**
  see packed cell volume.

- **PD**
  polydipsia

- **PDA**
  patent ductus arteriosis

- **PE**
  physical examination

- **PE (pulpal exposure)**
  opening of the pulp organ made of blood vessels, nerves, and cellular elements to the outside environment usually caused by trauma

- **peak milk**
  maximum daily milk yield during lactation. Good peak yield is 100-120 lbs and occurs between 60-90 days in milk.

- **paediatric administration set**
an administration set for intravenous fluid administration. The set has a spike to penetrate the container of fluids, a drip chamber and a long flexible tube that connects to the patient's catheter. The drip set drips 60 drops to deliver one ml of fluid. The drops form in the drip chamber through a rigid needle-like structure. This needle-in-the-drip chamber identifies a paediatric drip set.

- **pediculosis**
an infestation of lice.

- **pedigree**
cats that have been bred for a specific purpose or for strict physical characteristics, and have been bred along pure lines for many years without interbreeding.

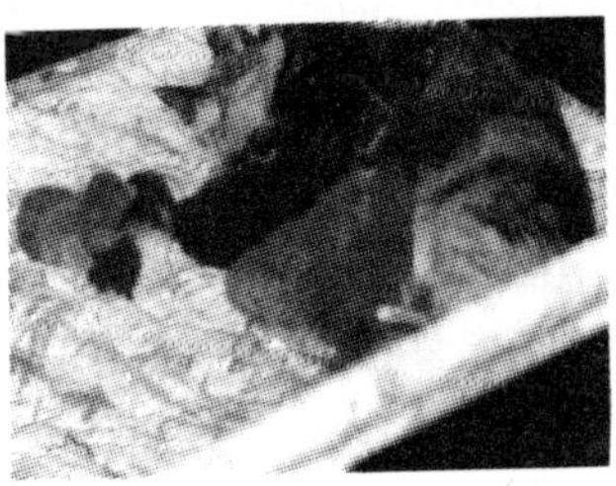

- **PEG tubes**
feeding tubes placed percutaneously using endoscopic guidance.

- **pelodera dermatitis**
rhabditic dermatitis. Larvae of the free living nematode, Pelodera strongyloides which penetrate the skin of animals.

- **pemphigus erythematosus (Abrev: PE)**
possibly an abortive form of pemphigus foliaceus. The clinical presentation is as a facial dermatitis.

- **pemphigus foliaceus**
a generalised scaling disease, with hair loss, and sometimes with the•formation of heavy crusts. Involvement of a nail bed leads to loss of the nail.

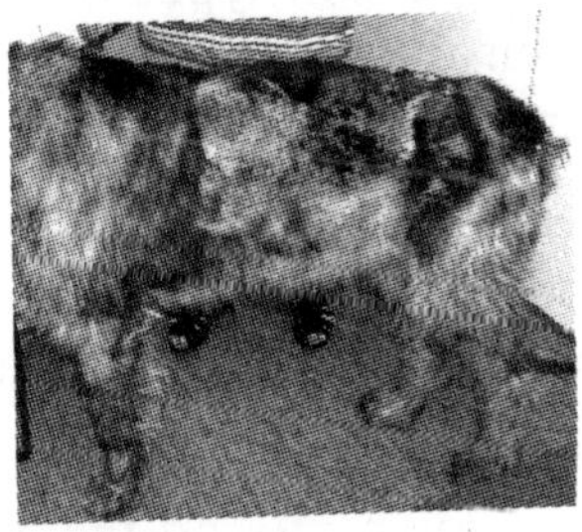

- **pemphigus foliaceus (Abrev: PF)**
the most common form of pemphigus recognised in the dog...also seen in the horse and other species.

- **pemphigus vegetans (Abrev: PVU)**
  a benign variant of pemphigus vulgaris with two classifications: the Neumann type which may begin and end as PVU and Hallopeau which is thought to be more of a benign form.

- **pen mating**
  a small number of females are penned with a male at regular intervals and are supervised during breeding.

- **penetration**
  the penis entering the female reproductive tract.

- **penicillinase**
  an enzyme produced by some bacteria which inactivates certain types of penicillin thus making the bacteria resistant to them.

- **penis**
  the male organ used to deposit semen in the female.

- **perianal**
  the region around the anus.

- **perianal fistula**
  a deep infection around the anus which often results in ulcers and deep draining tracts most commonly seen in German Shepherds.

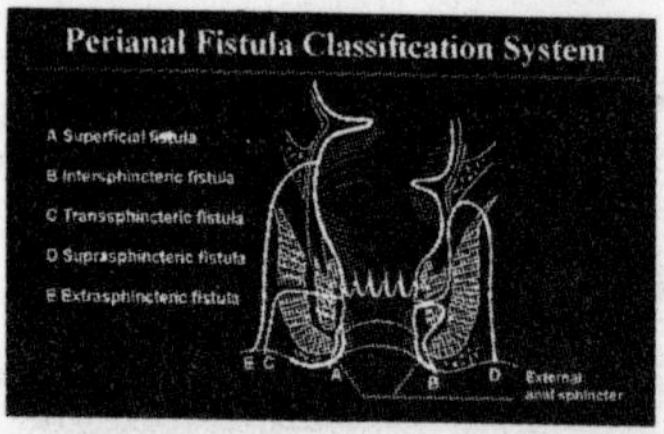

- **pericardium**
  a very thin tissue surrounding the heart. Abnormal fluid can accumulate between the heart and the pericardial membrane causing pericardial effusion.

- **perineal**
  the area between the anus and the genital organs.

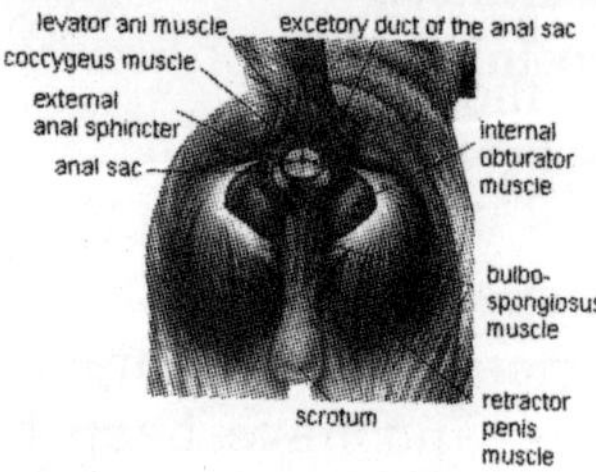

- **periostitis**
  inflammation of the tissue (periosteum) that overlies bone. Periostitis of the cannon bone is referred to as 'bucked shins', while periostitis of the splint bone is called a 'splint'.

- **peripheral IV catheter**
  a catheter placed in a smaller vein in a limb

(cephalic or saphenous). These catheters are relatively short in length.

- **peritoneal**
  the abdominal or belly cavity.
- **peritoneal cavity**
  the abdominal cavity between the viseral and parietal peritoneum.
- **peritonealdialysis**
  a process used to remove waste products from the body. Electrolyte fluids are administered into the abdomen, waste products of the body enter the fluids, and then the fluids are removed.
- **peritoneum**
  the membrane lining the wall of the abdominal cavity.
- **peritonitis**
  inflammation of the lining of the abdomen.
- **permethrin**
  a topical antiparasitic agent.
- **peroxidase-antiperoxidase staining**
  this technique uses an immuno histochemical procedure designed to demonstrate the presence of Ig or complement in a tissue section.
- **persistent pupillary membranes (Abrev: PPMs)**
  remnants of a blood vessels that once filled the anterior chamber and nourished the developing lens.
- **pet quality**
  a cat that does not meet the breed standard closely enough to be valuable to a breeding programme. Of course, pet quality cats are just as healthy and friendly as other cats.
- **PETA**
  People for the Ethical Treatment of Animals, an animal rights organisation.
- **pH**
  a measure of acidity or alkalinity. Values range from 0 (most acidic) to 14 (most alkaline or basic). A pH value of 7.0 is neutral (neither acidic nor alkaline).
- **phaeohyphomycoses**
  subcutaneous nodules, granulomatous lesions and draining tracts caused by Pythium sp.(Hyphomyces sp.), Dreschlera sp and other species.

- **Phagocyte**
  cell in the body which 'eats' damaged cells and foreign substances such as virus and bacteria. A macrophage is a type of phagocyte.

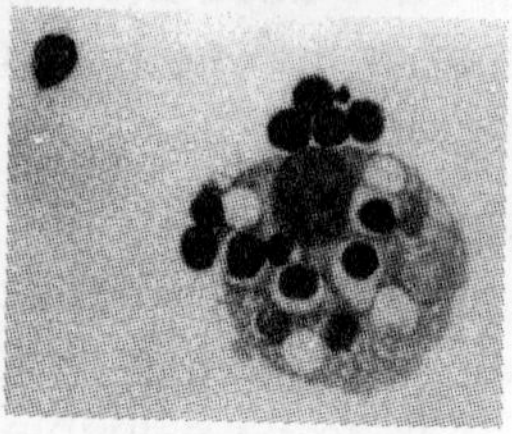

- **phagocytosis**
  the process of capture and destruction of foreign material. The two leading cells in this process are neutrophils and macrophages
- **phalanges**
  toes.
- **pharmacologic reactions to foods**
  an adverse reaction to food as a result of a naturally derived or added chemical that produces a drug-like pharmacological effect.
- **pharynx**
  back of the mouth. Throat.

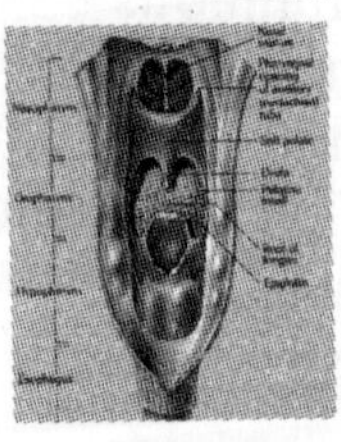

- **pheromone**
  chemical secreted by an animal and sensed by another animal of the same species, and often causing behaviour change in that animal.
- **phimosis**
  the penis cannot be extruded from the prepuce. Phimosis may be congenital due to a small preputial orifice or a persistent frenulum. Acquired inflammation or neoplasia can reduce the size of preputial orifice or increase the size of the penis causing phimosis.
- **photoperiod**
  the number of hours of light per 24-hour period.
- **photoreceptor layer**
  layer of the retina composed of the rods and cones.
- **photosensitivity**
  a condition in which the skin reacts abnormally to light, especially ultraviolet light or sunlight. It is usually caused by the interaction of light with certain chemicals in the skin such as antibiotics, other medications, hormones or toxins.

- **phthisis bulbi**
an eye that has degenerated after injury.

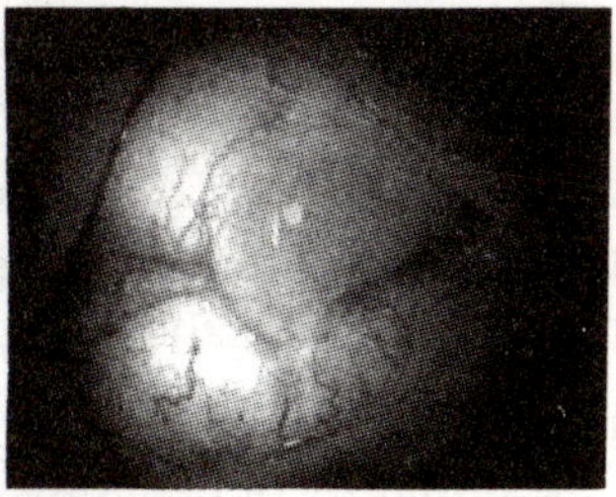

- **physiology**
the science dealing with the functions of animals.

- **physis**
plural physes. The 'growth plate' at the end of the long bones (such as the cannon bone) that lets the bone grow in length.

- **Phystochemical**
substances in plants which affect a body system and may promote health and decrease the risk of a disease such as cancer.

- **phystoestrogen**
substances which have an activity similar to oestrogens and are produced by plants.

- **pica**
chronic eating of non-food materials.

- **pigmentary keratitis**
the accumulation of pigment in the cornea in response to inflammation.

- **pin firing**
thermocautery used to increase blood flow to the leg to promote healing.

- **pinched muzzle**
snipy muzzle. Terminology usually employed to indicate an undesirable, overly refined muzzle. Such a muzzle is usually weakly structured and can appear over-chiselled and pointy. In some breeds, however, a pinched or snipy muzzle is to the liking (e.g., Lundehund).

- **pinking-up**
a lay term used to indicate pink nipples in a female animal which indicates increased blood flow to the nipples under the influence of progesterone.

- **pinnae**
the flap of the ear.

- **pinna-femoral reflex**
when the ear is rubbed, the dog scratches aggressively with the hind leg! Not a 'real'

reflex but is highly suggestive of scabies.

- **pinnal dermatitis**
  skin lesions on the ears.

- **pituitary gland**
  a hormone secreting (endocrine) gland at the base of the brain; it regulates growth as well as regulating the proper functioning of many other glands and processes.

Pituitary Gland

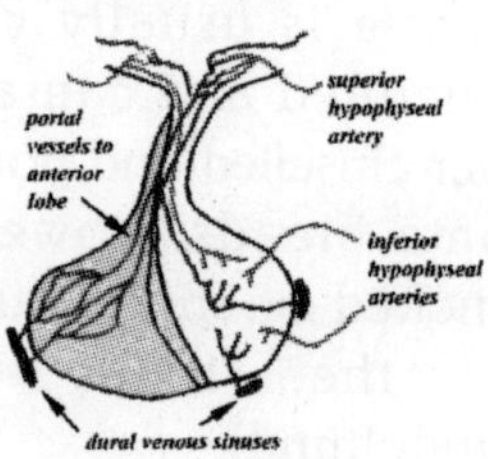

- **pizzle**
  prepuce.

- **placebo**
  a substance which is given that has no therapeutic value often called a 'dummy pill' or 'sugar pill'. Often given to half of the patients in a trial of a new drug, to better assess the effectiveness of the new drug.

- **placenta**
  after birth. An organ that allows for the mother to provide nutrition and remove wastes from the developing baby in the uterus.

- **plans**
  in a problem oriented record there are diagnostic plans, therapeutic plans and plans to inform the client.

- **plantar**
  pertaining to the sole of the foot or back of the hind limb from the hock down.

- **plantar ligament**
  the large ligament that is below and behind the hock joint.

- **plantigrade stance**
  standing and walking with the hocks on or almost touching the floor.

- **plaque**
  a build-up of bacteria, saliva and food on the teeth.

- **plasia**
  growth.

- **plasma**
  the clear part of blood that remains after blood is separated into cells and fluid before the blood clots. If the blood is allowed to clot then separated into cells and fluid, the fluid is then called serum.

- **plasma cell pododermatis**
  swelling and ulceration of the foot pads. Seen most frequently in cats.

- **plastron**
  the lower hard shell like structure which protects the abdomen of a turtle or tortoise.

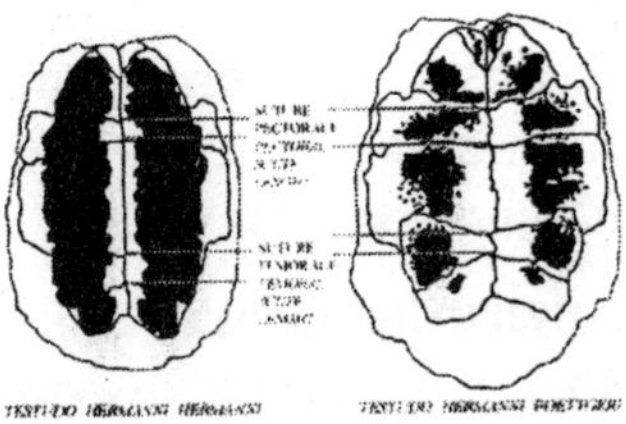

- **platelets**
  cellular components found in the blood which help clots to form. In the body, microscopically small vessels often break in the normal course of events. Platelets and a protein called fibrinogen 'plug' the break in the vessel and prevent blood from leaking out.

- **pluronic gel**
  topical application of an analgesic.

- **PM**
  1. pre-molar (tooth - followed by a number to indicate which one)
  2. post mortem

- **pneumonia**
  a serious disease characterised by lung inflammation.

- **pneumothorax**
  the abnormal accumulation of air in the chest cavity outside the lungs.

- **pocket technique**
  surgical technique for replacing a prolapse of the gland of the third eyelid.

- **pointed**
  a coat pattern consisting of a solid colour on the body and a darker colour on the ears, tail, face and legs.

- **pointer**
  a breed native to the British Isles, the Pointer is reportedly the first dog used to 'stand game', in the sense that we use the term today. The exact origin of the Pointer remains a topic of discussion. It was once held as common belief that the Pointer traced back to the pointers of Spain. This belief is still adamantly adhered to by many. An alternative theory states that the Pointer of Great Britain is a breed distinct from the Continental pointers, asserting that the various pointer breeds developed separately

but parallel to each other, regardless of whether or not the base stock was similar. What is certain is that the pointer did emerge as the premier workman of its kind. It is unquestionable that Spanish Pointer was infused into the Pointer's lines, but it remains undocumented whether or not the blood was received exclusively after the Pointer's type was fixed.

- **points**
extremes of the body comprising the mask, ears, legs and tail.

- **poison**
any substance that can cause an adverse effect when introduced into a biological system (not acting mechanically).

- **pole(s)**
the top of the head, between the ears.

- **poliosis**
whitening of the hair.

- **pollakiuria**
frequent passage of small amounts of urine. Pollakiuria is indicative of diseases of the lower urinary tract and genital tract.

- **polled**
breed where there has been a genetic selection for no horns. Some sheep breeds are horned in both sexes, in others only the males are horned and in yet others (the majority of breeds) neither sex is horned.

- **poly**
means several or too much such as polydactyly means having too many toes.

- **polyarteritis nodosa**
an inflammatory disease of small and medium sized arteries.

- **polyarthritis**
arthritis which involves two or more joints.

- **polyarthropathy**
inflammatory joint disease that involves multiple joints.

- **polyclonal antibody**
the term used to describe a mixture of Ig to a wide array of antigens.

- **polycystic kidney disease (Abrev: PKD)**
a disease in which kidney tissue is replaced by multiple cystic stuctures. There is an inherited form of polycystic

kidney disease in Persian cats.

- **polycythemia**
polycythemia is an increased number of circulating RBC. Most animals with increased PCV have relative polycythemia due to haemoconcentration. Splenic contraction can increase PCV by 10 to 15%. Absolute polycythemia is an increased total hemoglobin/ RBC mass with normal plasma volume. Absolute polycythemia can be a primary myeloproliferative disorder called polycythemia vera. The signs of polycythemia vera can include polyuria and polydipsia, bleeding from small capillary rupture, neurological disturbances caused by increased viscosity of blood.

- **polydactyl**
the presence of extra toes.

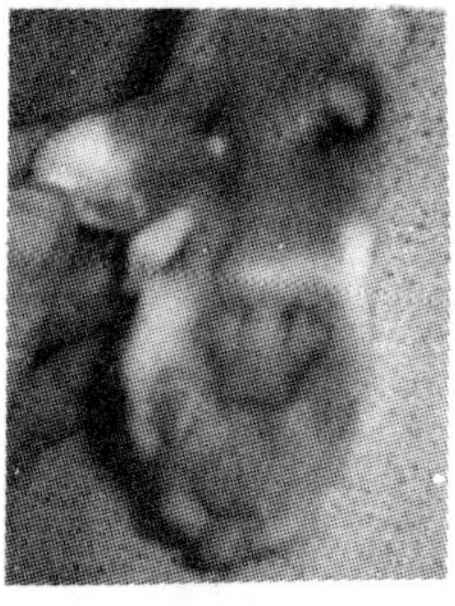

- **polydipsia (Abrev: PD)**
excessive thirst resulting in excessive drinking.

- **polyestrous**
during one sexual season, continuing to come into heat if not bred. Cats are polyestrous, dogs are not.

- **polymer**
a molecule made of repeating units (monomers). For example starch is a polymer of glucose molecules.

- **polymerase chain reaction (Abrev: PCR)**
a technique to rapidly produce many copies of a fragment of DNA.

- **polymyositis**
inflammation of several muscles at one time.

- **polyp**
a small growth from mucous membranes such as those lining the nasal cavity and intestinal tract.

- **polyphagia**
excessive ingestion of food.

- **polysaccharide**
a carbohydrate containing a large number of sugar groups. Starch is an example of a polysaccharide.

- **polyurethane**
  a type of plastic used to make, among other things, IV catheters.
- **polyuria (Abrev: PU)**
  urinating large amounts of urine.
- **polyvalent**
  a vaccine containing several antigens (multivalent).
- **pop**
  popliteal (lymph node)
- **portosystemic shunt, PSS**
  abnormal blood vessels in the liver preventing normal circulation and functioning of the liver.
- **portuguese water dog**
  robust and well-endowed with muscle and strength, the Portuguese Water Dog sports the conformation of a fine Olympic swimmer.
- **post coital**
  after sex.
- **post renal azotemia**
  an increase in nitrogen containing wastes in the blood due to an inability to excrete urine as a consequence of an obstruction to urine passage or to a ruptured bladder.
- **posterior**
  situated behind or toward the rear.
- **posterior chamber**
  space between the iris and lens.
- **posterior synechia**
  occurs when the inflamed iris sticks to the lens.
- **post-operative**
  after surgery.
- **postpartum**
  the period of time immediately following birth.
- **postprandial**
  the period of time immediately after eating.
- **potato dextrose agar**
  a fungal growth media that promotes rapid sporulation making identification possible at an earlier time than when using standard culture media.
- **povidine-iodine**
  a topical antibacterial available as a shampoo or in solution.
- **PP**
  periodontal pocket

- **PPI**
  parvovirus and parainfluenza: dog vaccine covering these diseases
- **PPP**
  pretty poor prognosis
- **praise**
  positive reinforcement that indicates satisfaction to your cat.
- **pre-anaesthetic**
  a drug given before general anaesthesia, usually a sedative or tranquilliser which is given to reduce apprehension and to allow the use of lower doses of the more potent anaesthetic agents.
- **pre-breeding evaluation**
  examination of potential breeding animals to assess their capability to produce offspring.
- **pred**
  prednisolone
- **predicted transmitting ability (Abrev: PTA)**
  genetic merit of parent transmitted to its progeny.
- **preemptive analgesia**
  the administration of analgesic drugs before the onset of a painful stimulus, administered to reduce the perception of pain.
- **pregnant**
  when a female animal is carrying unborn offspring.
- **premature**
  born too early.
- **premix**
  a uniform mixture of one or more microingredients and a carrier, used to facilitate uniform dispersion of micro-nutrients into a larger mixture.
- **prepotent**
  a cat who has such a strong genetic influence on its offspring that the offspring consistently resemble the parent. Most prepotent cats are line bred on one or more outstanding ancestors.
- **prepuce**
  the tissue that covers the penis. Sometimes called the sheath.
- **prerenal azotemia**
  an increase in nitrogen containing waste products in the blood caused by reduced renal blood flow as a consequence of hypovolemia or dehydration. Untreated prerenal azotemia can

progress to intrinsic renal disease.

- **prevalence**
  the proportion of sampled animals that display a condition of interest at a given point in time. It is a single measurement of each animal in a group. It is usually a static measure in which the time is short (1-7 days).

- **primary abnormality**
  morphological abnormalities of sperms that occur while the sperm are being produced in the testes.

- **primary closure**
  suturing the raw edges of the wound together.

- **primary oocyte**
  the immature egg as it is released from the ovary.

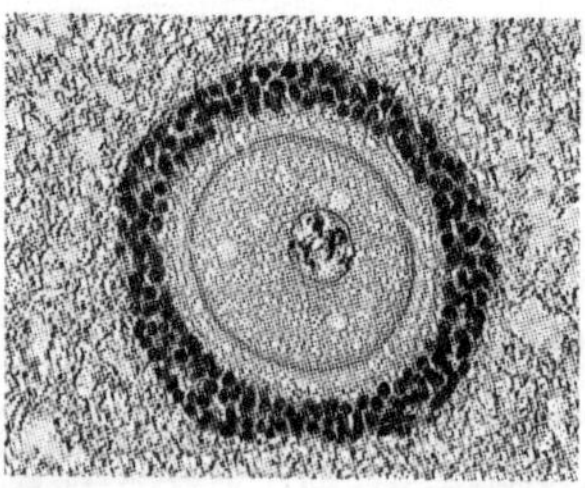

- **primary uterine inertia**
  ineffective or absent uterine contractions during parturition. Primary uterine inertia should be considered when a bitch is not able to start uterine contractions. This condition occurs most often in older bitches and/or bitches with hypocalemia and/or hypoglycemia.

- **prion**
  infectious protein. Scrapie in sheep, Creutzfeldt Jakob disease in humans, and Bovine Spongifor Encephalopathy in cattle (Mad Cow Disease)are all caused by prions.

- **prn**
  as needed (pro re nata - Latin)

- **prob**
  probably or problem

- **probiotics**
  a live microbial feed supplement which beneficially affects the host animal. Claims include reduced early mortality, increased growth rate, improved feed conversion, egg quality and animal health.

- **problem**
  a problem is anything that interferes with the patient's well being and requires further management or evalu-

ation or anything that the owner is concerned about

- **problem list**
  a list of what is wrong with a patient based on the information that is gathered from history, physical examination and the results of diagnostic tests.

- **problem oriented medical records (Abrev: POMR)**
  the POMR system is a logical system centred around the identification and resolution of the patient's problems. The problem oriented approach differs from other approaches in which a list of differential diagnoses are generated in the exam room, without giving much consideration to the possibility that not all the patient's problems are due to the same cause. Although the problem based approach is also intended to lead to a diagnosis, the problem based approach prevents the clinician from 'jumping to a diagnosis' with tunnel vision and potentially overlooking important aspects of the patients disease(s).

- **problem specific data base**
  the minimum amount of information that is planned to be collected for patients with specific types of problems. For example, a chest radiograph may be recommended to be preformed on all patients that were hit by a car.

- **procainamide**
  antiarrhythmic used in treatment of ventricular arrhythmias.

- **procalAmine**
  a pre-made solution used in partial parenteral solution.

- **proestrus**
  the stage of the estrus cycle right before an animal comes into heat.

- **progeny**
  offspring.

- **progesterone**
  the hormone produced by the corpus luteum which maintains pregnancy.

- **progestin implants for mares**
  it's an extralabel use of various cattle implants. Done in the neck region, seems to help for about 5-6 months, no hard data on any residual effects on fertility.

- **prognosis**
the forecasted outcome and recovery.

- **progress notes**
a written description in a patient's record that summarises data plans, treatment, rationelle for diagnostics and treatments, and the patient's response to treatment.

- **progressive retinal atrophy, PRA**
any of a number of inherited diseases of the eye leading to blindness. Generally starts with difficulty seeing in the dark followed by a loss of vision in the daylight. In the BMD it is an autosomal recessive trait.

- **prolactin**
hormone secreted by the pituitary gland that stimulates the growth of mammary tissue and the production of milk.

- **prolapse**
the abnormal position of an organ in which the organ pouches through an opening from which it does not normally protrude.

- **prolapsed rectum**
because of irritation or injury, the inner part of the rectum is pushed out so that it is visible as a pink mass protruding from the anal opening.

- **prop**
when a horse suddenly stops moving by digging its front feet into the ground.

- **proprioception**
maintenance of posture and movement through stimuli originating in the receptors in the joints, tendons, muscles, and labyrinth.

- **proptosis**
bulging of the eye out of the socket.

- **prostaglandin**
several types of chemicals made by cells which have specific functions such as controlling body temperature, stimulating smooth muscle, and influencing heat cycles.

- **prostaglandin analogue**
drugs used in the treatment of glaucoma. They cause extreme meiosis and may have an influence on the unconventional outflow of

aqueous. Lantoprost is available as a 0.005% topical solution.

- **prostaglandin F2 alpha**
a hormone that destroys the corpus luteum which in turn causes progesterone to decrease.

- **prostaglandin**
several types of chemicals made by cells which have specific functions such as controlling body temperature, stimulating smooth muscle, and influencing heat cycles.

- **prostate**
a accessory gland of the male that contributes to semen production.

- **prostatitis**
inflammation of the prostate gland.

- **prosthesis**
an artificial eye placed after enucleation for cosmetic purposes.

- **protease**
enzyme which breaks down protein.

- **protected fat**
a fat that has been treated or combined with another substance to prevent breakdown in the rumen.

- **protein**
naturally-occurring compounds containing nitrogen, carbon, hydrogen and oxygen, and sometimes sulfur or phosphorus. Proteins are made up of complex combinations of amino acids and are essential for animal growth, production and reproduction.

- **protein nitrogen units (Abrev: PNU)**
unit of strength for antigens used in intradermal skin testing. 100, 000 PNU = 1 mg protein.

- **protein supplement**
a feed or mixture of feeds containing 20% or more protein. Examples: soybean meal, canola meal.

- **prothrombin time (Abrev: PT)**
measurement of clotting time of plasma in the presence of excess tissue thromboplastin. Factors measured are fibrinogen, prothrombin, and factors V, VII, and X.

- **protozoans**
single celled animals invisible to the naked eye. Most

are free living and a few are parasites in animals or man.

- **proud flesh**
proud flesh is defined as an overabundance of granulation tissue, which is the normal tissue which grows in to fill a defect. It is composed mainly of fibroblasts and capillaries. When it overgrows above a plane level with the surrounding epithelium, it becomes more difficult for the adjacent skin to grow over the area.

- **proximal**
toward the body, i.e., the proximal cannon region is the upper portion of the cannon bone.

- **pruritus**
itchiness.

- **pseudohyperparathyroidism**
pseudohyperparathyroidism causes hypercalcemia and most commonly occurs in patients with lymphoma or tumours of the apocrine anal sac. Pseudohyperparathyroidism has been reported associated with other tumour types.

- **pseudomycetomas**
deep dermal or subcutaneous infections by dermatophytes. They present as nodules and draining lesions, that histologically are pyogranulomatous to granulomatous panniculitis. M. canis is the causative organism in the cat.

- **pseudopregnancy**
giving the appearance of being pregnant when not really pregnant. Signs may include weight gain, enlarged abdomen, mammary gland enlargement, and nesting behaviour. Pseudopregnancy is considered a normal occurrence in the bitch.

- **psittacine**
birds that belong to the order Psittaciformes. Common psittacines include budgies, cockatiels, lories, cockatoos, conures, amazons, African greys, lovebirds, senegals, andjardines.

- **PTS**
put to sleep (euthanase)

- **PU (pulpitis)**
inflammation of the pulp results in discoloration of the tooth

- **PU/PD**
  polyuria/polydipsia
- **puberty**
  when the female starts to have some reproductive activity.
- **pulled suspensory**
  suspensory ligament injury (suspensory desmitis) in which some portion of the fibres of the ligament have been disrupted and some loss of support of the distal limb may have occurred.
- **pulmonary**
  relating to the lungs.
- **pulmonary arteries**
  the large vessels leading from the heart to the lungs.
- **pulmonary edema**
  fluid accumulation in the lungs.
- **pulmonary emboli/embolism:**
  blood clot that travels to the blood vessels in the lung and obstructs them.
- **pulseless electrical activity (Abrev: PEA)**
  a new term for electrical-mechanical disassociation in which an ECG shows electrical activity of the heart but there is no associated mechanical activity (heartbeat).
- **punctum**
  holes in the edges of the eyelids through which tears enter the nasolacrimal ducts.
- **PUO**
  pyrexia of unknown origin
- **pupa**
  a dormant form of an insect (plural pupae). A larva spins a cocoon to protect itself, and becomes a pupa. The pupa does not feed but gradually changes form and becomes a new adult.
- **pupillary light response (Abrev: PLR)**
  the ability of the pupil to constrict in response to light.
- **purebred**
  a cat whose ancestors are all of the same breed, or whose ancestry includes crossbreeding that is allowed in the breed standard. For example, a purebred Bombay may also have Burmese cats in its background.
- **purulent**
  pus discharge.

- **pustule**
  small elevated area on the skin filled with pus.
- **px**
  1. physical examination or physical examination findings
  2. prognosis
- **pyelonephritis**
  a bacterial infection of the kidneys.
- **pyloroduodenal**
  an obstruction in the area where the stomach and small intestine meet.
- **pyoderma**
  skin infection with bacteria. Pyodermas involve coagulase positive bacteria, most commonly Staphylococcus intermedius.
- **pyometra**
  pus accumulation in the uterus, normally caused by bacterial infection.
- **recessive**
  requires a copy of the gene from both parents to exhibit the trait. Having only one copy of the gene makes the dog a carrier of the trait, and he will never exhibit the trait unless the gene is located on the 'X' or sex chromosome.
- **sarcomatumour**
  formed of connective tissue cells bone cartilage, muscle, blood vessel, or lymphoid tissue.
- **pyrexia**
  elevated temperature, fever.
- **pyriproxyfen**
  an insect growth regulator. Available combined with permethrin in a spray for use on adult dogs and a fogger or spray for household treatment.
- **pyuria**
  white blood cells in the urine.
- **PZI**
  protamine zinc insulin
- **q.d.**
  once a day. From latin: quaque die. Same as s.i.d. but not to be confused with q.i.d.
- **q.i.d.**
  four times a day. From latin: quater in die
- **QOL**
  quality of life
- **quarantine**
  any facility used to keep infected horses away from the general equine population.

- **quarter crack**
  a crack between the toe and heel, usually extending into the coronary band.
- **queen**
  a female cat. When used as a verb, 'to queen' describes a cat giving birth.

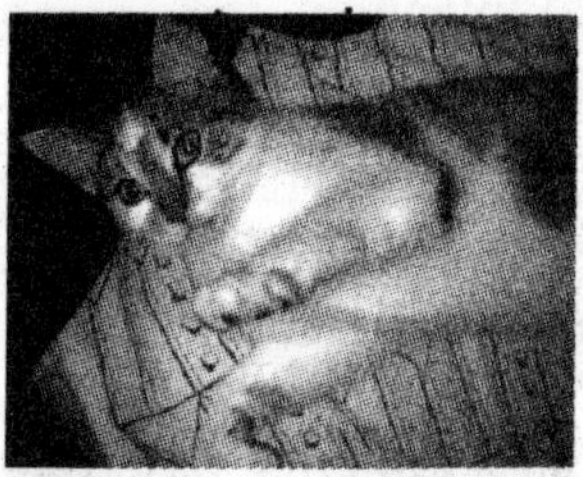

- **queening**
  in cats, the act of giving birth.
- **quick**
  the root inside a nail that feeds blood to the nail.
- **quick mix**
  a pre-made solution used in partial parenteral solution.
- **rotated tooth**
  usually secondary to tooth crowding, most commonly affected teeth are the maxillary second and third premolars

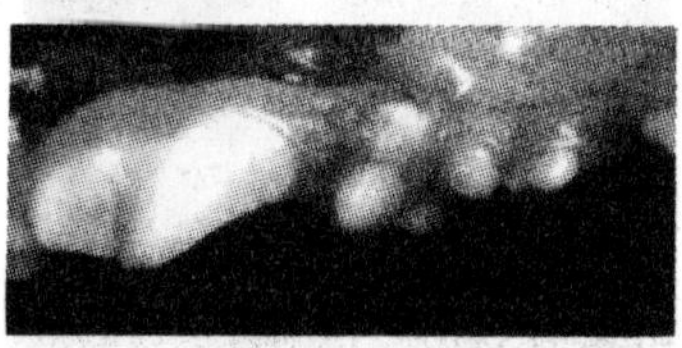

- **R/A**
  restoration amalgam

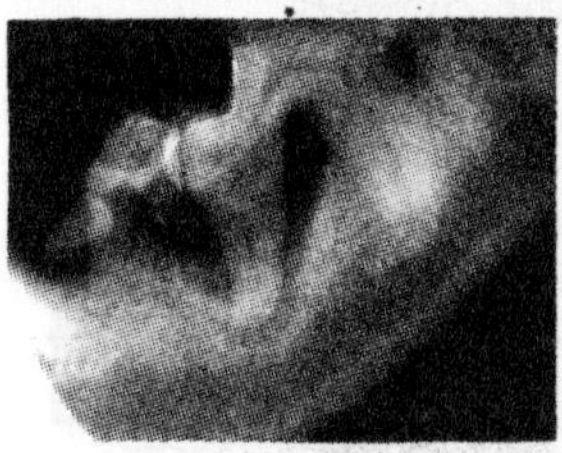

- **R/C**
  restoration composite
- **R/I**
  restoration glass ionomer
- **R/M**
  restoration metallic crown

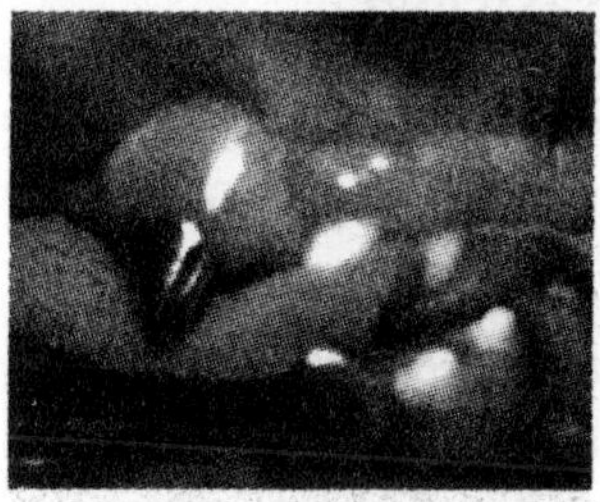

- **R/O**
  rule out
- **RA**
  right atrium
- **rabies**
  a fatal viral disease of warm blooded animals including man that affects the brain and is spread in the saliva of infected animals. Rabid animals have a temperament change. Wild creatures become bold enough to attack

human beings and domestic animals may turn on their owners.

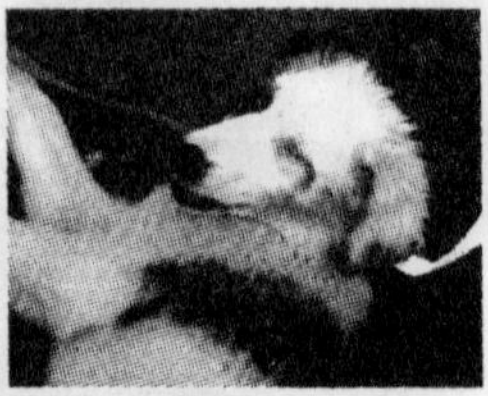

- **raddle**
marking crayon on breast of ram that will mark the rump of ewes that have been bred.

- **radial immuno diffusion (Abrev: RID)**
a test used to evaluate whether the newborn has received antibodies in colostrums.

- **radio-allergosorbent test (Abrev: RAST)**
test to measure specific serum IgE levels.

- **radiograph**
the image generated by an x-ray. Often the term x-ray is used incorrectly to refer to a radiograph.

- **radio immuno assay (Abrev: RIA)**
a method used to measure the concentration of some hormones.

- **radiology**
x-ray.

- **RAE**
right atrial enlargement

- **rainrot**
rainrot does have some resemblance to a fungus but it is 'not' a fungus. It is a bacterial infection. *Dermatophilus congolensis*, a filamentous bacterium is the causative agent.

- **ramp-up**
a period of time during which effective blood levels of a drug are building up.

- **ration**
the 24-hour feed allowance for an individual animal.

- **RBC**
red blood cell

- **RC 1W**
recheck in 1 week

- **RCM**
restrictive cardiomyopathy

- **RCT**
root canal therapy

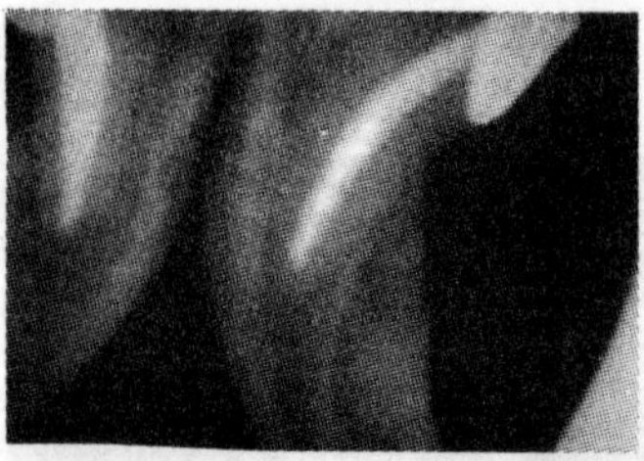

• **RD**
retained deciduous teeth
teeth that have not been shed when secondary (permanent) teeth erupt

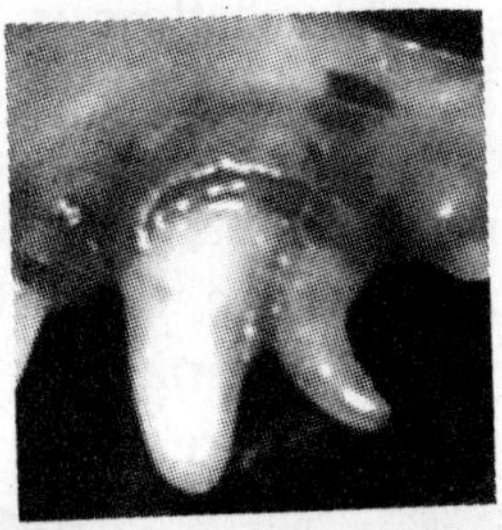

• **RDVM**
Referring Dr Veterinary Medicine

• **reagent grade**
a compound with the purity and quality that allows it to be used in a laboratory

• **receptive**
the female is accepting of being mounted and bred by a male.

• **receptivity**
when the female starts becoming receptive to the male and is ready to breed.

• **recombinant vaccine**
there are certain antigens on viruses and bacteria which are better at stimulating an antibody response by the animal than others. The genes for these antigens can be isolated, and made to produce large quantities of the antigens they code for. A recombinant vaccine contains these antigens, not the whole organism.

• **rectus muscles**
there are 4 rectus muscles that allow for movement of the globe: dorsal, ventral, lateral, and medial.

• **recumbency**
lying down.

• **redefined**
a problem is redefined if a more specific label can be applied. For example vomitting is redefined or updated to acute pancreatitis as laboratory results become available that support the diagnosis of pancreatitis.

• **redefined problem**
a patient's problem is redefined if it is updated to a higher level...for example, vomitting may be updated to uremia as the results of diagnostic tests become available and show an elevated BUN.

- **reflex ovulator**
only ovulating after being bred. Cats are reflex ovulators dogs are not.

- **registry**
a database of health information

- **regulation**
using insulin to maintain the blood glucose level of an animal within the acceptable range.

- **regurgitation**
backward movement of food from the oesophagus out the mouth.

- **rehydration solution**
a solution administered to a dehydrated animal to return its hydration state to normal. Most dehydrated dogs and cats have isotonic dehydration and are rehydrated with iostonic, isoionic solutions such as LRS or RS.

- **relaxin**
a hormone which is detectable when a fertilised egg is implanted, which usually occurs around day 21 following fertilisation.

- **renal**
pertaining to the kidneys.

- **renal blood flow (Abrev: RBF)**
the blood presented to the kidneys. The kidneys receive about 20 to 25% of cardiac output each minute. Renal blood flow is determined by blood volume, blood pressure and cardiac output. The kidneys can also autoregulate their blood flow within certain ranges of blood pressure.

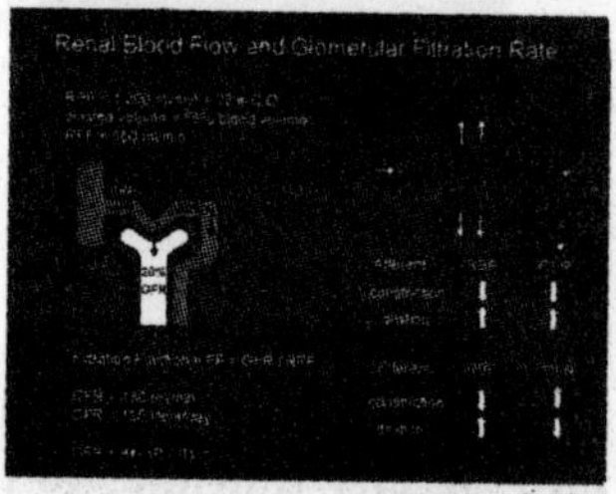

- **renal insufficiency**
the decreased ability of the kidneys to rid the body of wastes.

- **replacement**
a calf kept and/or raised at the dairy as a future replacement for a cow in the herd. Replacement rate should average between 25%-33% of the herd/year.

- **replacement females**
new females that have recently been introduced to a herd.

- **reproductive cycle**
  events that happen in the female such as ovulation, hormone production, receptivity, etc. In camelids the cycle does not follow regular time periods as it does in horses or cattle.

- **reservoir**
  where a disease causing organism lives and multiplies. Therefore the reservoir may not be the source of the organism.

- **reservoirs of the contagious mastitis**
  the cow herself, humans, flies, and others.

- **resistance**
  a term used to describe bacteria which have mutated or changed so that they are not affected by an antibiotic that previously killed them or slowed their growth. As more bacteria become resistant to various antibiotics, there are fewer antibiotics which will have an affect on them, thus newer and stronger antibiotics will need to be developed. Inappropriate use of antibiotics (using them too often, for too short a duration or in insufficient dose) may promote the development of resistance.

- **resolved**
  problems are resolved if they no longer exist either because they were treated or resolved spontaneously with the passing of time.

- **resorption**
  in pregnancy, a condition in which the foetus dies, and instead of being aborted, the foetal tissue dissolves within the uterus and is absorbed by the mother. The mother will show no outward signs of a foetal resorption.

- **respiratory**
  relating to breathing or the lungs.

- **respiratory depression**
  decrease in the rate or depth of respiration.

- **respiratory system**
  organ system responsible for gas exchange from nostrils to lungs.

- **respiratory transmission**
  the most common route of human exposure in countries where infection is controlled in animals and

where there is pasteurisation of milk.

- **resting membrane potential (Abrev: RMP)**
  the electrical charge of resting myocardial cells. Normally the RMP is -90 mV. Hyperkalemia elevates the RMP to a less negative state.
- **resuscitative fluid**
  a fluid used in cardiopulmonary resuscitation (CPR) in an attempt to restore circulation.
- **reticular activating formation**
  a collection of neurons in the brain that mediates many aspects of consciousness.
- **retina**
  the rear interior surface of the eyeball. The retina contains nerve cells referred to as rods and cones. The rods are sensitive to light and the cones to colour. The retina receives the light and colour and converts them into nerve impulses which go to the brain.
- **retinal dysplasia**
  a congenital anomalous development of the retina.
- **retinoids**
  synthetic derivatives of vitamin A.
- **retractor bulbi muscle**
  the muscle that pulls the eyeball back into the orbit.
- **retropulsion**
  pushing on the orbit to evaluate the ability to compress the soft tissue structures behind the orbit.
- **rex**
  re-examine
- **RF**
  right fore
- **RH**
  right hind
- **rhinotracheitis**
  a serious respiratory illness.
- **RI**
  re-examine/re-inspect
- **RI 7D**
  return in 7 days
- **ridgling ('rig')**
  a term describing either a cryptorchid or monorchid. Also spelled 'ridgeling.'
- **righting reflex**
  the ability to properly orient the body during a fall.

- **ring**

  an area at a show where one judge examines cats and awards prizes. A show may have several simultaneous rings.

- **ring bone**

  osteoarthritis of joints between the pastern bones ('high ring bone') or just above the coronet ('low ring bone').

- **ringer's solution**

  ringer's solution does not contain lactate. It contains a higher concentration of chloride compared to lactated Ringer's solution. Ringer's solution is considered an acidifying solution. This does not mean that it can cause metabolic acidosis, but it can assist a patient who has a metabolic alkalosis correct their own acid base abnormality.

- **ringworm**

  a type of fungal infection of the skin.

- **RL**

  right lower (eg. eyelid, lip)

- **RMRCVS**

  referring MRCVS

- **roan**

  a horse colour where the majority of the coat of the horse is a mixture of red and white hairs or brown and white hairs. The mane, tail and legs may be black, chestnut or roan unless white markings are present. Starting with foals of 1993, the colour classifications gray and roan were combined as 'roan or gray.'

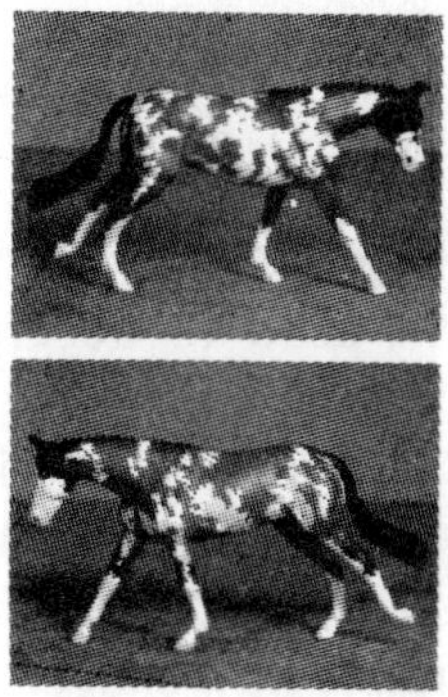

- **roaring (laryngeal hemiplegia)**

  a whistling sound made by a horse during inhalation while exercising. It is caused by a partial or total paralysis of the nerves controlling the muscles which elevate the arytenoid cartilages which thereby open the larynx. In severe cases, a surgical procedure known as 'tie-back surgery' (laryngoplasty) is performed, in which a suture is inserted through the cartilage to hold it out of the airway permanently. Paralysis almost exclusively occurs on the left side, most frequently in horses over 16 hands high.

- **rogue**
  ill-tempered horse.
- **rolling herd**
  the most recent 12 month herd milk production average.
- **rost**
  rostral
- **roughage**
  a term used to describe a feed high in fibre (greater than 18% crude fibre). Roughage tends to be bulky, coarse, and low in energy. Examples: hay, silage, straw.
- **roundworm**
  a parasitic worm resembling round spaghetti that may cause illness, particularly in young, old or weakened cats.

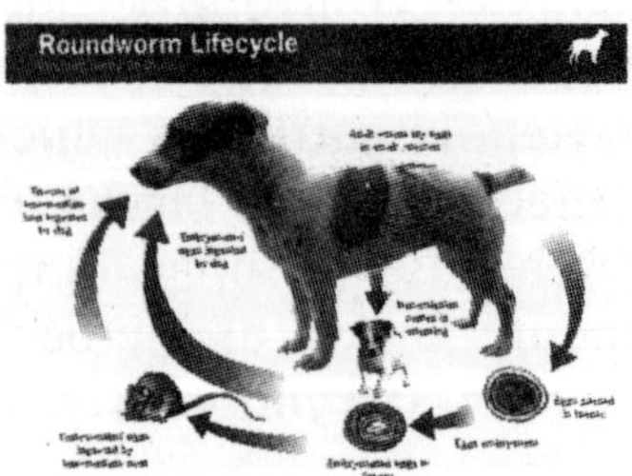

- **route of administration**
  the way a drug is administered to an animal i.e. orally, intramuscularly, intravenously.
- **route of infection**
  the manner in which an infectious agent gains access to the animal.
- **RPC**
  root planning closed
- **RPO**
  root planning open
- **RPT**
  repeat
- **RR**
  retained root
  areas where crown is no longer apparent but root(s) remain
- **RRM**
  restricted range of movement eg., in a joint
- **RRR**
  resting respiration rate
- **RS**
  remove sutures
- **RTA**
  road traffic accident
- **RU**
  right upper (eg. eyelid, lip)

- **ruff**
  Protruding or lengthened hair around the neck and chest.

- **rule-outs (Abrev: R/O)**
  rule-outs are also known as differential diagnoses and are possible causes for the problems displayed by a patient. For example, kidney failure is one rule out (or possible cause) for polyuria in a dog or cat.

- **ruminant**
  a cud-chewing animal having four stomach compartments. The rumen (first stomach), is a major site of microbial fermentation of feeds permitting breakdown of fibre. Examples: cattle, sheep, goats.

- **run down**
  abrasions of the heel.

- **RV**
  recheck

- **RV**
  right ventricle

- **RVE**
  right ventricular enlargement

- **supernumerary tooth**
  extra adult tooth in the arch. Most commonly located in the incisor and premolar areas. Supernumery teeth may cause overcrowding causing periodontal disease or traumatic occlusion

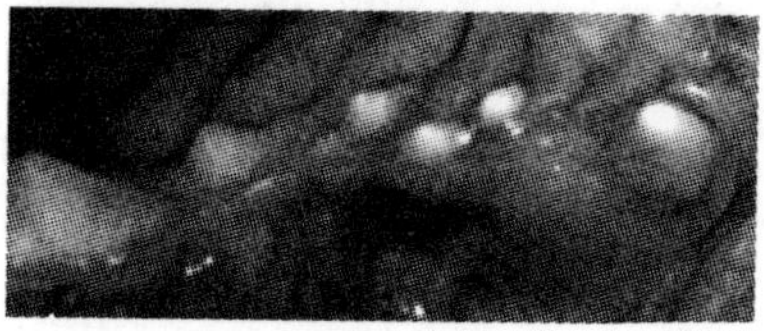

- **S&P**
  scale and polish (of teeth)

- **S.I.D.**
  Once a day. From latin semel in die

- **S/M**
  submandibular

- **S/O**
  stitches (or staples) out

- **S/R**
  suture removal

- **sabouraud's dextrose agar**
  the standard media for fungal culture.

- **sagittal**
  longitudinal view.

- **salmonella**
  major sign in affected horses is fetid and profuse diarrhoea. Fever, anorexia, and a significant neutropenia are also present. Origins – the

bacterium Salmonella spp. (there are over 2200 serotypes, most of them potential if not documented pathogens) Transmission is by contamination of food by faeces from an acutely affected animal, or by an inapparent carrier, some previously affected animals continue to shed the organism long after remission of clinical signs. Confirmation of infection is usually by faecal culture. Any disease which severely compromises the lining of the GI tract can resemble Salmonella.

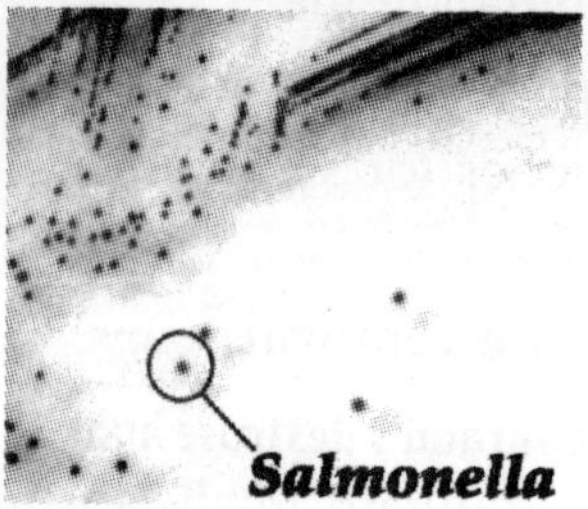

- **salmonella DT104**
an enteric bacteria that causes bloody diarrhoea, has resistance genes in its genome, and is zoonotic.

- **SALT(Abrev: ALT)**
serum alanine aminotransferase (SALT)or alanine aminotransferase (ALT). an enzyme found in hepatocytes (liver cells) released with cellular injury including cellular hypoxia.

- **sand crack**
see heel crack.

- **sanitiser**
a disinfectant of low toxicity used to reduce microbial contamination of food handling equipment.

- **SAP**
serum alkaline phosphatase. Also known as AP. An enzyme found in many tissues but most often elevated in serum in response to cholestasis and bone remodelling and glucocorticoid excess.

- **saprophytism**
organisms survive and persist in non-living or decaying organic matter. They are not usually parasitic, although may cause disease under certain circumstances – e.g. Aspergillus fumigatus and bovine abortion (fungal abortion).

- **sarcoid**
a tumour that occasionally occurs on the eyelids of horses.

- **sarcoma**
  cancer originating from fibrous tissues.
- **sarcoptes scabiei var. canis**
  the etiological agent of scabies.
- **sarcoptic mange**
  skin disease characterised by extreme itching, hair loss, and secondary infection. Usually widespread, but often seen on the belly and inner thighs. Can be treated, but spreads easily.
- **saturated fat**
  a completely hydrogenated fat. Saturated fats are solid at room temperature. Example: animal tallow.
- **saucer (fracture)**
  stress fracture of the front of the cannon bone that can be straight or curved.
- **savage**
  when a horse bites another horse or a person.
- **SBT**
  staffordshire bull terrier
- **SC or S/C**
  subcutaneous/subcuticular
- **scale**
  accumulation of loose fragments of the top layer of the skin.
- **Schiff-Scherringtonposture**
  a condition, caused by a lesion in the spinal cord, in which the front legs are held rigid and straight, and the rear legs are weak or paralysed. Sometimes, the neck may be hyper extended, with the head held up and over the back.
- **Schiotz tonometer**
  an indentation tonometer used to measure intraocular pressure based on how readily the cornea is 'indented' Schiotz indentation tonometer - IOP is calculated from how readily the cornea is 'indented'
- **Schirmer tear test**
  a test of the ability to produce tears.
- **scintigraphy**
  a technique where radio-labelled technetium is injected intravenously into a horse. A gamma camera is used to record uptake of the nucleotide in the tissues. It is particularly useful diagnostically to localize an area of inflammation in the musculoskeletal system. The most common radioisotope

used to image bones is technetium-99m.

- **sclera**
  the white part of the eye beneath the upper eyelid. The sclera normally has small blood vessels running across the surface.

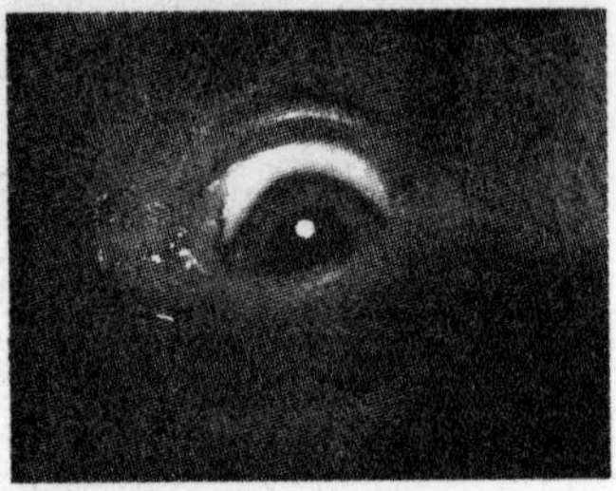

- **sclerosis**
  a hardening of tissue, usually the result of chronic inflammation.

- **scours**
  the discharge of more fluid than normal faecal matter from the bowel; often more frequently than normal.

- **scratching post**
  a free standing tower covered in burlap or other stiff material that cats use to safely rub their nails.

- **screenings**
  small, imperfect kernels, broken grains, hulls, weed seeds and other foreign material obtained from the cleaning of grain.

- **screw fixation**
  a procedure in which steel-alloy screws are surgically inserted to hold together a fractured bone.

- **scrotal hernia**
  the abnormal protrusion of part of an organ or tissue through the structures that normally contain it. An animal may be born with a hernia in which case it is congenital or it can get it can be acquired after birth.

- **scrotum**
  the skin sac that covers the testes.

- **scute**
  in turtles and tortoises, the plates which cover the bony portion of the shell. In snakes, the larger, thicker scales on the underside of the body which provide support, protection, and traction.

- **sclerotic dentin**
  shiny, transparent, dentin formed as a defence mechanism to chronic irritation.

- **supereruption**
condition where a tooth has the cemento enamel junction erupted more coronal than normal. Most common in the canines of older cats

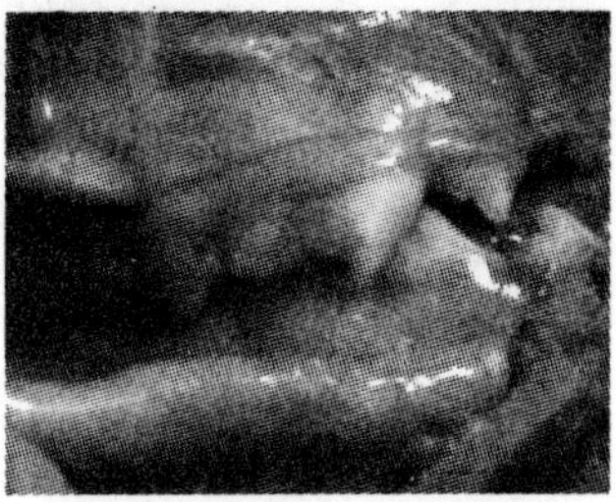

- **season**
a lay term used to refer to the beginning of proestrus.

- **seasonally polyestrous**
estrous cycles which are under the influence of light. The queen is a seasonally polyestrous animal.

- **sebaceous gland**
a gland in the skin which produces an oily substance.

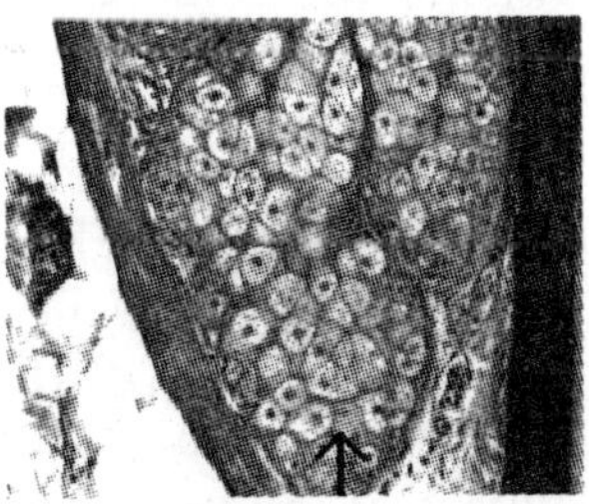

- **sebaceousadenitis**
inflammation of a sebaceous (oil-producing) gland. .In dogs, sebaceous glands are found on the top of the tail near its base, and at the junction of mucous membranes with skin. In cats, these glands are found on the chin, lip margins and the top of the tail.

- **seborrhea**
abnormal secretion of the sebaceous glands at the base of hair follicles causing anything from dandruff to greasy scales and crust.

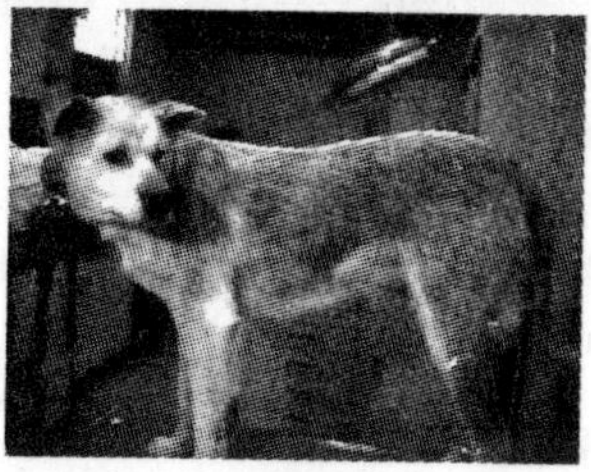

- **seborrhea, primary**
metabolic seborrhea. Scaling caused by endocrine disorders, aberrations in lipid availability, nutritional imbalances.

- **seborrhea, secondary**
scaling due to allergies, ectoparasite infestation, mycotic infections, immune-mediated disease.

- **sebum**
formed of diester waxes, cholesterol and free fatty

acids in sebaceous glands, which empty into the hair follicle or onto the skin.

- **second dam**
  grandmother of a horse. Also known as a 'granddam.'
- **second generation drugs**
  a description of medications developed from an earlier form of the medication. First generation medications were developed from the original form of the drug. Second generation medications are adaptations of first generation drugs. Third generation drugs are adaptations of second generation drugs.
- **secondary abnormality**
  morphologic abnormalities of sperm that develop while sperm are moving through the epididymus or occur as a result of handling sperm.
- **secondary infection**
  infection which occurs because the tissue and its natural defences have been damaged by another condition.
- **secondary oocyte**
  the egg after it has matured and is ready to be fertilised.
- **secondary response**
  the immune response produced by an animal who has previously encountered that specific antigen. Memory cells are responsible for this more efficient response. Also called anamnestic response.
- **secondary uterine inertia**
  ineffective or absent uterine contractions during parturition. Secondary uterine inertia may occur when a bitch is tired or exhausted from pushing to deliver and 'gives-up' on delivering puppies.
- **seizure**
  another term for convulsions.
- **seizure threshold**
  the level of stimulation at which a seizure is produced. Raising the seizure threshold makes it less likely a seizure will occur.
- **selective IGM deficiency**
  a deficiency in the production of the IgM antibody, one of the body's five classes of immunoglobulins, the proteins produced as antibodies to fight infection and toxins.

- **selective serotonin reuptake inhibitors (SSRIs)**
  medications which slow down the ability of nerve cells to absorb serotonin, a neurotransmitter (chemical that serves as a messenger between nerves). Example: Prozac.

- **selemectin**
  A neurotoxin recommended as a monthly topical 'pour on' insecticide. This product is also labelled for use against scabies, ear mites, internal parasites, and for tick control.

- **semen**
  the composite fluid ejaculated which includes sperm and supporting fluids.

- **semen extender**
  a substance added to semen to provide an appropriate environment and energy for the sperm to survive in vitro.

- **semi-longhair**
  a longhair that does not have an extremely long coat. For example, the Maine Coon is considered a semi-longhair, but the Persian is not.

- **seminal plasma**
  fluid produced by the prostate gland which is part of semen.

- **seminal vesicles**
  accessory sex glands in the male.

- **seminiferous tubules**
  the location in the testes in which sperm are produced.

- **seminoma**
  a testicular tumour that usually displays benign biological behaviour.

- **semipermeable membrane**
  a membrane that allows water and small molecules to pass through it but prevents passage of large molecules such as colloids. The peritoneal membrane lining the abdominal cavity is an example of a semi permeable membrane.

- **senile iris atrophy**
  atrophy of the constrictor muscle: poor pupillary light reflexes but normal vision. Pupil margin looks a bit moth-eaten and irregular.

- **sensible fluid losses**
  sensible fluid losses are those that can be easily detected and measured. Sen-

sible losses can occur through the urinary and gastrointestinal tracts. The loss of fluid through the GI tract is negligible in healthy dogs and cats but can be substantial through vomitting or diarrhoea. In the adult, healthy dog or cat, sensible loss is through urine and is about 12-20 ml/ lb/day. Loss of water through the urinary and GI tracts is usually accompanied by loss of electrolytes (in both health and disease) (an isotonic loss).

- **sensitive laminae**
  the area of the hoof that contains nerves and vessels.
- **sensitising soup**
  chemical mediators released by cells following tissue damage and inflammation that individually or collectively results in pain sensitivity.
- **sensory-discriminative dimension of pain**
  this dimension of pain gives the individual information about the location, onset, intensity, type and duration of pain.
- **separation anxiety**
  a behavioural condition in which the pet becomes anxious when separated from the owner. Dogs with separation anxiety tend to shadow their owners, greet them exuberantly when they return after being gone, and sometimes vocalise, chew destructively, and urinate or defecate when separated from their owners.
- **sepsis**
  the presence of infectious organisms in the blood.

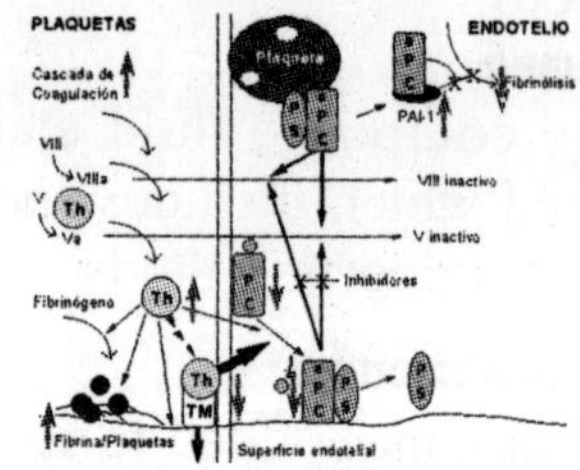

- **septic**
  a condition caused by an infection with bacteria or fungi or the toxins they produce.
- **septic arthritis**
  a bacterial infection in a joint causing inflammation.
- **septicemia**
  a disease affecting many organ systems due to toxins in

the blood which are released by bacteria or other micro-organisms. Signs include fever, pinpoint bruises on mucous membranes, and lesions in the joints, heart valves, eyes, or other organs.

- **seroconversion**
  a change in immune status from having no measurable antibodies against an infectious agent to development of measurable antibodies in the blood.

- **serology**
  laboratory testing for antibody- antigen reactions and antibody levels.

- **seroprevalence**
  the frequency of occurrence of exposure to an infectious agent based on measuring antibodies to the agent in the blood.

- **serotype**
  a subdivision of a species of micro-organisms (e.g. a bacteria) based upon its particular antigens.

- **serous**
  thin and watery.

- **sertoli cell**
  cells in the testicle which support the testosterone-producing cells. These cells can produce the female hormone, oestrogen.

- **sertoli cell tumour**
  a testicular tumour that may produce estrogens and cause signs of feminisation in the male dog.

- **serum**
  the clear part of blood that remains after blood is allowed to clot. Very similar to plasma except that plasma is the fluid part of blood when blood is separated into cells and fluid before the blood clots.

- **serum alanine aminotransferase (Abrev: SALT (ALT)**
  also known as alanine aminotransferase (ALT). An enzyme found in hepatocytes (liver cells) released with cellular injury including cellular hypoxia.

- **serum alkaline phosphatase Abrev: SAP (AP)**
  also known as alkaline phosphatase (AP). An enzyme found in many tissues but most often elevated in serum in response to cholestasis, bone remodelling or glucocorticoid excess.

- **service dogs**
service dogs, also known as mobility dogs, are trained to assist a physically disabled person. The dogs help the individual accomplish many everyday activities. They are also trained in a number of safety procedures, should the need arise.

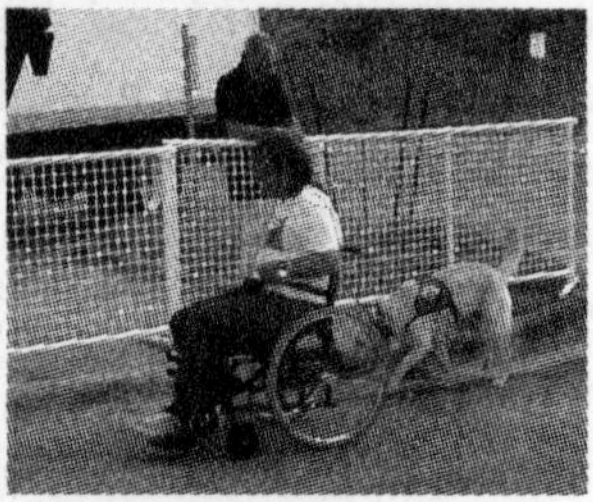

- **service/conception**
number of AI or natural services needed to achieve pregnancy (conception). Goal is 2-2.5 Svc/con.

- **sesamoid (fracture)**
fracture of the sesamoid bone. Fractures can be small chips or involve the entire bone. Surgical repair is often done by arthroscopy.

- **sesamoid bones**
two small bones (medial and lateral sesamoids) located above and at the back of the fetlock joint. Four common fractures of the sesamoids are apical (along the top of the bone), abaxial (the side of the sesamoid away from the ankle joint), mid-body (sesamoid broken in half) and basilar (through the bottom) fractures.

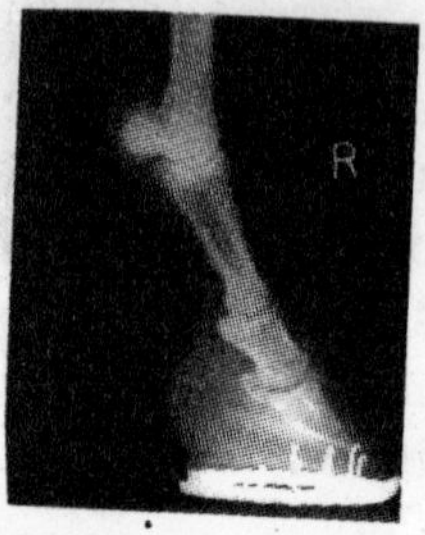

- **sesamoiditis**
inflammation of the sesamoid bones.

- **setters**
setters or 'couchers' preceded our modern spaniels. These dogs couch, or creep slow and low to the ground, in scenting their winged quarry. Today's setters are among the most beautiful of the gundogs. England's Gordon Setter and English Setter, Ireland's Irish Setter, and France's Èpagneul Français, are among them. The earliest setters, such as the Llewellyn, Laverak, and the Èpagneul Ecossais, contribute to the gene pool of both

our contemporary setters and spaniels.

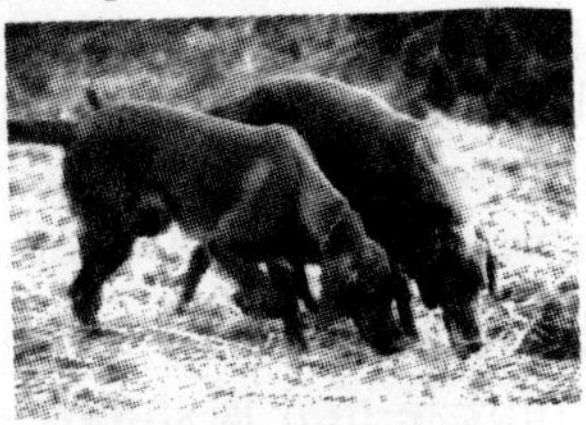

- **sex allowance**
female horses (fillies and mares), according to their age and the time of year, are allowed to carry three to five pounds less when meeting males.

- **shaded**
a coat pattern consisting of a single colour that varies from light to dark shading across the length of each hair.

- **shadow roll**
a (usually sheepskin) roll that is secured over the bridge of a horse's nose to keep it from seeing shadows on the track and shying away from or jumping them.

- **shaker foal/botulism**
causative agent is Clostridium botulinum. Produces seven different toxins, which act by binding irreversibly to presynaptic neurons. Horses either ingest the toxin from foodstuffs, or absorb it from organisms producing it in contaminated wounds or in damaged gut tissue. Sources of ingested toxin are commonly rodent carcasses in cured hay, silage, or improperly cured hay. Signs: rapidly progressing flaccid paralysis, tremors, hind limb weakness, progressing to paralysis of pharyngeal area, tongue, etc. Often an inability to swallow is the first sign noted. Animals become recumbent, there is paralysis of respiratory muscles. Therapy: administration of antitoxin. However, this will not help neurons where toxin has already bound. Supportive care. Horses which receive antitoxin before reaching the stage of recumbency have a better prognosis. Vaccination of pregnant mares with botulism toxoid may be employed in endemic areas to prevent the development of 'shaker foal' syndrome, which is caused by ingestion of spores and subsequent

growth of organisms and toxin production in the gut.

- **SHD**
  short haired domestic (non-pedigree cat)
- **shearing**
  mechanical removal of fleece. Done yearly and in some breeds more frequently.
- **shedding (of organisms)**
  a term used to describe the release of organisms (bacteria, protozoa, viruses) into the environment from an infected animal. The organisms may be in the stool, urine, respiratory secretions, or vaginal discharges. The 'shedding' animal may or may not be showing symptoms of disease.
- **shed row**
  stable area. A row of barns.
- **shipping fever**
  a complex seen in cattle, especially feedlot cattle, where the stress of shipping weakens their immune system and they develop viral and then opportunistic bacterial infections.
- **shock**
  a physical state often caused by severe injury, and characterised by depressed physical response (blood pressure, heart rate, etc.).
- **short muzzle**
  a muzzle that is stubby and shorter than half the length of the skull, typical of the brachycephalic breed (e.g., Pug, Bulldog, Shih Tzu).

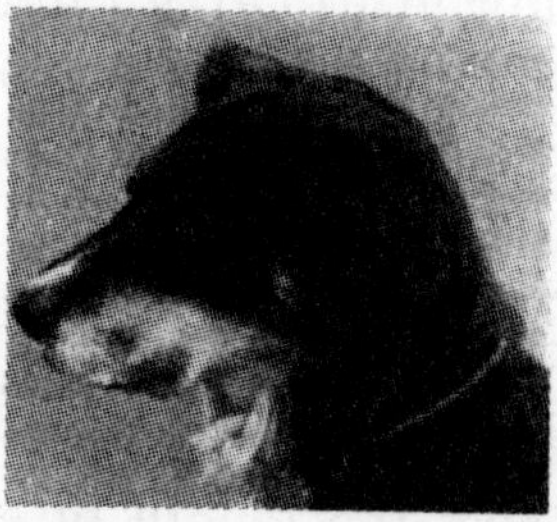

- **shorthair**
  a cat with a relatively short coat. The coat may be very close-lying and sleek, or it may be thick and plush.
- **shot reactions**
  neither phenylbutazone nor penicillin have any efficacy in treatment of allergic reactions. Bute may decrease inflammation, but it does not treat anaphylaxis. Injectable penicillin can cause a fairly dramatic amount of swelling and dis-

comfort, not to mention the occasional anaphylactic or procaine reaction. DMSO is used intravenously in cases of ischemic damage. You have to dilute it to avoid haemolysis of red cells which occurs if it is infused full-strength.

- **SI**
  1. small intestine
  2. self inflicted
- **SIBO**
  small intestinal bacterial overgrowth
- **sickle hock**
  sickle hock is a term used to describe a conformation fault in the hind leg—an overtly forward curve to the hocks, so the leg ends up set under the horse more than is desirable.
- **sid**
  once daily
- **sig**
  signalment
- **signalment**
  this is the physical description of the animal including species, breed, sex, neuter status, age and colour and/or markings.
- **silage**
  pickled forage, a feed that is harvested at 30-60% dry matter and allowed to ferment as a means of preservation.
- **silage additives**
  substances added during the ensiling process to enhance the correct and rapid fermentation of the feed.
- **silicone**
  a polymer of alternating oxygen and silicon atoms combined with other organic groups. Catheters made of silicone are relatively inert and cause less stimulation of clot formation compared to other materials.
- **simple (fracture)**
  a fracture along a single line which does not penetrate the skin
- **simultaneous ventilation compression CPR**
  for every compression, you give the patient a simultaneous ventilation. The ventilatory rate is very high and matches the chest compression rate.

- **sire**
  1. the breeding male, also called a stud.
  2. to beget foals.

- **SIT**
  self-inflicted trauma.

- **skin cytology**
  examination, with a microscope, of a skin scraping or material from swabbing the skin. The material maybe stained and checked for the presence of yeast, bacteria, tumour cells, etc.

- **skin scraping**
  scraping some material from the surface of the skin and looking at it under a microscope, e.g., to check for skin mites.

- **skin turgor**
  skin elasticity. Skin turgor is used to assess hydration.

- **skull**
  all of the many bones of the head, including those of the face and lower jaw and those that surround the brain. The skull and the head are not synonymous, nor does the skull consist only of the bony area that surrounds the brain. In the dog fancy, however, the term skull is sometimes used to refer exclusively to the brain surround, while face is used to include the bony matter thereof. Often we come across the term back skull or top skull. These two terms are synonymous, and both refer to the brain surround, the cavum cranii.

- **skull types**
  it is interesting that although the actual size of the canine skull varies from the tiny Chihuahua to the massive Dogue de Bordeaux, with a myriad of shapes and stops in between, the actual 'type' of skull can be categorized into three general classes (based on the base-to-width ration), with but a handful more of specialized skull divisions used in the dog fancy. This is astonishing because the canine skull actually varies more in size and shape than that of any other animal species. The three basic skull classifications are: the brachycephalic, dolichocephalic, and mesaticephalic. The brachycephalic skull is broad at its base but short in its length. The extant breed

with the largest skull is the Dogue de Bordeaux, whose skull is of the brachycephalic type. Other brachycephalic dogs include the Pug and the Bulldog. The dolichocephalic skull is narrow at its base yet long in its length. Examples include many sighthounds, such as the Afghan Hound, Whippet, and Greyhound. Mesaticephalic skulls are balanced in width and length. Many gundogs, including the Brittany and the Vizsla, have mesaticephalic skulls.

- **slab (fracture)**
  a fracture in a bone in a joint that extends from one articular surface to another. Most often seen in the third carpal bone of the knee.

- **slipped**
  a breeding term meaning spontaneous abortion.

- **slit-lamp biomicroscopy**
  provides magnification and depth for examination of the eyelids, puncta, conjunctiva, sclera, cornea, anterior chamber, iris, lens, and anterior vitreous.

- **smooth muscle**
  the type of muscle found in internal organs such as the stomach and intestines.

- **sn**
  sneezing

- **snip**
  small patch of white hairs on the nose or lips of a horse.

- **snipy**
  used mostly in a derogatory sense, it refers to a weak, often narrow, construction to the foreface, mostly the muzzle and jaw, but can refer to the entire foreface in breeds that require a strong, solid construction in this area. Snipiness is the characteristic of a snippy foreface or muzzle.

- **snow nose**
  loss of pigmentation on the nose, usually in winter.

- **SOAP**
  SOAP's are progress notes recorded in a medical record. S = subjective information O = objective information A = assessment of information P = plans for diagnoses, treatment or client information.

- **socks**
  solid white markings extending from the top of the hoof to the ankles.

- **solid**
  a coat pattern consisting of a single colour.

- **solid horse**
  contender.

- **soluble intake protein (Abrev: SIP)**
  portion of the protein intake that is completely soluble in rumen fluid and rapidly utilized by bacteria. Soluble protein forms part (or all) of the degradable intake protein (DIP) value of a feed.

- **soluble carbohydrate**
  also, soluble fibre. Easily digested carbohydrates like starch.

- **somatic**
  relating to the wall of the body as distinguished from the viscera.

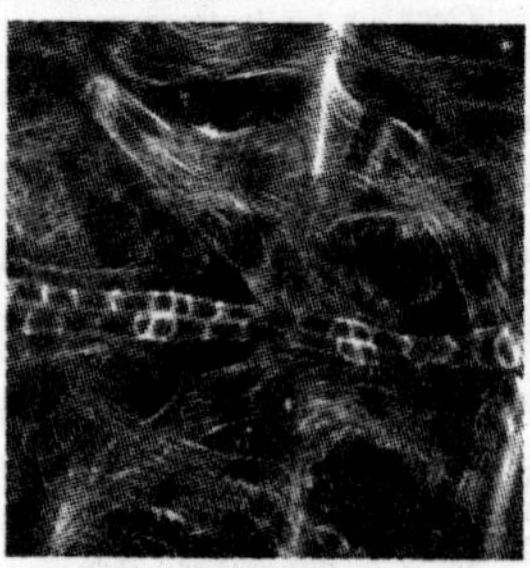

- **somatic cell count**
  an indicator of mastitis, the accumulation of cells, chiefly leukocytes, in the milk in response to an antigen. Goal: greater than 95% of all cows with counts less than 200, 000 cells/ml milk, and a bulk tank (herd average) count of <200, 000 cells/ ml.

- **somato sensory**
  sensory signals from tissues. Somatic usually refers to input from body tissue other than viscera.

- **somnolence**
  sleepiness, a condition of semi consciousness approaching coma.

- **somogyi effect**
  a condition in which the blood glucose level increases if too much insulin is given. It occurs when insulin causes the blood glucose level to go so low it stimulates the production of other hormones in the body such as epinephrine which promote the breakdown of glycogen (the chemical compound which the body uses to store glucose) and increases the blood glucose

level above normal. It is also called rebound hyperglycemia or insulin-induced hyperglycemia.

- **source-oriented record**
  a record keeping system in which all data of a similar type are clustered together, e.g. all laboratory reports and together.

- **spay**
  sterilisation by surgical removal of the ovaries and uterus of a female animal.

- **species**
  a biological classification that combines organisms sharing common characteristics and are able to mate and produce fertile offspring.

- **specific pathogen free pigs (Abrev: SPF pigs)**
  the pigs are taken surgically at birth and reared in a pig free environment so they have no contact with other pigs and no opportunity to catch a disease.

- **specific treatment**
  treatment that will eliminate or modify the primary cause of a disease process. For example, surgical removal of a tumour.

- **speedy cut**
  injury to the inside of the knee or hock caused by a strike from another foot.

- **sperm**
  spermatozoa. The male structure that fertilises an egg.

- **spermatogenesis**
  formation of sperm in the testes.

- **spermatozoa**
  sperm. The male structure that fertilises an egg.

- **speuter**
  an agglomeration of spay and neuter. Another word for alter.

- **sphincter**
  a ring like band of muscle that constricts a passage or closes an opening e.g. the anal sphincter constricts to close the anus and relaxes when the animal is passing stool. The urethral sphincter closes the urinary bladder.

- **spillover**
  what spillover means is that rabies viral variant isolated

from a rabid animal will be the variant from the terrestrial wildlife reservoir in that area. That is why if you have a rabid raccoon in Montana it will be spill over from a skunk because that is the only wildlife reservoir that maintains the virus in that area.

- **spinal myelopathy**
  disease of the myelin, or covering (sheath) of the spinal nerves (the spinal cord).

- **spinoreticular**
  a tract in the spinal cord leading to behavioural responses that help the individual determine whether a painful input is tolerable or not. Also conveys visceral pain.

- **spinothalamic**
  a tract in the spinal cord which conveys impulses associated with pain and temperature sensation, and tactile sensation. Somatic pain pathway.

- **spiral (fracture)**
  fracture that spirals around bone.

- **spirochete**
  a type of bacteria which is long, slender and assumes a spiral shape. Leptospira species and the bacteria that causes Lyme disease (Borrelia burgdorferi) are spirochetes.

- **spit box**
  a generic term describing a barn where horses are brought for post-race testing. Tests may include saliva, urine and/or blood.

- **spit the bit**
  a generic term for an exhausted horse.

- **spitting off**
  when the female is no longer receptive to the male indicating she has ovulated.

- **splay-legged**
  a condition in newborn pigs that involves a muscle weakness so they are unable to stand and bear their weight.

- **spleen**
  part of the immune system of an animal. A large tongue-shaped organ in the abdomen containing many lymphocytes. The spleen filters blood and removes damaged cells. It can also manufacture new blood

cells if the animal's bone marrow is damaged.

- **splint**
  1. either of the two small bones that lie along the sides of the cannon bone. 2. the condition where calcification occurs on the splint bone causing a bump. This can result from response to a fracture or other irritation to the splint bone. A common injury is a popped splint.
- **sporotrichosis**
  cutaneous nodules; draining, ulcerative tracts caused by Sporothrix schenckii. Lesions may be focal or disseminated.
- **spotted**
  a coat pattern with many dark, rounded spots, particularly at the rear of the body.
- **spray**
  the behaviour, commonly seen in the tom cat, of urinating everywhere (typically on the walls, floor, etc) to establish territory.
- **spraying**
  when a Cat (usually a male) sprays urine to mark its territory.
- **springer or fresh**
  cow/heifer that has recently calved.
- **sq**
  subcutaneous
- **squamate**
  scaly-bodied reptile including lizards and snakes.
- **ss**
  skin scrape
- **ssri**
  selective serotonin reuptake inhibitors: Medications which slow down the ability of nerve cells to absorb serotonin, a neurotransmitter(chemical that serves as a messenger between nerves).example: Prozac.
- **stades procedure**
  a surgical procedure for correcting upper eyelid entropion.
- **stage 1**
  this is the stage of cervical dilation and lasts 6-8 hrs in the bitch and queen.
- **stage 2**
  this is the stage of foetal expulsion in the labour of a bitch or queen and lasts 3-6 hrs.

- **stage 3**
this is the stage of placental expulsion in the labour of a bitch or queen and lasts 5-15 min.

- **stall walker**
horse that moves about its stall constantly and frets rather than rests.

- **stallion**
a male horse used for breeding.

- **stallion season**
the right to breed one mare to a particular stallion during one breeding season.

- **stallion share**
a lifetime breeding right to a stallion; one mare per season per share.

- **stanchion barn**
stall barn where cows are chained within their stalls.

- **standard drip sets**
an administration set for intravenous fluid administration. The set has a spike to penetrate the container of fluids, a drip chamber and a long flexible tube that connects to the patient's catheter. The end of the drip set vary by manufacturer, requiring anywhere from 10-20 drops to comprise a millilitre.

- **staphylococcus, staph**
a type of bacteria. Normally found on the skin and upper respiratory tract, but can occasionally cause localised suppurating infection.

- **staple**
a group of wool fibres.

- **star**
any of a number of white markings on the forehead. (The forehead is defined as being above an imaginary line connecting the tops of the eyes.)

- **stasis**
in the gastro intestinal tract, a condition in which the food does not move through normally, but remains in one section, e.g., food does not pass from the stomach into the intestine.

- **status epilepticus**
a condition in which the animal exhibits one severe (Grand Mal) seizure right after another, with no time to recover in-between.

- **stayer**
a horse that can race long distances.

- **stenosis**
  a narrowing of a tubular structure. For example the intestine may stricture interfering with movement of food through the intestine.
- **stenosis (aortic)**
  obstruction of the blood flowing from the left ventricle to the aorta.
- **stenosis (mitral)**
  narrowing of the mitral valve that separates the left atrium and the left ventricle.
- **stenosis (pulmonary artery)**
  narrowing of the outflow from the lungs.
- **stenosis (subaortic)**
  narrowing of the aorta just below the semilunar valves. Severity increases with age.
- **stereoscopic vision**
  the ability to see in three dimensions.
- **sterilisation**
  a process, often surgical, that prevents animals from being able to reproduce.
- **sterilise**
  to destroy all micro organisms; usually not possible with chemical disinfectants, and requires physical disinfections.
- **sternal**
  laying down on the chest and belly.
- **stifle**
  the large joint above the hock which is made up by the femur, the patella and the tibia.
- **sto**
  speak to owner
- **stockings**
  solid white markings extending from the top of the hoof to the knee or hock.
- **stomatitis**
  inflammation of the mouth including the gums and tongue.
- **stones**
  a mass, usually formed from mineral salts, occurring within the hollow organs: kidney, gallbladder, urinary bladder.
- **stop**
  located between the eyes, the stop is the sloping down of the skull at this area. The angle of the drop as well as the pronouncement of the area varies among breeds.

Generally speaking, brachycephalic dogs have a pronounced stop wile dolichocephalic dogs have a slight stop. Mesaticephalic dogs tend to have either defined or average stops.

- **storage diseases**
  diseases in which cells of the body accumulate (store) a substance that causes the cells to malfunction. For example cells may store too much fat or sugar.

- **strangles**
  strangles - Bacterial Streptococcus equi. Spread by direct contact with nasal secretions or pus from draining submandibular abscesses. These can be indirectly spread via buckets, pitchforks, stomach tubes, hands, etc.
  Signs— usually occur 3-4 days after exposure, initially, fever, anorexia, swollen submandibular lymph nodes, which rupture and drain infectious material, purulent nasal discharge, confirmation by culture of abscess material or nasopharyngeal swab. Horses showing the early signs of infection (fever, depression) should be promptly isolated. If caught before lymph node abscessation has progressed to any marked extent, these animals can be treated with penicillin.
  Horses which have already developed abscesses are better left off antibiotics in uncomplicated cases, as antibiotics tend to prolong the course of the disease. Mature abscesses should be lanced and warm compresses and flushing hasten their resolution.
  Exposed but asymptomatic horses 'may' benefit from preventative treatment with antibiotics, but this is of benefit 'only' in cases where they will not still be exposed after antibiotics are discontinued. Most cases of strangles are messy and gross and so forth, but not usually fatal.

- **stranguria**
  straining to urinate.

- **strategic worming**
  worming during the times of year that infection is most likely to occur.

- **stratum corneum**
the outer layer of skin.

NORMAL SKIN

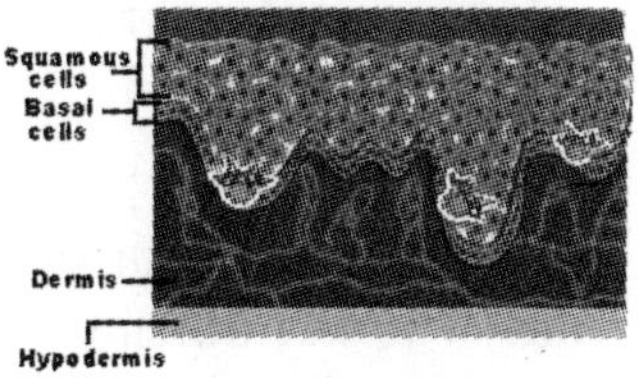

- **stress (fracture)**
a fracture produced by the stress created by a repetitive loading cycle on the bone, commonly found in athletic training. Usually seen in the front of the cannon bone as a severe form of bucked shins. Also seen in the tibia and causes a hard-to-diagnose hind limb lameness.

- **stress-induced hyperglycemia**
a condition in cats in which the blood glucose level becomes abnormally high when the animal is stressed e.g. in the veterinarian's office.

- **stria**
streaks in the cornea caused by the cornea stretching from increased pressure.

- **stricture**
similar to stenosis. Narrowing of a tubular structure.

- **strip**
to remove residual milk from the mammary gland (udder).

- **stripe**
a white marking running down a horse's face, starting under an imaginary line connecting the tops of the eyes.

- **stroma**
thickest layer of the cornea.

- **structural carbohydrates**
complex carbohydrates (fibre)including cellulose, hemicellulose, lignin and pectin that form the plant cell wall. Measured in the laboratory as neutral detergent fibre (NDF).

- **struvite**
a chemical compound, magnesium ammonium phosphate, which is made by the body and can form crystals and stones in the urinary bladder.

- **stud**
the breeding male also called a sire.

- **stud book**
a record for the breeding particulars of dogs of recognized breeds. Each registry

has an official stud book which represents a breed's ancestry since its induction into the registry.

- **stud cat**
  a whole male cat that is part of a breeding program.

- **subalbinotic**
  animals with blue irises.

- **subcorneal**
  just under the stratum corneum.

- **subcorneal pustular dermatosis (Abrev: SPD)**
  a rare condition characterised by the formation of pustules which are subcorneal in location.

- **subcutaneous (Abrev: SC or SQ)**
  giving a drug, fluid or vaccine under the skin.

- **subluxation**
  a partial dislocation of a joint in which the bones become out of alignment but the joint itself is still intact.

- **subq.**
  subcutaneous. Given beneath the skin.

- **substrate**
  relative to the husbandry of reptiles, amphibians, and small mammals, the substrate is the material that lines the bottom of a cage.

- **subunit vaccine**
  a vaccine that use parts of a pathogen rather than the whole organism.

- **suckling**
  a foal in its first year of life, while it is still nursing.

- **sudden acquired retinal degeneration syndrome (Abrev: SARDS)**
  acute (2 days-2 weeks) degeneration of the photoreceptors followed by the other retinal layers affecting both eyes simultaneously.

- **suffering**
  an unpleasant emotional state, but the external expression of suffering through behaviour is distress.

- **sulfonamides**
  a class of antibiotics which contain sulphur. They are bacteriostatic (they stop the growth (reproduction) of bacteria, but do not kill them).

- **sulk**
  when an animal refuses to extend itself.

- **superfecundation**
  having a litter with more than one father (or breeding).

- **superficial cells**
  epithelial cells from the vagina which are also called cornified or anucleated cellsa and are the largest of the epithelial cells present during estrus. If 80-90% of the cells in the smear are superficial cells that can be used as an indication to start breeding.

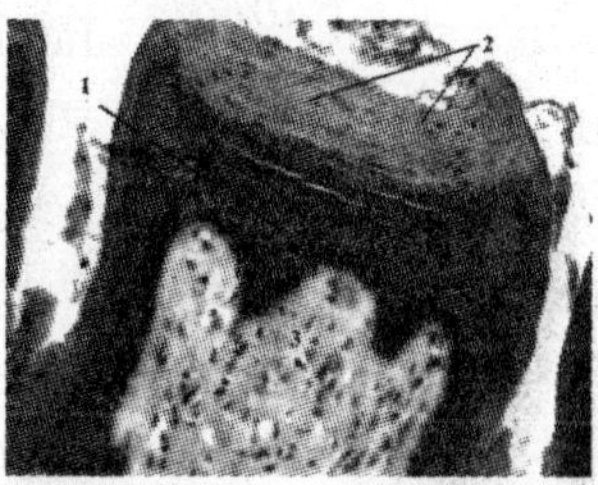

- **superficial flexor tendon**
  present in all four legs, but injuries most commonly affect the front legs. Located on the back (posterior) of the front leg between the knee and the foot and between the hock and the foot on the rear leg. The function is to flex the digit (pastern) and knee (carpus) and to extend the elbow on the front leg and extend the hock on the rear leg. Functions in tandem with the deep flexor tendon.

- **superficial intermediate cells**
  epithelial cells exfoliated from the vagina during late proestrus to early estrus. They are larger than parabasal cells and have small nuclei and irregular/folded borders.

- **superior check ligament**
  fibrous band of tissue that originates above the knee and attaches to the superficial flexor tendon. Primary function is support of this tendon. Accessory ligament of the superficial flexor tendon.

- **supplement**
  feed or feed mixtures rich in one or more of protein, energy, vitamins, minerals or antibiotics. Combined with other feeds to produce a more complete feed.

- **supportive treatment**
  supportive treatment corrects or modifies abnormalities that occur secondary to a disease process. For example fluid and electrolyte therapy for a patient with hypoadrenocorticism.

- **supraventricular tachycardia**
  a condition in which the heart beats very rapidly because of signals coming from the atria (chambers of the heart that receive the blood) or near the junction of the atria with the ventricles (the chambers of the heart that pump the blood to the body or lungs).
- **surgical scrubs**
  povidone iodine or chlorhexidine surgical scrub for cleaning.
- **suspensory ligament**
  originates at the back of the knee (front leg) and the back of the top part of the cannon bone (hind leg), attaching to the sesamoid bones. The lower portion of the ligament attaches the lower part of the sesamoid bones to the pastern bones. Its function is to support the fetlock. The lower ligaments that attaches the sesamoid bone to the pastern bones are the distal sesamoidean ligaments.
- **SVECCS**
  society for veterinary emergency medicine and critical care.
- **svelte**
  describes a cat's body type characterised by a fine bone structure and narrow shape.
- **swayback**
  horse with a prominent concave shape of the backbone, usually just behind the withers (saddle area).
- **swb**
  salt water bathing
- **sweet feed**
  a commercial feed sweetened with molasses to improve palatability.
- **sx**
  surgery
- **symbiosis**
  parasitic state in which the parasite and animal survive in a beneficial relationship – e.g. bacteria within the rumen.
- **symblepharon**
  adherence of the conjunctiva to the cornea.
- **sympathomimetic**
  producing effects similar to the 'flight or fight' response, which means the body is alerted to a danger of some sort and prepares to basically run or fight. Sym-

pathomimetic effects include increased heart rate, sweating, and increased blood pressure.

- **symptomatic treatment**
  symptomatic treatment eliminates or suppresses clinical signs without affecting or knowing the underlying cause of the sign. For example antiemetics to suppress vomitting.

- **synapse**
  the location at which a nerve impulse is transmitted from one neuron to another.

- **synchronous diaphragmatic flutter**
  a contraction of the diaphragm in synchrony with the heart beat after strenuous exercise. Affected horses have a noticeable twitch or spasm in the flank area which may cause an audible sound, hence the term 'thumps.' Most commonly seen in electrolyte-depleted/exhausted horses. The condition resolves spontaneously with rest.

- **syncope**
  the temporary loss of consciousness; fainting.

- **synergist**
  an agent that enhances the action of another.

- **synergistic**
  two or more drugs which enhance the effectiveness of each other.

- **synovial**
  pertaining to a joint made up of bone ends covered with cartilage, ligaments, a cavity filled with synovial fluid (joint fluid), and an outside fibrous capsule e.g. hip joint, elbow joint.

- **synovial fluid**
  fluid made by the synovial cells that lubricates joints .

- **synovial joint**
  a movable joint that consists of articulating bone ends covered by articular cartilage held together with a joint capsule and ligaments and containing synovial fluid in the joint cavity.

- **synovial sheath**
  the inner lining of a tendon sheath that produces synovial fluid. Allows ease of motion for the tendons as they cross joints.

- **synovitis**
  inflammation of a synovial structure, typically a synovial sheath.

- **systemic**
  proliferation of histiocytes invading the skin and lymph nodes. Can go into remission for years, or progress to the malignant form. Can be treated, but not cured.

- **systemic**
  body-wide process (e.g. systemic infection).

- **systemic lupus erythematosis, sle**
  an autoimmune disease in which the immune system sees its own body as foreign matter. Characterised by polyarthritis, hemolytic anemia, skin disease, among many other symptoms.

- **T**
  thoracic (vertebra - usually followed by a number to denote which one)

- **T cell**
  also called T lymphocytes. The type of lymphocyte which is responsible for cell mediated immunity. T cells may directly kill a cell or produce chemicals called lymphokines that activate macrophages which will kill the cell.

- **T cytotoxic cells (Abrev: TC cells)**
  their function is to use perforins and cytotoxins to destroy target cells that are carrying foreign proteins on their surface.

- **t.i.d**
  three times a day from latin: ter in die

- **tabby**
  a coat pattern consisting of two or more colours in a striped pattern.

- **tachycardia**
  an abnormally high heart rate.

- **tachypnea**
  rapid breathing.

- **tacrolimus**
  a compound with similar actions as cyclosporine (inhibition of IL-2 through inhibition of calcineurin). Available as a topical ointment (0.1%)

- **tagamet**
  a medication used to treat ulcers.

- **tail enders**
  cow producing low levels of milk at the end of their lactation.
- **TAN-SAL**
  tannic acid solution used as a topical drying agent.
- **tapering muzzle**
  wedge-shaped muzzle, also called pointed muzzle.
- **tapetum**
  a highly reflective layer located in the dorsal half of the choroid in most domestic species (pig and llama being exceptions).
- **tapetum lucidum**
  mirror-like layer of cells behind the cat's retina. these cells reflect light for good night vision.
- **tapeworm**
  a long, flat, white parasite that inhabits the intestinal tract and causes illness; this infection can spread to humans.
- **tarsal plate**
  a plate of cartilage that gives rigidity to the eye.
- **tarsorrhaphy**
  suturing together of the eyelid margins partially or totally to make the palpebral fissue smaller or to protect the cornea.
- **tarsus**
  the ankle (rear leg) of dogs and cats; also called the hock.
- **tartar**
  a build-up of bacteria, saliva and food on the teeth which becomes mineralised, forming a hard coating and eventually causing gum disease and tooth loss.
- **tattoo**
  a permanent, indelible mark on the inside of the upper lip used to identify the horse.
- **tb**
  tabby
- **tb/w**
  tabby and white
- **teaser**
  a male horse used at breeding farms to determine whether a mare is ready to receive a stallion.
- **teaser bitch**
  a bitch which is used to excite a male dog in order to collect a semen sample for semen analysis or artificial insemination.

- **teaser ram**
  a ram incapable of inseminating the ewe (e.g. vasectomised).

- **teat orifice**
  the opening at the bottom of the teat where milk exits. This opening serves as a potential route for bacteria to enter the teat.

- **telogen**
  the resting phase of the hair cycle before it is shed.

- **temporo mandibular joint**
  the joint between the lower jaw and the skull.

- **tendon**
  cords of strong, white (collagen) elastic fibres that connect a muscle to a bone or other structure and transmit the forces generated by muscular contraction to the bones.

- **terrestrial rabies**
  rabies in terrestrial mammals, mammals that walk on the ground like a skunk or raccoon.

- **tertiary hyperparathyroidism**
  tertiary hyperparathyroidism is a relatively uncommon event occurring in some chronic renal failure patients, which may result in a moderate increase in calcium.

- **testes**
  structures that produce sperm.

- **testicles**
  same as testes. An organ that produces sperm.

- **testicular degeneration**
  the deterioration of the testicular tissue with resultant decrease in function.

- **testicular hypoplasia**
  testicles that are smaller than normal.

- **testosterone**
  the male sex hormone produced by the testes.

- **tetanus shot**
  the standard 'tetanus shot' is tetanus toxoid, which induces an immune response from the host. Active immunity. Tetanus antitoxin, usually given to animals with no or unknown vaccination history, is the purified antibody taken from a hyper immunised animal, and is called 'passive immunity.'

- **tgo**
  to go home
- **thermography**
  diagnostic technique utilizing instrumentation that measures temperature differences. Records the surface temperature of a horse. Unusually hot or cold areas may be indicative of some underlying pathology (deviation from the normal).
- **third generation drugs**
  a description of medications developed from an earlier form of the medication. First generation medications were developed from the original form of the drug. Second generation medications are adaptations of first generation drugs. Third generation drugs are adaptations of second generation drugs.
- **thoracic pump theory**
  CPR performed in patients over 7 kg positioned in dorsal recumbency likely uses the thoracic pump theory which says that when the chest is compressed, the heart underneath the chest wall is not directly compressed but rather the chest compression is causing an increase in intrathoracic pressure. The increase in intrathoracic pressure collapses veins, prevents retrograde blood flow back towards the abdomen and compresses arteries which pushes blood forward towards the heart and brain. The heart is just acting as a passive conduit and doesn't change shape very much at all.
- **thorax**
  another term for chest.
- **thoroughpin**
  swelling of the synovial sheath of the deep flexor tendon above the hock.
- **three-in-one formula**
  a formula for partial parenteral nutrition that can be tailored to the individual patients by compounding the formula. Most, if not all, commercial solutions provide amino acids and dextrose but don't typically provide lipids.
- **thrombocytopenia**
  a lower than normal number of platelets in the blood. Platelets, which are actually fragments of specific types

of cells, are necessary for blood to clot. Signs of thrombocytopenia include bruising and bleeding from the nose, into the gastrointestinal tract, etc.

- **thrombocytopenic purpura**
is a disease characterised by the formation of platelet clots in the microcirculation (very small vessels)--. Exact cause is unclear but thought to be due to infections, inherited conditions or immunologic abnormalities. Results in bleeding with a low platelet count, anaemia, neurologic symptoms kidney disease and fever.

- **thromboemboli**
a blood clot which forms in a blood vessel, then breaks loose into circulation and may lodge and obstruct other blood vessels.

- **thrombophlebitis**
inflammation of a vein associated with thrombus formation. The thrombus may break loose as a thromboembolis and then plug other blood vessels.

- **thrombosis**
the formation of blood clots in blood vessels.

- **thumps**
synchronous diaphragmatic flutter. The diaphragm contracts in the rhythym of the heartbeat. Usually due to an electrolyte disturbance, which presumably alters the membrane potential of the phrenic nerve, causing it to depolarise along with the electrical impulse which is propagated during cardiac muscle depolarisation.

- **thymus gland**
located in the thoracic inlet/cranial mediastinum. 'Cranial' in the context of anatomic description means towards the head, as opposed to 'caudal', which is, surprise, towards the tail. Thymus gland shrinks as the horse ages.

- **thyroid**
the largest of the hormone secreting (endocrine) glands located in the neck; it regulates metabolism.

- **thyroid (hyper)**
excessive production of thyroid hormones, often seen in older dogs, causing excessive thirst, weight loss, increased appetite and restlessness.

• **thyroid**
decreased production of thyroxine, causing poor coat, weight gain, mental dullness, fatigue, cold intolerance, and infertility.

• **thyrotropin releasing hormone**
hormone produced by the hypothalamus that stimulates the pituitary gland to produce thyrotropin (thyroid stimulating hormone; TSH) which in turn stimulates the thyroid gland to produce thyroid hormone. Also called TSH-releasing factor or TSH-releasing hormone.

• **ticked**
a coat pattern consisting of banded hairs.

• **ticking**
light hairs that are scattered among darker coloured hairs or spatterings of lighter hairs among darker coloured hairs.

• **tid**
three times daily

• **tie-back surgery**
a procedure (laryngoplasty) used to suture the arytenoid cartilage out of the airway.

• **tissue**
a group of specialised cells that together perform a particular function, e.g., muscle tissue, nerve tissue, bone

• **titer**
a measurement of the amount of antibodies in the blood. The test to measure antibodies is usually performed by making a number of dilutions of the blood and then measuring at what dilution there is sufficient antibody to react in the test. For example, a titer of 1:8 (one to eight) means the blood can be diluted to one part blood and seven parts saline and still produce a positive reaction in the test. The higher the titer (1:16 is higher than 1:8), the more antibody is present. (NOTE: The word titer may also be used when discussing the amount of antigen present e.g. a high titer vaccine has a large number of virus particles.)

• **t-l**
thoraco-lumbar

• **tli**
trypsin-like immunoreactivity

- **tmj**
temporo-mandibular joint
- **tn or tn**
temperature normal
- **tnt**
toe nail trim
- **TNTC**
too numerous to count. Used primarily to describe the number of red or white cells observed per high power field when performing a urinalysis.
- **toe crack**
a crack near the front of the hoof.
- **toe-in**
a conformation flaw in which the front of the foot faces in and looks pigeon-toed, often causing the leg to swing outward during locomotion ('paddling').
- **toe-out**
a conformation flaw in which the front of the foot faces out, often causing the leg to swing inward during locomotion ('winging').
- **tolerance**
specific unresponsiveness to a given antigen
- **tolerance levels**
1/1000th the level where birth defects were induced by a drug and 1/100th the level where other side effects were induced.
- **tom**
Un-neutered male cat.
- **tonometry**
measuring pressure in the eyeball.
- **tonopen tonometer**
an applanation tonometer used to caloculate IOP from the force required to flatten (applanate) the cornea.
- **topical**
to be used on the skin.
- **topskull**
dome or crown.
- **torsion**
twisting of a body part. For example, a retained testicle may twist, cutting off its blood supply.
- **tort**
tortoise shell
- **tort/w**
tortoiseshell and white
- **tortie**
a combination of the Tortoiseshell and the Tabby

pattern that is also known by the name 'Patched Tabby'.

- **tortoiseshell**
  a coat pattern consisting of a mosaic blend of black and orange.

- **total body water**
  total body water accounts for ~ 60 to 70% of an animal's body weight. Total body water is distributed across interconnected compartments. 2/3 of total body water is located within cells and 1/3 in extra cellular locations including plasma and interstitial locations

- **total digestible nutrients (Abrev: TDN)**
  a term describing the energy value of feedstuffs, comparable to DE in accuracy. TDN over- estimates the energy value of roughages in comparison to grains.

- **total mixed ration (Abrev: TMR)**
  a ration where all feed ingredients (mineral, vitamins, grains) are mixed in a nutritionally balanced ration.

- **total parenteral nutrition (Abrev: TPN)**
  providing 100% of a patient's caloric needs by the intravenous route through a central catheter.

- **total protein (Abrev: TP)**
  all the proteins in the blood stream including albumin, immunoglobulins and other globulins. TP can be measured with a refractometer or by chemical methods.

- **toxemia**
  a poisoning sometimes due the absorption of bacterial products (endotoxins) formed at a local source of infection.

- **toxicity**
  potency; amount of a poison that will cause an adverse effect.

- **toxicology**
  the study of poisons (toxicants).

- **toxins**
  poisons either from the environment or wastes accumulating in the blood due to organ failure. E.G. uremic wastes are those toxins that accumulate in the blood when the kidneys fail.

- **toxoid**
  inactivated toxin from a particular bacteria that is injected and generates antibodys to the toxin.
- **tpn**
  total parenteral nutrition
- **TPR**
  a common medical abbreviation for temperature, pulse, and respiration.
- **tprn**
  temperature, pulse and respiration all normal
- **trachea**
  a synonym for the windpipe.
- **tracheo bronchitis**
  inflammation of the trachea and bronchi.
- **trait**
  an inherent physical or mental characteristic; a distinguishing quality; a peculiarity.
- **tranquilliser**
  a drug that calms an animal without affecting consciousness.
- **trans abdominal ultra sonography**
  passing sound waves through the belly to see internal organs and structures.
- **transdermal**
  absorption of a drug across the intact skin.
- **transient**
  temporary
- **transient diabetes**
  a period where the animal does not require exogenous insulin. This period can last weeks, months, or years. Transient diabetes is not uncommon in cats, but it usually never occurs in dogs.
- **transitional cell carcinoma (Abrev: TCC)**
  a tumour originating from the transitional epithelium lining the urinary tract. The most common location for development of transitional cell carcinoma tumours is in the trigone of the urinary bladder.
- **transmissibility/contagiousness**
  capacity of parasite to spread between animals – e.g. Salmonella dublin is regard as highly contagious between heifers and calves via faeces.

- **transplacental**
  transplacental means crossing the placenta. The placenta is the in-utero connection between the mother and the foetus. Transplacental means something (a drug, antibodies, an infectious agent, etc.) crosses from the mother to the foetus before birth. This can be good in the case of antibodies that protect the newborn from disease early in life or bad if it is an infectious agent that transfers from mother to baby.

- **transport host**
  an animal or insect which carries an immature parasite from one mammalian host to another.

- **transrectal ultrasonography**
  placing the ultrasound probe into the rectum in order to more clearly recognize internal organs and structures.

- **transverse**
  cross sectional view of a structure.

- **travasol**
  an amino acid solution used in TPN and PPN.

- **trichiasis**
  normal hair from around the eyes is directed towards the eye, causing irritation.

- **trichogram**
  this is a hair 'plucks'. The trichogram is useful to evaluate the integrity of hair shafts and also serves as a test for demodicosis and dermatophytosis.

- **tricuspid valve defect**
  a defect in the heart valve that separates the right atrium and the right ventricle.

- **tricyclic antidepressant**
  a class of antidepressants which work by decreasing the amount of certain chemical transmitters taken up by specific nerve cells. The tricyclic antidepressants include clomipramine, amitriptyline and fluoxetine (Prozac) and are often used to treat behavioural problems in small animals.

- **tris-EDTA solution**
  a combination of EDTA, tromethane [hydroxymethyl] aminomethane) and sodium dodecyl sulfate used intreatment of Pseudomonas otitis.

- **tubal ligation**
a sterilisation process that ties the fallopian tubes, preventing the release of eggs.

- **tubing**
inserting a nasogastric tube through a horse's nostril into its stomach for the purpose of providing oral medication.

- **tumor**
abnormal growth or swelling; term often used to designate cancer.

- **tup**
a male sheep.

- **tupping**
putting the rams and ewes together for mating.

- **twbc**
total white blood cells

- **twds**
towards

- **twitch**
a restraining device usually consisting of a stick with a loop of rope or chain at one end, which is placed around a horse's upper lip and twisted, releasing endorphins that relax a horse and curb its fractiousness while it is being handled.

- **tying up (acute rhabdomyolysis)**
a form of muscle cramps that ranges in severity from mild stiffness to a life-threatening disease. A generalised condition of muscle fibre breakdown usually associated with exercise. The cause of the muscle fibre breakdown is uncertain. Signs include sweating, reluctance to move, stiffness and general distress.

- **type I diabetes**
a form of diabetes in which so little insulin is produced that supplemental insulin must be given for the animal to live. Also called insulin dependent diabetes mellitus (IDDM).

- **type II diabetes**
a type of diabetes mellitus in which blood glucose levels are higher than normal but they are not immediately life threatening and the animal can survive without supplemental insulin. Also called non-insulin dependent diabetes mellitus (NIDDM).

- **u/a or ua**
urinalysis

- **uga**
  under general anaesthetic
- **ula**
  under local anaesthetic
- **ulcer**
  a rupture in the body's tissue, skin or membrane; usually associated with the stomach lining and its subsequent pain and injury.
- **ultrasound/ultrasonography**
  a technique used to get the image of a deep structure within the body by directing ultrasound waves at it and recording the reflections (echoes) from it.
- **umbilical cord**
  the tubular structure that connects the foetus to the placenta and carries nutrients to the foetus and removes its wastes.
- **umbilicus**
  the area of the body where the umbilical cord is attached; the belly button.
- **unaltered**
  an intact male or female cat with full reproductive abilities.
- **unavailable protein/heat damaged protein**
  portion of the protein irreversibly bound to the fibre fraction in feedstuffs. It is usually a small fraction of the total protein, but can be greatly increased by heat.
- **undegradable intake protein (Abrev: UIP)**
  portion of ingested protein that escapes rumen degradation and is digested directly in the other stomachs or small intestine; generally a more expensive source of protein. Commonly referred to as 'bypass' protein.
- **undercolour**
  the colour of the hair closest to the skin.
- **unilateral**
  involving one side.
- **unsaturated fat**
  any fat that is not completely hydrogenated. Unsaturated fats are liquid at room temperature. Examples: corn oil, vegetable oil.
- **untried**
  a stallion that has not been bred.

- **ununited anconeal process, uap**
  the anconeal process never unites with the ulna, can detach and form a loose body in the joint, called a joint mouse.

- **unwind**
  gradually withdrawing a horse from intensive training.

- **upright silo**
  storage unit for high moisture feed, generally silage.

- **urate**
  a chemical compound which contains uric acid and is made by the body and can form crystals and stones in the urinary bladder. Uric acid is a waste product from the breakdown of certain proteins.

- **urea**
  waste product of protein metabolism that is removed from the body by the kidneys.

- **urease**
  an enzyme that breaks down urea. Urea is a waste product of protein metabolism that is removed from the body by the kidneys.

- **ureter**
  a small tubular structure leading from the kidney to the bladder. There are 2 ureters, one from each kidney. (Modified: 10/18/1999)

- **urethra**
  the tubular structure that transports urine from the urinary bladder to the outside and in the male, carries semen to the outside.

- **urinary bladder**
  the sac-like structure that holds urine until the animal passes the urine.

- **urinary incontinence**
  a phrase used to describe the inability to control urination.

- **urinary obstruction**
  a blockage in the urinary system most often occurring in the urethra, the tube that leads from the urinary bladder to the outside of the body.

- **urinary retention**
  a condition in which the urinary bladder does not rid itself of all urine it contains during the process of urination.

- **urination**
  to pass urine.
- **urine**
  liquid wastes.
- **urine specific gravity (Abrev: USG)**
  the weight of urine compared to an equal volume of water. In general, the greater the USG, the more concentrated is the urine.
- **uro-vagina**
  presence of urine in the vagina.
- **urt**
  upper respiratory tract
- **urti**
  upper respiratory tract infection
- **urticaria**
  an allergic reaction of the skin characterised by reddened irregular, elevated patches and severe itching. Also called hives.
- **us**
  1. urine sample
  2. ultrasound
- **uterine inertia**
  ineffective or absence of uterine contractions during delivery.
- **uterine prolapse**
  a side effect that may occur after a difficult birth where the uterus comes out the birth canal.
- **uterine torsion**
  twisting of an organ, in this case, twisting of the uterus.
- **uterine tubes**
  tubes that connect the ovarian bursa to the uterus. Eggs are transported through these tubes to the uterus.
- **uteroverdin**
  a green pigment present in the placenta attached to the endometrium of a bitch. As placental separation occurs during whelping the pigment is discharged.
- **uterus**
  the female organ in which the foetus develops.
- **uti**
  urinary tract infection
- **uvea**
  the vascular layer of the eye comprised of the iris, ciliary body, and choroid.
- **uveitis**
  inflammation of the eye.

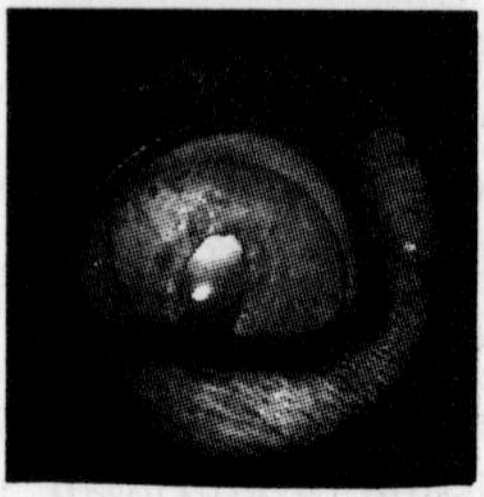

- **uveodermatologic syndrome**
  depigmentation of the skin and hair, and of the nose, lips, eyelids, footpads and anus.

- **vital pulpotomy**
  surgical amputation of the dental pulp coronal to the cemento enamel junction, and restoration of the reduced crown

- **v&d or v/d +**
  vomitting and diarrhoea

- **V.M.D.**
  veterinary medical doctor.

- **v/d -**
  no vomitting, no diarrhoea

- **v+**
  vomitting

- **v++**
  moderate vomitting

- **v+++**
  severe vomitting

- **vacc**
  vaccinate or vaccine

- **vaccination**
  the act of giving a vaccine.

- **vaccine**
  an injection that helps the body build immunity to disease.

- **vaccine failure**
  a term used to describe a condition in which an animal who was vaccinated against a disease still gets the disease. In truth, there is usually nothing wrong with the vaccine but for some reason the animal's immune system did not adequately react to it.

- **vagina**
  the part of the female reproductive tract connected to the vulva on one end and the cervix on the other.

- **vaginal cytology**
  taking samples of the epithelial cells lining the vagina in order to help determine the state of the bitches cycle. The appearance of the cells changes in response to estrogen.

- **vaginal prolapse**
  prolapse of the vagina through the lips of the vulva. Vaginal prolapse most

often occurs during proestrus or early estrus, during the time of estrogen stimulation.

- **vaginitis**
  inflammation of the vagina.

- **van or van pattern**
  a colour pattern which restricts colour to the head and the tail, leaving the body and most of the extremities white. Most standards for this pattern allow for no more than two small spots of colour on the body. The name comes from the Turkish Van breed, which always exhibit this pattern.

- **vascular**
  relating to blood vessels, both arteries and veins.

- **vasculitis**
  inflammation of blood vessels.

- **vasectomy**
  a sterilisation process that removes a male cat's sperm transporting connective tubes.

- **vasoconstriction**
  a decrease in the diameter of blood vessels.

- **vasodilator**
  agent which dilates, or increases the diameter of blood vessels.

- **vasopressin**
  an extremely potent vasoconstrictor. It may replace the use of epinephrine in treatment of refractory ventricular fibrillation.

- **vasopressor**
  a drug that stimulates the contraction of the muscle in the walls of capillaries and arteries causing vasoconstriction and an increase in blood pressure.

- **VCAPP**
  veterinary and comparative anatomy, pharmacology and physiology.

- **VCS**
  veterinary clinical sciences.

- **vector**
  a carrier, in the case of recombinant vaccines, a 'safe' virus used to introduce immunogenic DNA into the host animal during vaccination.

- **VEE (venezuelan equine encephalomyelitis)**
  a highly contagious disease affecting the central ner-

vous system that can cause illness or death in horses and humans.

- **vein**
  a blood vessel that carries blood back to the heart. The pressure in veins is lower than in arteries. Veins contain less oxygen and nutrients than arteries and contain waste products that they carry to the lungs or other organs for disposal.

- **venacava**
  either of two large veins carrying blood to the right atrium of the heart. The cranial venacava brings blood from the head region, front legs, and upper chest to the heart; the caudal(or posterior) venacava carries blood from the areas of the abdomen and hind legs to the heart.

- **venereal**
  sexually transmitted. Transmissible venereal tumours occur on the genital organs; penis or vagina, and are transmitted from dog to dog by sexual contact.

- **venous**
  referring to the system of veins.

- **vent**
  the outside opening of the cloaca, which is a common passage way for faeces, urine, and reproduction.

- **ventilator**
  a device that is used to control breathing.

- **ventral**
  down; toward the belly.

- **ventricle**
  the heart has 4 chambers; the two chambers that make up the bottom of the heart are the ventricles. Fluid filled spaces in the brain are also called ventricles.

- **ventricular arrhythmia**
  a heart condition in which the heart beats irregularly and/or at an abnormal rate because of signals coming from the ventricles (chambers of the heart that pump the blood).

- **verminous pneumonia**
  pneumonia caused by worms.

- **vertebrae**
  the segments of the backbone. Each vertebrae is separated from adjacent ver-

tebrae by a spongy structure called a disk.

- **vertebrate**
animal with a vertebral column (spine). Includes such animals as fish, birds, turtles, reptiles, amphibians, and mammals.

- **vertical transmission**
ways an infection is spread from a parent to its offspring.

- **vesicle**
small elevated area on the skin filled with a clear fluid.

- **vestibular**
pertaining to balance. The inner ear and the cerebellum of the brain are responsible for maintaining balance.

- **vestibulum**
the area of the female genital tract between the vulva and the vestibular sphincter that opens into the vagina cavity and has on it's floor the opening of the urethra.

- **veterinarian surgeon**
an animal doctor.

- **vicryl rapide**
an absorbable suture which breaks down in about 2 weeks.

- **villi**
microscopic projections which cover the intestine, greatly increasing the surface area and therefore, increasing the ability to absorb nutrients. Singular: Villus.

- **virgin**
never been bred.

- **virucide**
a substance that kills viruses.

- **virulence**
the ability of an organism to cause disease.

- **virus**
the smallest form of life, invisible with an ordinary microscope. An infectious unit that enters and uses cells of plants or animals for replication. Some viruses cause disease in animals or plants.

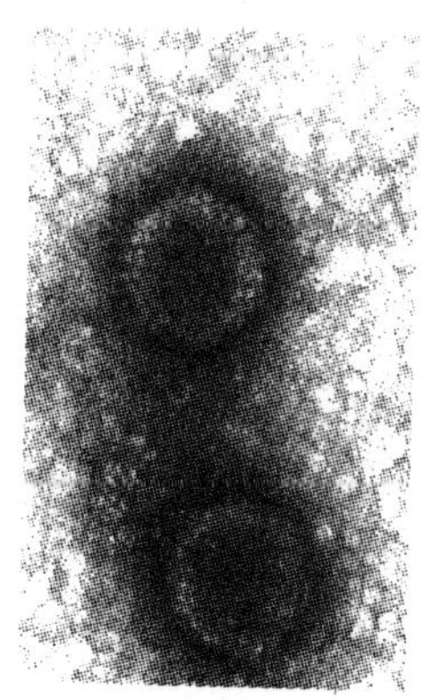

- **viscera**
  a general term for the abdominal organs which are also called viscera. viscerocutaneous pertaining to the internal organs and skin.

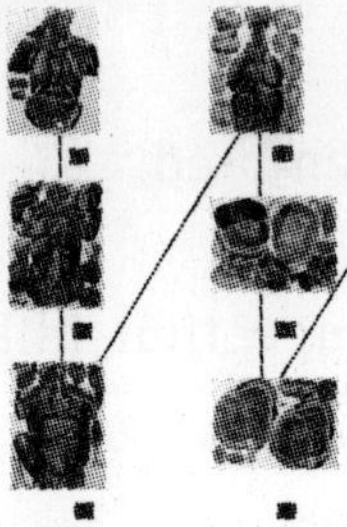

- **viscosity**
  thickness of a fluid, e.g. molasses is more viscous than water.
- **vital signs**
  the signs of life which are pulse, respiration, and temperature.
- **vitamins**
  organic compounds that function as parts of enzyme systems essential for many metabolic functions.
- **vitiligo**
  depigmentation.
- **vitreocentesis**
  obtaining a sample of fluid from the vitreous for cytology or culture.
- **vitreous**
  clear, jellylike substance filling the vitreous chamber, the most posterior cavity in the eye, comprising two-thirds of the volume of the eye. Maintains the shape of the globe.
- **vivonex**
  a hypoallergenic elemental diet.
- **VMB**
  very much better
- **VMI**
  very much improved
- **VMP**
  veterinary microbiology and pathology.
- **vocal folds**
  the membranes attached to the arytenoid cartilages in the larynx. Vibration produces vocalisation.

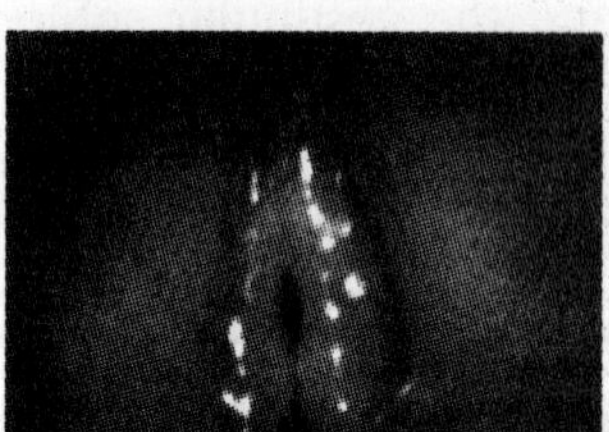

- **volatile fatty acids (Abrev: VFA)**
  by products of digestion in the rumen that make an acidic environment and

keep pathogenic bacterial populations down.

- **volvulus**
  twisting of the stomach or intestine, which often has the effect of cutting off the blood supply to it.

- **vomeronasal organ**
  sensory organ also called 'Jacobson's organ,' which detects pheromones.

- **vomitting**
  the cardiac sphincter, at the junction of the oesophagus and stomach, doesn't open for things to work in reverse, and two—the stomach is almost entirely within the ribcage, making the requisite muscular effort which accompanies vomitting in other species almost impossible.

- **Von Willebrand's disease**
  deficiency of coagulation factor VIII causing prolonged bleeding time. This can be an autosomal dominant trait, but Bernese Mountain Dogs have Type I, which is an autosomal recessive trait.

- **von willebrand's factor**
  a blood factor that promotes platelet adhesion.

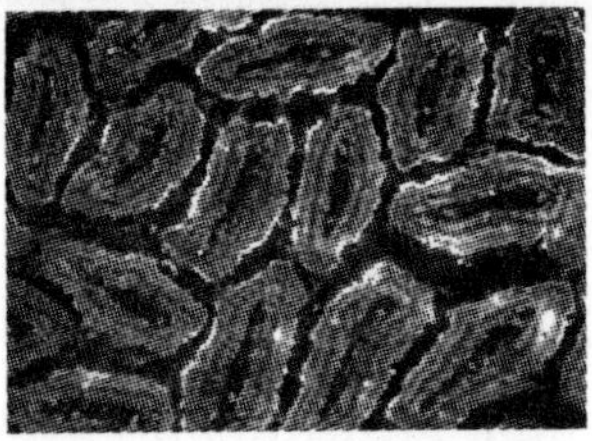

- **vulva**
  the opening into the female genital tract from the outside of the animal.

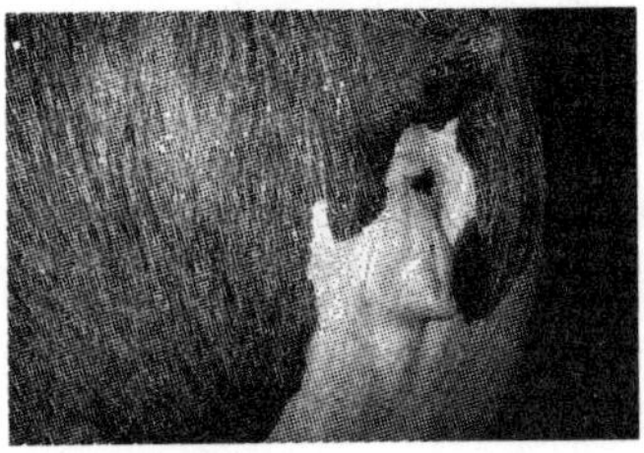

- **worn tooth**
  usually secondary to abrasion from grinding or wearing away of tooth substance by mastication

- **walking dandruff**
  common name for Cheyletiella infestation.

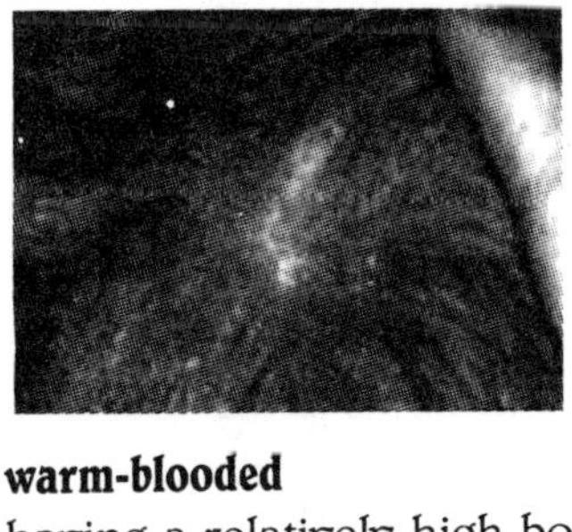

- **warm-blooded**
  having a relatively high body temperature that is regulated

internally and is independent of the environmental temperature. Mammals and birds are warm-blooded.

- **wart**
  benign growth caused by a virus.

- **wasting**
  loss of muscle mass due to decreased food intake or increased metabolic rate.

- **water soluble vitamins**
  includes B complex vitamins and vitamin C. Not normally supplemented for ruminants after two months of age because rumen microbes are able to manufacture enough to meet the animal's requirements.

- **wry bite or wry mouth**
  a skeletal defect where the midline of the maxilla does not line up with the midline of the mandible

- **WBC**
  white blood cell. There are several types of WBCs including, neutrophils, lymphocytes, eosinophils and monocytes.

- **wean**
  to persuade kittens that are totally reliant on their mother's milk for sustenance to start taking solid food.

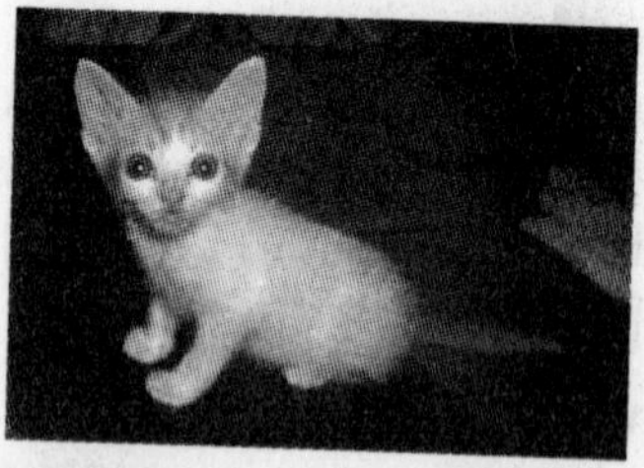

- **weaner**
  lamb after weaning to 12 months. No exact age but approx from 10 to 12 months.

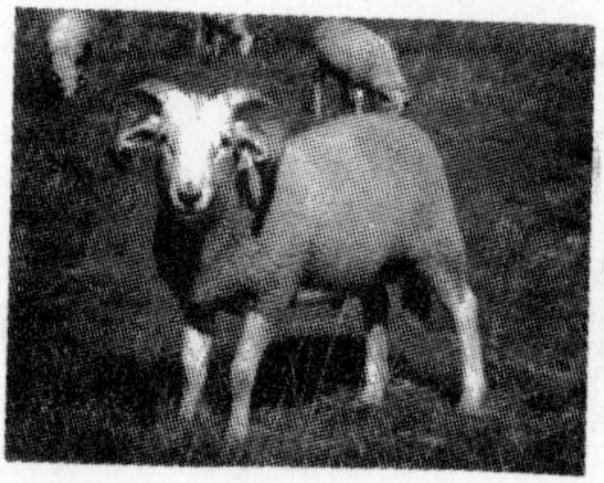

- **weanling**
  a foal that is less than one-year-old that has been separated from its dam.

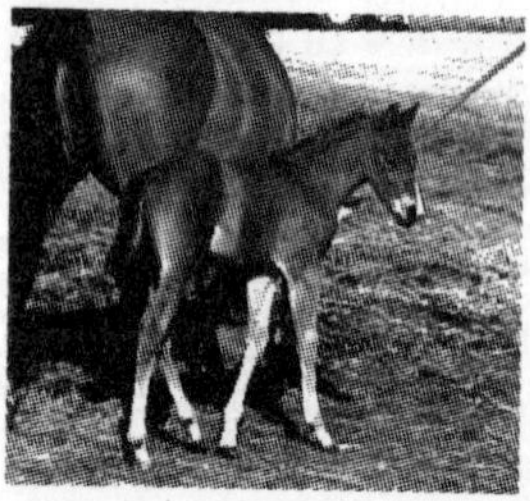

- **weight-averaged molecular weight**
  the sum of the number of molecules at each number-

averaged molecular weight divided by the total number of molecules in solution. The weight-averaged molecular weight gives an indication of how long a solution will exert an oncotic effect. Generally, the larger the weight-averaged molecular weight, the longer it lasts.

- **weight-for-age**
  an allowance condition in which each entrant is assigned a weight according to its age. Females usually receive a sex allowance as well.

- **wet cow average**
  average milk production by lactating cows. Goal is 70 to 80 lbs/day, 21, 000-24, 000 per year.

- **wether**
  a castrated male sheep.

- **wear facet**
  a flattened highly polished area on the tooth's surface from chronic wear

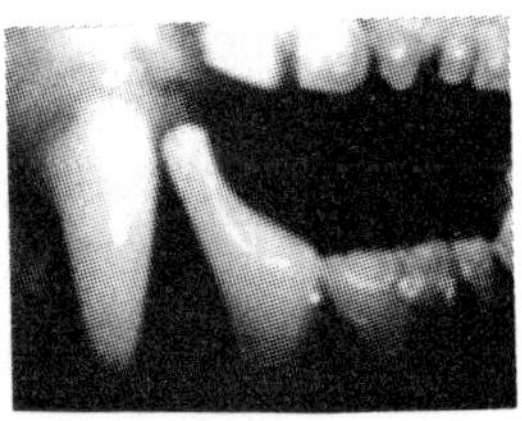

- **wheal**
  a circumscribed raised lesion of edemma of the dermas. A large number of wheals is urticaria.

- **whelping**
  in dogs, the act of giving birth.

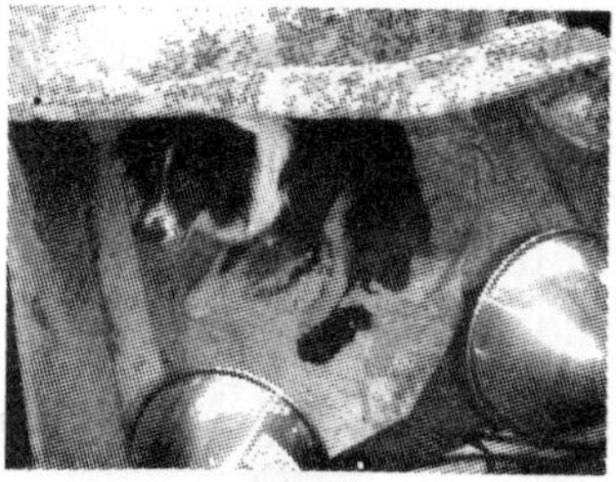

- **whisker break**
  an indentation in the upper jaw.

- **whisker pad**
  the thickened, or fatty pads around the whisker area.

- **white**
  a horse colour, extremely rare, in which all the hairs are white. The horse's eyes are brown, not pink, as would be the case for an albino.

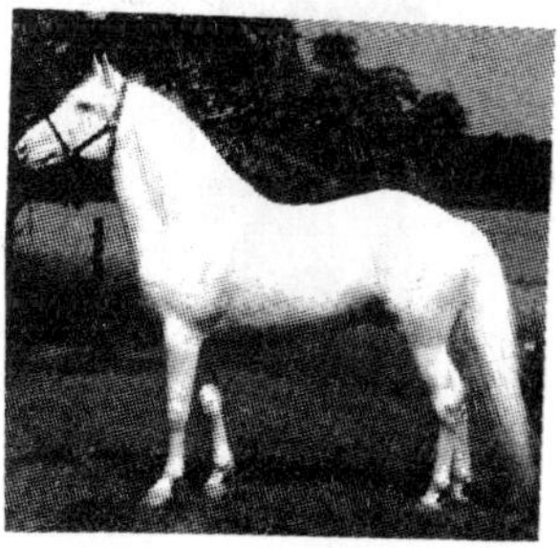

- **white blood cells (WBCs)**

cells in the blood whose major role is to defend the body against invading organisms such as bacteria, viruses, and fungi. There are different types of leukocytes lymphocytes are part of the immune system; monocytes, eosinophils and neutrophils eat or engulf organisms; basophils contain histamine and are involved in inflammatory reactions.

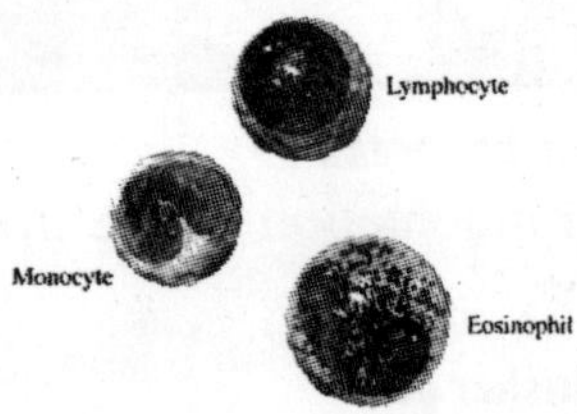

- **white line**

when looking at the sole of the foot, the thin area between the insensitive outer hoof wall (insensitive laminae) and the inner sensitive laminae.

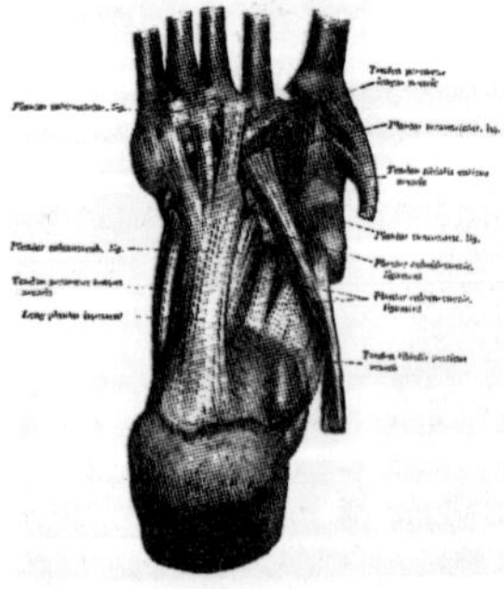

- **white muscle disease**

another name for a selenium deficiency.

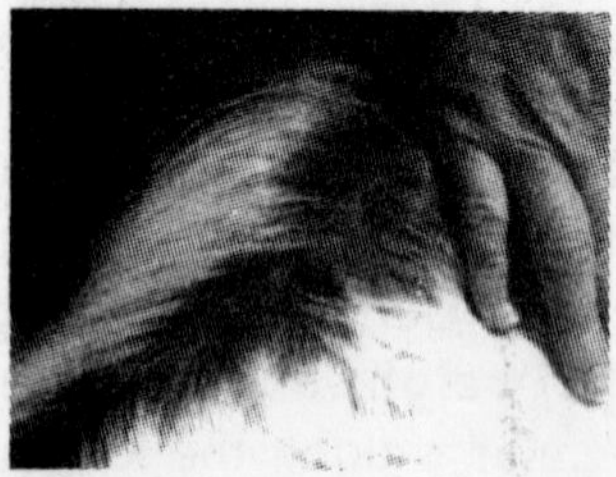

- **whole**

not neutered or spayed.

- **wind up**

sensitisation of the central nervous system in response to sustained pain. With sustained pain, new receptors (NMDA receptors)are formed in the central nervous system. These receptors use a very fast neurotransmitter and cause a marked increase in the amount of pain transmitted to the brain. They also prevent opioids from working to their full effectiveness.

- **window of susceptibility**

a time period in the life of a young animal in which the maternal antibodies are too low to provide protection against a certain disease but too high to allow a vaccine to work and produce immunity.

- **windpuffs**

windpuffs are a filling of the joint capsule of the fetlock.

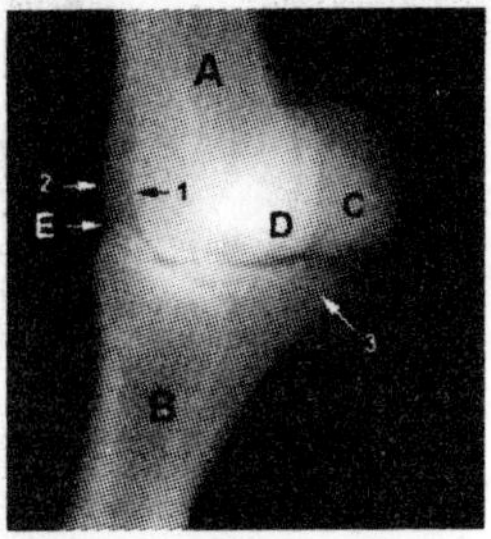

- **winstrol/steroids**

winstrol is a synthetic anabolic steroid. The therapeutic use of these compounds is to help build lean body mass and to inhibit the breakdown of muscle protein in debilitated animals. Their common use is a quick 'training' tool.

- **witches milk**

goats sometimes come into milk without having been bred, and the term is used to describe that condition.

- **withdrawal periods**

the amount of time it takes for a drug to be broken down in the body until it is at a level safe for human consumption.

- **withdrawal time**

time meat must be withheld from sale following treatment to avoid sale of residue laden meat.

- **withers**

the highest point of the shoulders, immediately behind the neck.

- **withholding period**

the time after a drug is administered, before the animal can be marketed (or the milk used for human consumption).

- **withholding time**

time milk must be withheld from sale following treatment to avoid appearance of residues in milk.

- **WMD**

white meat diet

- **WNL**

within normal limits

- **WO**

weeks old (following a number)

- **wobbler syndrome**

neurological disease clinically associated with general a non-coordination and muscle weakness. Can be caused by an injury to the spinal cord in the area of the cervical (neck) vertebrae or is associated with malformation of the cervical vertebrae.

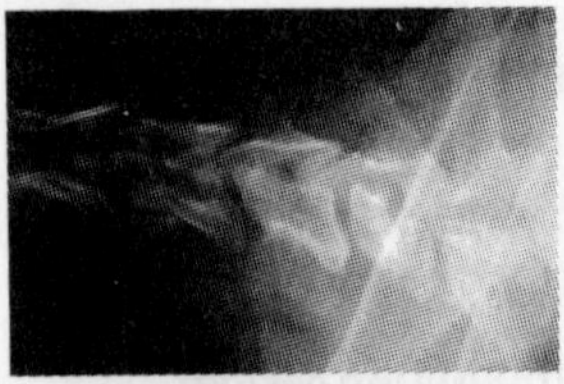

Surgical techniques for the management of cervical spondylopathy (Wobbler syndrome) have been compared

- **wood's light**
  an ultraviolet light filtered through nickel oxide. Of the common dermatophytes, only M. canis fluoresces, 25 to 50% of the time.

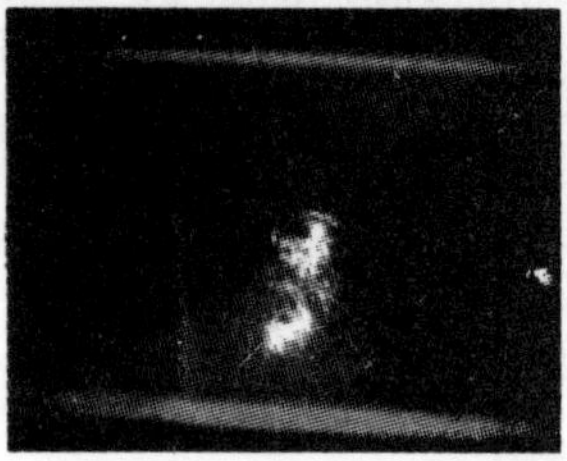

- **wt**
  weight
- **wt!!**
  overweight
- **x**
  extracted tooth
- **x/12**
  x months
- **x/24**
  x hours
- **x/52**
  x weeks
- **x/60**
  x minutes
- **x/7**
  x days
- **xeroradiography**
  a costly type of x-ray procedure using specially sensitised screens that give higher resolution on the edges of bone and better visualization of soft tissue structures.
- **xr or xr**
  X-ray
- **X-ray**
  the X-ray is the high energy beam that produces a 'picture' of a body part which is called the radiograph. Radiographs are commonly, but incorrectly, referred to as X-rays.

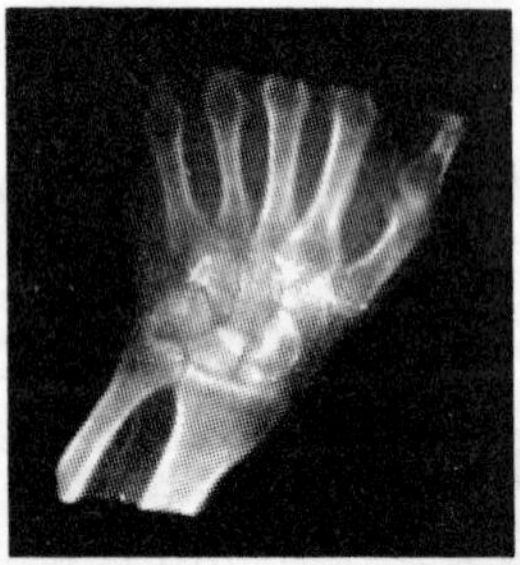

- **yearling**
  sheep 12 to 24 months of age.

- **yeast**
a single cell fungi which improves feed digestion by stimulating microbial activity and stabilizing digestive tract pH. Products packaged as 'yeast' consist of cells only; 'yeast culture' includes live yeast cells plus growth media.

- **yersinia pestis**
etiologic agent of plague.

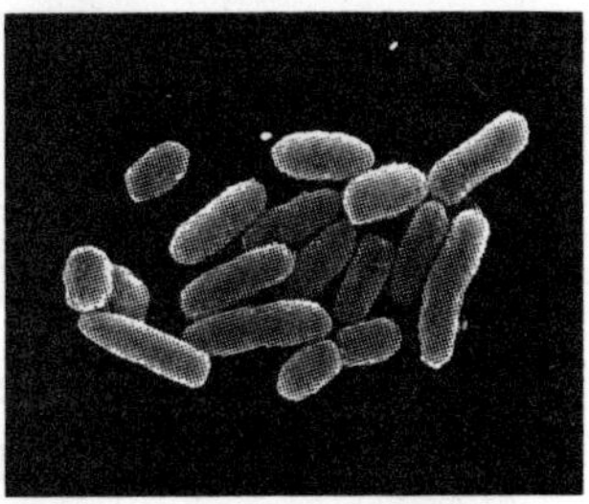

- **yo**
years old (following a number)

- **zantac**
a medication used to treat ulcers.

- **zona pellucida**
the envelope surrounding the egg or ovum.

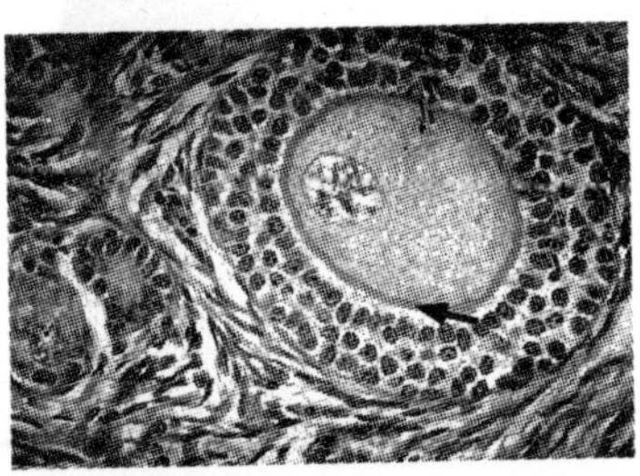

- **zoonoses**
a biologically heterogeneous group of infectious diseases.

- **zoonosis**
a disease that can be transmitted from animals to people.

- **zoonotic disease**
infectious diseases naturally transmitted from vertebrate animals to humans. Some of these diseases can be harboured in a vertebrate animal but there might be a vector involved in transmission, so that is still a zoonotic disease because it is harboured in a vertebrate animal. Additionally the disease may be food or water borne, so you don't need to have direct contact with an animal to acquire a zoonotic disease.

- **zoonotic infection**
refers to infectious microorganisms that have the potential to cause disease in humans. Public Health is the study of zoonotic infections.

Note

Note

Note

Note

Note